S0-AYC-020

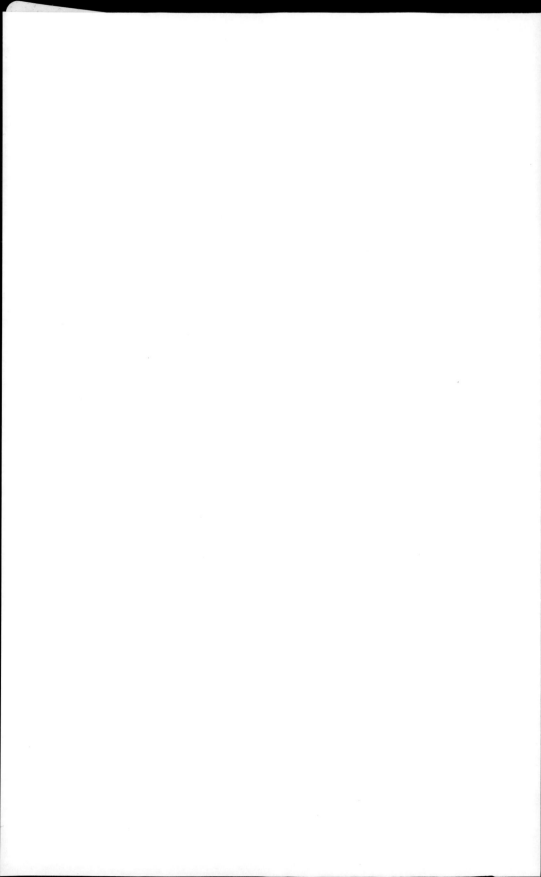

EYE CARE
SOURCEBOOK

SIXTH EDITION

Health Reference Series

EYE CARE SOURCEBOOK

SIXTH EDITION

Basic Consumer Health Information about Vision and Disorders Affecting the Eyes and Surrounding Structures, Including Facts about Hyperopia, Myopia, Presbyopia, Astigmatism, Cataracts, Macular Degeneration, Glaucoma, and Other Disorders of the Cornea, Retina, Macula, Conjunctiva, and Optic Nerve

Along with Guidelines for Recognizing and Treating Eye Disorders, Advice about Protecting the Eyes, Tips for Living with Vision Impairment, a Glossary of Terms Related to the Eye Disorders, and a Directory of Resources for Further Information

OMNIGRAPHICS

615 Griswold St., Ste. 520, Detroit, MI 48226

* * *

OMNIGRAPHICS
Kevin Hayes, Managing Editor

* * *

ISBN 978-0-7808-1794-4
E-ISBN 978-0-7808-1795-1

Library of Congress Cataloging-in-Publication Data

Title: Eye care sourcebook

Other titles: Ophthalmic disorders sourcebook

Description: Sixth edition. | Detroit, MI : Omnigraphics, [2020] | Series: Health reference series | Revision of: Ophthalmic disorders sourcebook. 2nd ed. c2003. | Includes bibliographical references and index. | Summary: "Provides basic health information about vision and disorders affecting the eyes and surrounding structures, along with facts about various eye disorders, guidelines for recognizing and treating eye emergencies, advice about protecting the eyes, and tips for living with low vision. Includes glossary, index, and other resources"-- Provided by publisher.

Identifiers: LCCN 2020000347 (print) | LCCN 2020000348 (ebook) | ISBN 9780780817944 (library binding) | ISBN 9780780817951 (ebook)

Subjects: LCSH: Eye--Diseases--Popular works. | Eye--Care and hygiene--Popular works.

Classification: LCC RE51 .O64 2020 (print) | LCC RE51 (ebook) | DDC 617.7--dc23

LC record available at https://lccn.loc.gov/2020000347

LC ebook record available at https://lccn.loc.gov/2020000348

This book is printed on acid-free paper meeting the ANSI Z39.48 Standard. The infinity symbol that appears above indicates that the paper in this book meets that standard.

Printed in the United States

Table of Contents

Part 2. Understanding and Treating Refractive, Eye Movement, and Alignment Disorders

Part 3. Understanding and Treating Disorders of the Cornea, Conjunctiva, Sclera, Lens, Iris, and Pupil

Part 4. Understanding and Treating Disorders of the Macula, Optic Nerve, Retina, Vitreous, and Uvea

Part 5. Eye Injuries and Disorders of the Surrounding Structures

Part 6. Congenital and Other Disorders That Affect Vision

Part 7. Vision Impairment Rehabilitation and Recent Research

Preface

ABOUT THIS BOOK

According to the Centers for Disease Control and Prevention (CDC), about 4.2 million Americans over 40 years of age suffer from uncorrectable vision impairment and about 1.02 million are blind as of 2012. It is predicted that the numbers could double by 2050. The most common causes of vision loss among adults in order of prevalence are cataracts, diabetic retinopathy, glaucoma, and age-related macular degeneration. Often these impairments can develop gradually and few are aware of the warning signs of serious eye disorders. The effects of many of these disorders could be lessened or eliminated entirely with regular comprehensive eye exams and early detection which can help diagnose emerging vision problems before vision loss is noticeable.

Eye Care Sourcebook, Sixth Edition explains how the eyes work and offers suggestions for maintaining healthy eyes. Information about disorders affecting the eyes' refractive ability, ability to move, and alignment is provided. It also includes facts about various disorders that affect different parts of the eyes and surrounding structures such as cornea, conjunctiva, sclera, lens, iris, pupil, macula, optic nerve, retina, vitreous, and uvea. Signs and symptoms of these disorders are explained along with diagnosis and treatment procedures. It describes congenital and hereditary disorders that affect vision, and infectious diseases and other disorders with eye-related complications. It also provides suggestions to help prevent eye injuries. The book concludes with a summary of tips for living with vision impairment, a glossary of terms related to eye disorders, and a directory of resources for further help and information.

HOW TO USE THIS BOOK

This book is divided into parts and chapters. Parts focus on broad areas of interest. Chapters are devoted to single topics within a part.

Part 1: Eye and Eye-Care Basics explains how the eyes work and offers suggestions for maintaining healthy eyes. It discusses common pediatric and age-related vision concerns and describes the most common methods of diagnosing vision and other eye-related problems. Statistical data on vision disorders is also provided.

Part 2: Understanding and Treating Refractive, Eye Movement, and Alignment Disorders describes common disorders affecting the eyes' refractive ability, ability to move, and alignment, including astigmatism, hyperopia, myopia, presbyopia, amblyopia, Brown syndrome, nystagmus, and strabismus. It provides details about the different types of eyeglasses and contact lenses and describes how to fit them and care for them properly. It concludes with a discussion of the most common types of refractive surgery.

Part 3: Understanding and Treating Disorders of the Cornea, Conjunctiva, Sclera, Lens, Iris, and Pupil discusses various disorders that affect cornea, conjunctiva, sclera, lens, iris, and pupil such as corneal injury, keratitis, corneal dystrophies, cataracts, conjunctivitis, dry eye, episcleritis, leukocoria, pinguecula, and Peters anomaly. It also gives information about corneal transplant.

Part 4: Understanding and Treating Disorders of the Macula, Optic Nerve, Retina, Vitreous, and Uvea provides information about various disorders that affect macula, optic nerve, retina, vitreous, and uvea. It details the signs and symptoms of these disorders and explains how they are diagnosed and treated.

Part 5: Eye Injuries and Disorders of the Surrounding Structures discusses how to recognize and treat eye injuries, including chemical burns, foreign objects in the eye, and blowout fractures. It includes a description of recommended forms of workplace and sports eye protection. It also discusses the most common disorders of the eyelids and tear ducts and also gives an insight into digital eyestrain.

Part 6: Congenital and Other Disorders That Affect Vision describes the most common hereditary and other congenital disorders affecting vision, including achromatopsia, color blindness, WAGR syndrome, etc. It provides information about how stroke and diabetes can affect the eyes. Fungal infections that affect the eyesight and other eye-related complications are also discussed.

Part 7: Vision Impairment Rehabilitation and Recent Research defines what is meant by the terms "low vision" and "legal blindness," and provides tips for coping with vision loss. It provides details about mobility aids and new technologies that assist people with vision impairment. It talks about

Social Security available for people with vision disorders. Information about vision-related research is also provided.

Part 8: Additional Help and Information includes a glossary of terms related to eyes and eye disorders and a directory of resources for further help and support.

BIBLIOGRAPHIC NOTE

This volume contains documents and excerpts from publications issued by the following U.S. government agencies: Agency for Healthcare Research and Quality (AHRQ); Center for Parent Information & Resources (CPIR); Centers for Disease Control and Prevention (CDC); Federal Occupational Health (FOH); Genetic and Rare Diseases Information Center (GARD); Genetics Home Reference (GHR); National Cancer Institute (NCI); National Center for Biotechnology Information (NCBI); National Eye Institute (NEI); National Highway Traffic Safety Administration (NHTSA); National Human Genome Research Institute (NHGRI); National Institute of Arthritis and Musculoskeletal and Skin Diseases (NIAMS); National Institute of Diabetes and Digestive and Kidney Diseases (NIDDK); National Institute of Environmental Health Sciences (NIEHS); National Institute of Neurological Disorders and Stroke (NINDS); National Institute on Aging (NIA); National Institutes of Health (NIH); Occupational Safety and Health Administration (OSHA); Office of Disease Prevention and Health Promotion (ODPHP); U.S. Department of Energy (DOE); U.S. Department of Justice (DOJ); U.S. Department of Veterans Affairs (VA); U.S. Environmental Protection Agency (EPA); U.S. Equal Employment Opportunity Commission (EEOC); U.S. Food and Drug Administration (FDA); U.S. Library of Congress (LOC); and U.S. Social Security Administration (SSA).

It may also contain original material produced by Omnigraphics and reviewed by medical consultants.

ABOUT THE *HEALTH REFERENCE SERIES*

The *Health Reference Series* is designed to provide basic medical information for patients, families, caregivers, and the general public. Each volume provides comprehensive coverage on a particular topic. This is especially important for people who may be dealing with a newly diagnosed disease or a chronic disorder in themselves or in a family member. People looking for preventive guidance, information about disease warning signs, medical statistics, and risk factors for health problems will also find answers to their questions in the *Health Reference Series*. The *Series*, however, is not intended to serve as a tool for diagnosing illness, in prescribing treatments, or as a substitute for the physician–patient relationship. All people concerned about medical symptoms or the possibility of disease are encouraged to seek professional care from an appropriate healthcare provider.

A NOTE ABOUT SPELLING AND STYLE

Health Reference Series editors use *Stedman's Medical Dictionary* as an authority for questions related to the spelling of medical terms and *The Chicago Manual of Style* for questions related to grammatical structures, punctuation, and other editorial concerns. Consistent adherence is not always possible, however, because the individual volumes within the *Series* include many documents from a wide variety of different producers, and the editor's primary goal is to present material from each source as accurately as is possible. This sometimes means that information in different chapters or sections may follow other guidelines and alternate spelling authorities. For example, occasionally a copyright holder may require that eponymous terms be shown in possessive forms (Crohn's disease vs. Crohn disease) or that British spelling norms be retained (leukaemia vs. leukemia).

MEDICAL REVIEW

Omnigraphics contracts with a team of qualified, senior medical professionals who serve as medical consultants for the *Health Reference Series*. As necessary, medical consultants review reprinted and originally written material for currency and accuracy. Citations including the phrase "Reviewed (month, year)" indicate material reviewed by this team. Medical consultation services are provided to the *Health Reference Series* editors by:

Dr. Vijayalakshmi, MBBS, DGO, MD
Dr. Senthil Selvan, MBBS, DCH, MD
Dr. K. Sivanandham, MBBS, DCH, MS (Research), PhD

OUR ADVISORY BOARD

We would like to thank the following board members for providing initial guidance on the development of this series:

- Dr. Lynda Baker, Associate Professor of Library and Information Science, Wayne State University, Detroit, MI
- Nancy Bulgarelli, William Beaumont Hospital Library, Royal Oak, MI
- Karen Imarisio, Bloomfield Township Public Library, Bloomfield Township, MI

- Karen Morgan, Mardigian Library, University of Michigan-Dearborn, Dearborn, MI
- Rosemary Orlando, St. Clair Shores Public Library, St. Clair Shores, MI

HEALTH REFERENCE SERIES UPDATE POLICY

The inaugural book in the *Health Reference Series* was the first edition of *Cancer Sourcebook* published in 1989. Since then, the *Series* has been enthusiastically received by librarians and in the medical community. In order to maintain the standard of providing high-quality health information for the layperson the editorial staff at Omnigraphics felt it was necessary to implement a policy of updating volumes when warranted.

Medical researchers have been making tremendous strides, and it is the purpose of the *Health Reference Series* to stay current with the most recent advances. Each decision to update a volume is made on an individual basis. Some of the considerations include how much new information is available and the feedback we receive from people who use the books. If there is a topic you would like to see added to the update list, or an area of medical concern you feel has not been adequately addressed, please write to:

Managing Editor
Health Reference Series
Omnigraphics
615 Griswold St., Ste. 520
Detroit, MI 48226

Part 1 | **Eye and Eye-Care Basics**

Chapter 1 | How the Eyes Work

ANATOMY OF THE EYEBALL

The eye consists of a retinal-lined fibrovascular sphere which contains the aqueous humor, the lens and the vitreous body as illustrated in Figure 1.1.

The retina is the essential component of the eye and serves the primary purpose of photoreception. All other structures of the eye are subsidiary and act to focus images on the retina, to regulate the amount of light entering the eye or to provide nutrition, protection or motion. The retina may be considered as an outlying island of the central nervous system (CNS), to which it is connected by a tract of nerve fibers, the optic nerve.

As in the case of the brain and the spinal cord, the retina is within two coats of tissue which contribute protection and nourishment. On the outside of the sphere, corresponding to the dura mater, a layer composed of dense fibrous tissue serves as a protective envelope, the fibrous tunic. The posterior part of the fibrous tunic, the sclera, is white and opaque. Although it retains its protective function, the anterior portion, the cornea, is clear and transparent.

Immediately internal to the sclera, and between it and the retina, lies the uvea, a vascular tunic analogous to the pia-arachnoid of the central nervous system. Primarily, the uvea provides nutrients to the eye. The posterior portion of the uvea is the choroid, a tissue composed almost entirely of blood vessels. A second portion of the

This chapter contains text excerpted from the following sources: Text under the heading "Anatomy of the Eyeball" is excerpted from "The Eye and Visual Nervous System: Anatomy, Physiology and Toxicology," National Institute of Environmental Health Sciences (NIEHS), April 1982. Reviewed March 2020; Text under the heading "How Your Eyes Help You to See" is excerpted from "How the Eyes Work," National Eye Institute (NEI), July 16, 2019.

uvea, the ciliary body, lies just anterior to the choroid and posterior to the corneoscleral margin and provides nutrients by forming intraocular fluid, the aqueous humor. In addition, the ciliary body contains muscles which provide a supporting and focusing mechanism for the lens. The most anterior portion of the uveal tract, the iris, is deflected into the interior of the eye. The iris acts as a diaphragm with a central rounded opening, the pupil, which dilates to allow more light to the retina in dim lighting and constricts in bright lighting. The iris also has some degree of nutritive function, since it acts to help regulate the fluid flow in the eye.

The lens, the focusing mechanism of the eye, is located immediately behind the iris and is supported from the ciliary body by a suspensory ligament, the zonule. The space between the iris and the lens is called the "posterior chamber." The anterior chamber consists of the space between the iris and the cornea. Behind the lens is the vitreous, a gel-like, transparent body which occupies the space between the lens and the retina.

THE CORNEA

The cornea, the window of the eye, is unique because of its transparency. Corneal transparency is dependent on a special arrangement of cells and collagenous fibrils in an acid mucopolysaccharide environment, to an absence of blood vessels, and to deturgescence (the state of relative dehydration of corneal tissue). Any toxin interfering with any one of these factors may result in corneal opacification.

Structure of the Cornea

As illustrated in Figure 1.2, the cornea is composed of five distinct layers: (1) epithelium, (2) Bowman's membrane, (3) stroma, (4) Descemet's membrane and (5) endothelium. In addition, a tear film always covers the cornea of a healthy eye.

The tear film. The tear film is made up of three layers. The portion immediately next to the epithelium is rich in glycoprotein produced by the goblet cells of the conjunctival epithelium; a middle, watery layer is secreted by the lacrimal glands; an outside oily layer is produced by the meibomian glands and the glands of Moll

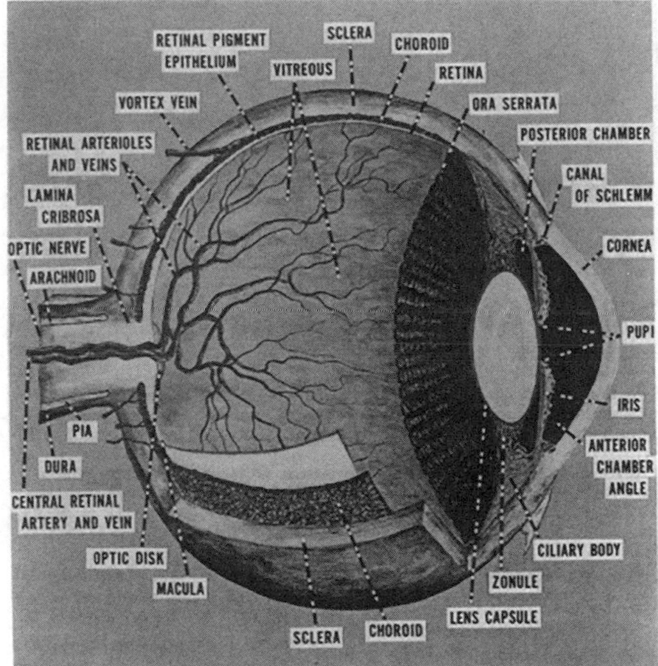

Figure 1.1. The Internal Structure of the Eye

and Zeis of the lid. The tear film is essential for the maintenance of the proper optical qualities of the cornea and its deficiency may result in corneal damage.

Corneal epithelium. The corneal epithelium consists of five or six layers of cells which rest on a basement membrane. It is replaced by growth from its basal cells with perhaps greater rapidity than any other stratified epithelium.

Bowman's membrane. Bowman's membrane is not a true basement membrane but is a clear acellular layer which is a modified portion of the superficial stroma. It is a homogenous layer without cells and has no capacity to regenerate if injured.

Corneal stroma. The stroma makes up approximately 90 percent of the thickness of the cornea. It consists of alternating lamellae of collagenous tissue parallel to the surface of the cornea. The corneal cells, or keratocytes, are relatively few and lie within the collagen lamellae.

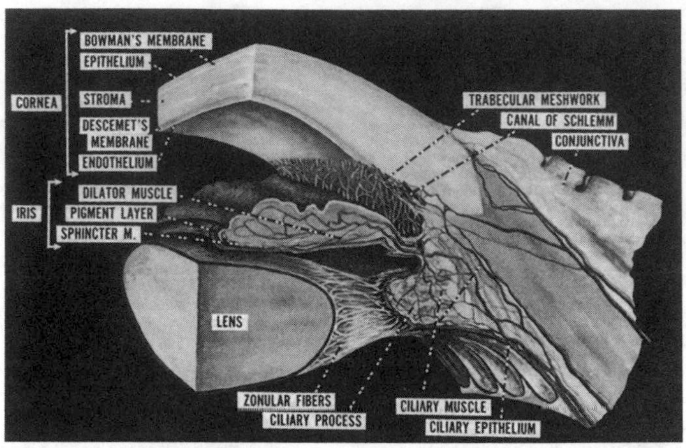

Figure 1.2. Structure of the Anterior Compartment of the Human Eye

Descemet's membrane. Descemet's membrane is a strong, homogeneous true basement membrane. It is produced by the endothelial cells and can be regenerated if injured. Descemet's membrane is elastic and is more resistant than the remainder of the cornea to trauma and disease.

Corneal endothelium. The corneal endothelium consists of a single layer of flattened cuboidal cells. The endothelium does not regenerate and is essential for maintaining dehydration of corneal tissue. Therefore, chemical or physical damage to the endothelium of the cornea is far more serious than epithelial damage. Destruction of the endothelial cells may cause marked swelling of the cornea and result in loss of its transparency.

THE SCIERA

The sclera is hydrated and has large collagen fibrils arranged haphazardly; therefore, it is opaque and white rather than clear. The sclera has three layers: the episclera, the outer layer; the sclera; and the melanocytic layer, the inner lamina fusca. The episclera, a highly vascular connective tissue, attaches Tenon's capsule to the sclera. The sclera proper is relatively avascular and contains considerable elastic tissue. The sclera is approximately 1 mm thick posteriorly and gradually thins to about 0.3 mm just posterior to the insertions of the recti muscles. Therefore, these sites posterior to the insertion of the muscles are the areas of the eye which are most liable to rupture with trauma to the globe.

THE RETINA

The sensory retina covers the inner portion of the posterior two-thirds of the wall of the globe. It is a thin structure which in the living state is transparent and of a purplish-red color due to the visual purple of the rods. The retina is a multilayered sheet of neural tissue closely applied to a single layer of pigmented epithelial cells. The sensory retina is attached only at two regions; the anterior extremity is firmly bound to the pigment epithelium at its dentate termination, the ora serrata. Posteriorly, the optic nerve fixes the retina to the wall of the globe. This potential space between the sensory retina and the retinal pigment epithelium may fill with fluid and result in retinal detachment. The fluid usually comes from the vitreous and enters the subretinal space through a tear or hole in the retina (rhegmatogenous or tear-induced retinal detachment). Less commonly, fluid may leak from blood vessels and cause an exudative retinal detachment.

The retina is 0.1 mm thick at the ora serrata and 0.23 mm thick at the posterior pole. It is thinnest at the fovea centralis, the center of the macula. The fovea may suffer irreparable damage in a brief period of separation from its only blood supply, the underlying choriocapillaris, during retinal detachment.

Composition of the Sensory Retina

The sensory retina is composed of highly organized tissue consisting of nine histologic layers resting on pigment epithelium. From the outside of the eye the layers are in the following order: (1) the layer of rods and cones; (2) the external limiting membrane; (3) the outer nuclear layer; (4) the outer plexiform layer; (5) the inner nuclear layer; (6) the inner plexiform layer; (7) the ganglion cell layer; (8) the nerve fiber layer; (9) the internal limiting membrane.

Retinal Pigment Epithelium

The pigment epithelium consists of a single layer of cells which is firmly attached to the basal lamina of the choroid and loosely attached to the rods and cones. Microvilli form the apical parts of the cells and project among the rods and cones. The pigment granules consist of melanoprotein and lipofuscin.

The functions of the pigment epithelium are not completely understood. It produces pigment which acts to absorb light. Also, it has phagocytic functions and provides mechanical support to the processes of the photoreceptors.

Photoreceptor Cells of the Retina

The rods and cones, the light receptive elements of the retina, transform physical energy into nerve impulses. Transformation of light energy depends on alteration of visual pigments contained in the rods or cones. Rhodopsin, a derivative of vitamin A, is the visual pigment of the rods. Rhodopsin is composed of retinal (vitamin A aldehyde) bound to a large protein, opsin. The retinal is the same in both rods and cones but the protein moiety differs. Light isomerizes the retinal from the 1 1-cis to an all-trans shape, releasing the retinal from the opsin. The chemical sequence following the isomerization of retinal produces a transient excitation of the receptor which is propagated along its axon. The bipolar cell transmits this information to the inner plexiform layer where it is modified through connections between amacrine, bipolar, and ganglion cells. The ganglion cells pass this analyzed information to the brain.

AQUEOUS HUMOR

Aqueous humor, contained in the anterior compartment of the eye, is produced by the ciliary body and drained through outflow channels into the extraocular venous system. The aqueous circulation is a vital element in the maintenance of normal intraocular pressure (IOP) and in the supply of nutrients to avascular transparent ocular media, the lens, and the cornea. Circulatory disturbance of the aqueous humor leads to abnormal elevation of the IOP, a condition known as "glaucoma," which can ultimately lead to blindness.

Aqueous Humor Formation

Formation of aqueous humor is dependent upon the interaction of complex mechanisms within the ciliary body, such as blood flow, transcapillary exchange, and transport processes in the ciliary epithelium. Maintenance of the IOP is controlled by a delicate equilibration of aqueous humor formation and outflow; aqueous formation and ocular blood flow are in turn influenced by the IOP.

Formation of Aqueous by the Ciliary Epithelium

The ciliary epithelium is composed of two layers, the outer pigmented and the inner nonpigmented epithelium. ATPase is responsible for sodium transport to the posterior chamber and for aqueous formation. It is found predominantly in the nonpigmented epithelium.

Chemical analysis of the aqueous humor indicates that this fluid is not a simple dialysate or ultrafiltrate of the blood plasma. Continuous aqueous production by the ciliary processes requires an active mechanism demanding metabolic energy. Aqueous humor formation is thereby thought to be due to a secretory mechanism in the ciliary epithelium together with ultrafiltration from the capillaries in the ciliary processes. The secretory mechanism involves active transport of electrolytes, coupled fluid transport, and carbonic anhydrase action.

Aqueous Humor Circulation and Drainage

The anterior ocular compartment containing aqueous humor consists of two chambers of unequal volume, the anterior and posterior chambers (Figure 1.2). Communication between the anterior and posterior chambers occurs through the pupil. The aqueous humor is secreted by the ciliary processes into the posterior chamber from which it flows into the anterior chamber. It is drained from the anterior chamber into the extraocular venous systems through porous tissue in the iridocorneal angle and Schlemm's canal (in man and primates) or venous plexus (in lower mammals). This drainage system is called the "conventional drainage route." In man and primates, some aqueous leaves the eye by bulk flow via the ciliary body, suprachoroid, and sclera to the episcleral space; this route is called the "uveoscleral drainage route" or "unconventional route."

THE LENS

The lens is a biconvex, transparent, and avascular structure. It is suspended behind the iris by the zonule of Zinn, a suspensory ligament, which connects it with the ciliary body. The lens capsule is a semipermeable membrane which will admit water and electrolytes. A subcapsular epithelium is present anteriorly. Subepithelial lamellar fibers are continuously produced throughout life. The nucleus and cortex of the lens are made up of long concentric lamellae each of which contains a flattened nucleus in the peripheral portion of the lens near the equator.

Function of the Lens

The lens acts to focus light rays upon the retina. To focus light from a near object, the ciliary muscle contracts, pulling the choroid forward and releasing the tension on the zonules. The elastic lens capsule then molds the pliable lens into a more spherical shape with greater refractive power. This process is known as "accommodation." With age, the lens becomes harder and the ability to accommodate for near objects is decreased.

Composition of the Lens

The lens consists of about 65 percent water and about 35 percent protein (the highest protein content of any tissue of the body). Potassium is more concentrated in the lens than in most body tissues and ascorbic acid and glutathione are both present in the lens. It contains no nerve fibers or blood vessels; therefore, its nutrition is derived from the surrounding fluids. Mechanical injury to the lens or damage from altered nutrient concentration in the aqueous may result in cataract formation.

THE VITREOUS

The vitreous is a clear, avascular, gel-like body which comprises two-thirds of the volume and weight of the eye. It fills the space bounded by the lens, retina, and optic disc. Its gelatinous form and consistency are due to a loose syncytium of long-chain collagen molecules capable of binding large quantities of water. The vitreous is about 99 percent water; collagen and hyaluronic acid make up the remaining 1 percent.

THE VISUAL PATHWAY

The visual pathway from the retina may be divided into six levels: (1) the optic nerve, (2) the optic chiasm, (3) the optic tract, (4) the lateral geniculate nucleus, (5) the optic radiation and (6) the visual cortex.

Anatomy of the Optic Nerve

The optic nerve consists of about 1 million axons arising from the ganglion cells of the retina. The nerve fiber layer of the retina is comprised of these axons and they converge to form the optic nerve. The orbital portion of the nerve travels within the muscle cone to enter the bony optic foramen to gain access to the cranial cavity. The optic nerve is made up of visual fibers (80%) and afferent pupillary fibers (20%).

The Optic Chiasm

After a 10 mm intracranial course, the optic nerves from each eye join to form the optic chiasm. At the optic chiasm the nasal fibers, constituting about three-fourths of all the fibers, cross over to run in the optic tract of the opposite side.

The Optic Tract

In the optic tract, crossed nasal fibers and uncrossed temporal fibers from the chiasm are rearranged to correspond with their position in the lateral geniculate body. All of the fibers receiving impulses from the right visual field are projected to the left cerebral hemisphere; those from the left field to the right cerebral hemisphere. Each optic tract sweeps around the hypothalamus and cerebral peduncle to end in the lateral geniculate body with

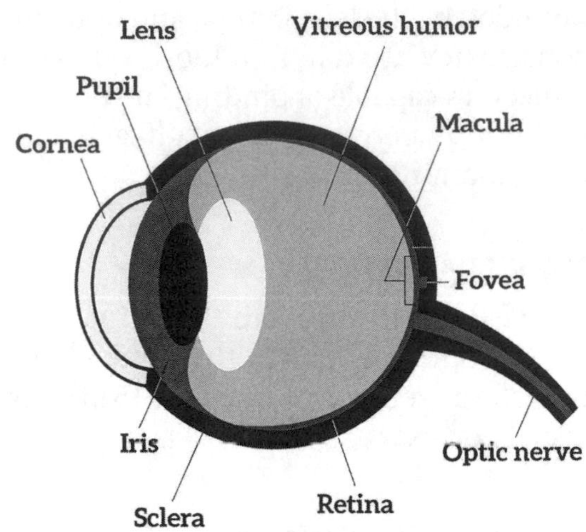

Figure 1.3. Working of the Eyes

a smaller portion carrying pupillary impulses continuing to the pretectal area and superior colliculi.

The Lateral Geniculate Nucleus

The visual fibers synapse in the lateral geniculate body. The cell bodies of this structure give rise to the geniculocalcarine tract (GCT), the final neuron of the visual pathway.

The Optic Radiation

The GCT passes through the posterior limb of the internal capsule and then fans into the optic radiation which traverses parts of the temporal and parietal lobes en route to the occipital cortex.

The Visual Cortex

Optic radiation fibers representing superior retinal quadrants terminate on the superior lip of the calcarine fissure, and those representing inferior retinal quadrants end in the inferior lip. The macula is represented in a large region posteriorly, and retinal areas close to the macula are represented more anteriorly.

HOW YOUR EYES HELP YOU TO SEE

All the different parts of your eyes work together to help you see. First, light passes through the cornea (the clear front layer of the eye). The cornea is shaped similar to a dome and bends light to help the eye focus. Some of this light enters the eye through an opening called the "pupil." The iris (the colored part of the eye) controls how much light the pupil lets in. Next, the light passes through the lens (a clear inner part of the eye). The lens works together with the cornea to focus light correctly on the retina.

When light hits the retina (a light-sensitive layer of tissue at the back of the eye), special cells called "photoreceptors" turn the light into electrical signals. These electrical signals travel from the retina through the optic nerve to the brain. Then the brain turns the signals into the images you see.

Your eyes also need tears to work correctly.

Chapter 2 | Keep an Eye on Your Vision Health

Going to the doctor, going to the dentist—all are part of taking care of your health. But going to the eye doctor? Also important! Eye exams at every age and life stage can help keep your vision strong. Many people think their eyesight is just fine, but then, they get that first pair of glasses or contact lenses and the world comes into a clear view—everything from fine print to street signs.

Improving your eyesight is important—about 11 million Americans age 12 years of age need vision correction—but it is just one of the reasons to get your eyes examined. Regular eye exams are also an important part of finding eye diseases early and preserving your vision.

ONLY YOUR EYE DOCTOR KNOWS FOR SURE

Eye diseases are common and can go unnoticed for a long time—some have no symptoms at first. A comprehensive dilated eye exam by an optometrist or ophthalmologist (eye doctor) is necessary to find eye diseases in the early stages when treatment to prevent vision loss is most effective.

During the exam, visual acuity (sharpness), depth perception, eye alignment, and eye movement are tested. Eye drops are used to make your pupils larger so that your eye doctor can see inside your eyes and check for signs of health problems. Your eye doctor may even spot other conditions, such as high blood pressure or diabetes, sometimes even before your primary-care doctor does.

This chapter includes text excerpted from "Keep an Eye on Your Vision Health," Centers for Disease Control and Prevention (CDC), July 26, 2018.

VISION CARE CAN CHANGE LIVES

Early treatment is critically important to prevent some common eye diseases from causing permanent vision loss or blindness.

- Cataracts (clouding of the lens), the leading cause of vision loss in the United States
- Diabetic retinopathy (causes damage to blood vessels in the back of the eye), the leading cause of blindness in American adults
- Glaucoma (a group of diseases that damages the optic nerve)
- Age-related macular degeneration (AMD) (the gradual breakdown of light-sensitive tissue in the eye)

Of the estimated 61 million U.S. adults who are at high risk for vision loss, only half of them visited an eye doctor in the past 12 months. Regular eye care can have a life-changing impact on preserving the vision of millions of people.

START EARLY

Though people tend to have more vision problems as they get older, children need eye exams to ensure healthy vision, too. But less than 15 percent of preschool children get an eye exam and less than 22 percent receive vision screening. A vision screening can reveal a possible vision problem, but cannot diagnose it. A comprehensive dilated eye exam is needed to diagnose eye diseases.

Amblyopia (reduced vision due to the eye and brain not working together properly) is the most common cause of vision loss in children—2 to 3 out of 100 children. Amblyopia needs to be treated promptly to help prevent vision loss.

REGULAR EYE EXAMS

Children's eyes should be checked regularly by an eye doctor or pediatrician. The U.S. Preventive Services Task Force (USPSTF) recommends vision screening for all children at least once between three and five years of age to detect amblyopia or risk factors for the disease.

People with diabetes should get a dilated eye exam every year.

Some people who are at higher risk for glaucoma and should get a dilated eye exam every two years include:

- African Americans 40 years and older
- All adults older than 60, especially Mexican Americans
- People with a family history of glaucoma

OTHER REASONS TO SEE YOUR EYE DOCTOR

If you have any of the following eye problems, do not wait for your next appointment—visit your eye doctor as soon as possible:

- Decreased vision
- Draining or redness of the eye
- Eye pain
- Double vision
- Floaters (tiny specks that appear to float before your eyes)
- Circles (halos) around lights
- Flashes of light

DIABETES AND YOUR EYES

Diabetic retinopathy is a common complication of diabetes. High blood sugar damages the blood vessels in the retina (a light-sensitive part of the eye), where scarring can cause permanent vision loss.

Diabetic retinopathy is also one of the most preventable causes of vision loss and blindness. Early detection and treatment can prevent or delay blindness due to diabetic retinopathy in 90 percent of people with diabetes, but 50 percent or more of them do not get their eyes examined or are diagnosed too late for effective treatment.

People with diabetes are also at a higher risk for other eye diseases, including glaucoma and cataracts. If you have diabetes, an eye exam every year is necessary to protect and preserve your eyesight and eye health.

Chapter 3 | Maintaining Eye Health

Chapter Contents

Section 3.1 | **Simple Tips for Healthy Eyes**

This section includes text excerpted from "Simple Tips for Healthy Eyes," Centers for Disease Control and Prevention (CDC), June 6, 2019.

Your eyes are an important part of your health. You can do many things to keep them healthy and make sure you are seeing your best. Follow these simple guidelines for maintaining healthy eyes well into your golden years.

HAVE A COMPREHENSIVE DILATED EYE EXAM

You might think your vision is fine or that your eyes are healthy, but visiting your eye-care professional for a comprehensive dilated eye exam is the only way to really be sure. When it comes to common vision problems, some people do not realize they could see better with glasses or contact lenses. In addition, many common eye diseases, such as glaucoma, diabetic eye disease, and age-related macular degeneration (AMD), often have no warning signs. A dilated eye exam is the only way to detect these diseases in their early stages.

During a comprehensive dilated eye exam, your eye-care professional places drops in your eyes to dilate or widen the pupil to allow more light to enter the eye, the same way an open door lets more light into a dark room. This process enables your eye-care professional to get a good look at the back of the eyes and examine them for any signs of damage or disease. Your eye-care professional is the only one who can determine if your eyes are healthy and if your vision at its best.

MAINTAIN YOUR BLOOD SUGAR LEVELS

Ninety percent of blindness caused by diabetes is preventable. Ask your healthcare team to help you set and reach goals to manage your blood sugar, blood pressure, and cholesterol—also known as the "ABCs of diabetes."

- **A1C.** The goal set for many people is less than seven percent for this blood test, but your doctor might set different goals for you.

- **Blood pressure.** High blood pressure causes heart disease. The goal is less than 140/90 mmHg for most people, but your doctor might set different goals for you.
- **Cholesterol.** Low-density lipoproteins (LDL) or "bad" cholesterol builds up and clogs your blood vessels. High-density lipoproteins (HDL) or "good" cholesterol helps remove the "bad" cholesterol from your blood vessels. Ask what your cholesterol numbers should be.

KNOW YOUR FAMILY'S EYE HEALTH HISTORY

Talk to your family members about their eye health history. It is important to know if anyone has been diagnosed with an eye disease or condition since many are hereditary.

EAT RIGHT TO PROTECT YOUR SIGHT

You may have heard that eating carrots are good for your eyes. But eating a diet rich in fruits and vegetables particularly dark leafy greens such as spinach, kale, or collard greens—is important for keeping your eyes healthy, too. Research has also shown that eating fish high in omega-3 fatty acids, such as salmon, tuna, and halibut, also increases the benefits to your eyes.

MAINTAIN A HEALTHY WEIGHT

Being overweight or obese increases your risk of developing diabetes and other systemic conditions, which can lead to vision loss, such as diabetic eye disease or glaucoma. If you are having trouble maintaining a healthy weight, talk to your doctor.

WEAR PROTECTIVE EYEWEAR

Wear protective eyewear when playing sports or doing activities around the house. Protective eyewear includes safety glasses and goggles, safety shields, and eye guards specially designed to provide the correct protection for the activity in which you are engaged. Most protective eyewear lenses are made of polycarbonate, which is 10 times stronger than other plastics. Many eye-care providers sell protective eyewear, as do some sporting goods stores.

QUIT SMOKING OR NEVER START

Smoking is as bad for your eyes as it is for the rest of your body. Research has linked smoking to an increased risk of developing AMD, cataract, and optic nerve damage, all of which can lead to blindness.

BE COOL AND WEAR YOUR SHADES

Sunglasses are a great fashion accessory, but their most important job is to protect your eyes from the sun's ultraviolet (UV) rays. When purchasing sunglasses, look for the ones that block out 99 to 100 percent of both UV-A and UV-B radiation.

GIVE YOUR EYES A REST

If you spend a lot of time at the computer or focusing on any one thing, you sometimes forget to blink and your eyes can get fatigued. Try the 20-20-20 rule: Every 20 minutes, look away about 20 feet in front of you for 20 seconds. This short exercise can help reduce eyestrain.

CLEAN YOUR HANDS AND YOUR CONTACT LENSES—PROPERLY

To avoid the risk of infection, always wash your hands thoroughly before putting in or taking out your contact lenses. Make sure to disinfect contact lenses as instructed and replace them as appropriate.

PRACTICE WORKPLACE EYE SAFETY

Employers are required to provide a safe work environment. When protective eyewear is required as a part of your job, make a habit of wearing the appropriate type at all times, and encourage your coworkers to do the same.

Section 3.2 | **Smoking and Eye Health**

This section includes text excerpted from "Vision Loss, Blindness, and Smoking," Centers for Disease Control and Prevention (CDC), March 22, 2018.

Smoking is as bad for your eyes as it is for the rest of your body. If you smoke, you can develop serious eye conditions that can cause vision loss or blindness. Two of the greatest threats to your eyesight are:

- Macular degeneration
- Cataracts

Macular degeneration also called "age-related macular degeneration" (AMD), is an eye disease that affects the central vision. You need a central vision to see objects clearly and for common tasks, such as reading, recognizing faces, and driving.

There are two forms of AMD: dry AMD and wet AMD. Macular degeneration always begins in the dry form, and sometimes progresses to the more advanced wet form, where vision loss can be very rapid if left untreated.

Cataracts cause blurry vision that worsens over time. Without surgery, cataracts can lead to serious vision loss. The best way to protect your sight from damage associated with smoking is to quit or never start smoking.

SYMPTOMS OF EYE DISEASES RELATED TO SMOKING

You may think your eyes are fine, but the only way to know for sure is by getting a full eye exam. AMD often has no early symptoms, so getting an eye exam is the best way to spot this eye disease early. An eye specialist will place special drops in your eyes to widen your pupils. This offers a better view of the back of your eye, where a thin layer of tissue (the retina) changes light into signals that go to the brain. The macula is a small part of the retina that you need for sharp, central vision.

When symptoms of AMD do occur, they can include:

- Blurred vision or a blurry spot in your central vision
- The need for more light to read or do other tasks

- Straight lines that look wavy
- Difficulty in recognizing faces

Eye injections are often the preferred treatment for wet AMD. Your doctor can inject a drug to stop the growth of these blood vessels and stop further damage to your eyes. You may need injections on a regular basis to save your vision.

HOW DOES SMOKING AFFECT YOUR EYES?

Smoking causes changes in the eyes that can lead to vision loss. If you smoke:

- You are twice as likely to develop AMD compared with a nonsmoker
- You are two to three times more likely to develop cataracts compared with a nonsmoker

HOW CAN YOU PREVENT VISION LOSS RELATED TO SMOKING?

If you smoke, stop. Quitting may lower your risk for both AMD and cataracts. If you already have AMD, quitting smoking may slow the disease. AMD tends to get worse over time. Quitting smoking is something within your control that may help save your sight. Other healthy habits may also help protect your eyes from cataracts and AMD:

- Exercise regularly.
- Maintain normal blood pressure and cholesterol levels.
- Eat a healthy diet rich in green, leafy vegetables and fish.
- Wear sunglasses and a hat with a brim to protect your eyes from sunlight.

HOW IS A CATARACT TREATED?

The symptoms of an early cataract may improve with new eyeglasses, brighter lighting, antiglare sunglasses, or magnifying lenses.

When glasses and brighter lighting do not help, you may need surgery. A doctor will remove the cloudy lens and replace it with an artificial lens. This clear, plastic lens becomes a permanent part of your eye.

HELP FOR VISION LOSS

Coping with vision loss can be frightening, but there is help to make the most of the vision you have left and to continue enjoying with your friends, family, and special interests. If you have already lost some sight, ask your healthcare professional about low-vision counseling and devices such as high-powered lenses, magnifiers, and talking computers.

Section 3.3 | Eye Cosmetic Safety

This section includes text excerpted from "Using Cosmetics Safely," U.S. Food and Drug Administration (FDA), November 15, 2017.

GENERAL TIPS

Follow these safety guidelines when using cosmetics products of any type:

- Read the label. Follow all directions and heed all warnings.
- Wash your hands before you use the product.
- Do not share makeup.
- Keep the containers clean and tightly closed when not in use, and protect them from temperature extremes.
- Throw away cosmetics if there are changes in color or smell.
- Use aerosols or sprays cans in well-ventilated areas. Do not use them while you are smoking or near an open flame. It could start a fire.

EYE MAKE-UP TIPS

There are special safety guidelines for using cosmetics in the eye area. Be sure to keep these practices in mind:

- Do not use cosmetics near your eyes unless they are meant for your eyes. For example, do not use lip liner on your eyes.

- Do not add saliva or water to mascara. You could add germs.
- Throw away your eye makeup if you get an eye infection. The makeup could have become contaminated.
- Do not dye or tint your eyelashes. The U.S. Food and Drug Administration (FDA) has not approved any products for permanent dyeing or tinting of your eyelashes or eyebrows.

UNDERSTANDING COSMETIC LABELS

Being familiar with the product you are using is important. Be sure to read the entire label, including the list of ingredients, warnings, and tips on how to use the product safely. Also, be aware of the following terms that you may see on the label:

- **Hypoallergenic.** Do not assume that the product will not cause allergic reactions. The FDA does not define "hypoallergenic."
- **Organic or natural.** The source of the ingredients does not determine how safe it is. Do not assume that these products are safer than products made with ingredients from other sources. The U.S. Department of Agriculture (USDA) defines what it means for cosmetics to be labeled "organic." However, there is no formal USDA or FDA definition for "natural."
- **Expiration dates.** The law does not require cosmetics to have an expiration date. However, a cosmetic product may go bad if you store it the wrong way—for example, in a place that is too warm or too moist. Marking the container with the date you open a cosmetic may help you keep track of the age of your cosmetics.

REPORT PROBLEMS TO THE FDA

The law does not require cosmetics to be approved by the FDA before they are sold in stores. However, the FDA does monitor consumer reports of adverse events with cosmetic products.

Please notify the FDA if you experience a rash, redness, burn, or another unexpected reaction after using a cosmetic product. Also, please contact the FDA if you notice a problem with the cosmetic product itself, such as a bad smell, color change, or foreign material in the product.

Follow these steps:

- Stop using the product.
- Call your healthcare provider to find out how to take care of the problem.
- Report problems to the FDA in either of these ways:
  - Contact MedWatch, the FDA's Safety Information and Adverse Event Reporting Program (AERS):
    - By phone: 800-FDA-1088 (800-332-1088)
    - Online: File a voluntary report
  - Contact the Consumer Complaint Coordinator in your area.

Section 3.4 | **Protecting Your Vision: Facts and Fiction**

This section includes text excerpted from "Protecting Your Vision: Facts and Fiction," U.S. Food and Drug Administration (FDA), January 26, 2014. Reviewed March 2020.

Whether you are nearsighted, farsighted, or have 20/20 vision, it is important to take good care of your eyes. May is Healthy Vision Month, and a good time to examine the facts—and fiction—surrounding healthy vision.

IT IS LEGAL TO MARKET DECORATIVE CONTACT LENSES AS OVER-THE-COUNTER PRODUCTS—AND THEY ARE SAFE TO WEAR, EVEN IF AN EYE DOCTOR HAS NOT EXAMINED THEM ON YOU FIRST

Fiction. Decorative contact lenses are medical devices regulated by the U.S. Food and Drug Administration (FDA). Places that advertise them as cosmetics or sell them without a prescription are breaking the law. Moreover, an eye doctor (ophthalmologist or optometrist) must examine each eye to properly fit the lenses and evaluate how your eye responds to wearing contact lenses. A poor fit can cause serious eye damage.

LASER POINTERS AND TOYS CONTAINING LASERS CAN CAUSE PERMANENT EYE DAMAGE

Fact. According to Dan Hewett, a health promotion officer at FDA's Center for Devices and Radiological Health (CDRH), "A beam shone directly into a person's eye can injure it in an instant, especially if the laser is a powerful one." In fact, when operated unsafely, or without certain controls, the highly-concentrated light from lasers—even those in toys—can be dangerous, causing serious eye injuries and even blindness. And not just to the person using a laser, but to anyone within the range of the laser beam.

EATING LOTS OF CARROTS IS GOOD FOR YOUR VISION

Fact. Carrots are good food for healthy eyesight because they contain carotenoids, which are precursors of vitamin A. Carotenoids is a nutrient important to your eyes. However, a well-balanced diet can contain lots of foods that offer similar benefits, such as other dark colored fruits and vegetables such as peas and broccoli. Eating a well-balanced diet also helps you maintain a healthy weight, which makes you less likely to develop obesity-related diseases such as type 2 diabetes, the leading cause of blindness in adults.

SITTING TOO CLOSE TO MOVIE, TELEVISION, AND COMPUTER SCREENS WILL DAMAGE YOUR EYES

Fiction. According to the American Academy of Ophthalmology (AAO), watching televisions, including flat screens, cannot cause your eyes any physical harm. The same is true for using the computer too much or watching 3-D movies. The AAO says your eyes may feel more tired if you sit too close to the TV or spend a lot of time working at the computer, but you can fix that by giving your eyes a rest.

IT IS OKAY TO USE AN OVER-THE-COUNTER EYE RELIEVER EVERY DAY

Fiction. According to FDA's Wiley Chambers, M.D., doctors do not recommend long-term use of redness-alleviating drops. Although initially, they help to constrict the blood vessels in the eyes (getting the so-called "red" out), continued use leads to a rebound effect. After continued use, the drops can become the reason that your eyes are red. It is best to use them just for a day or two, Chambers says.

SMOKING INCREASES YOUR RISK OF DEVELOPING MACULAR DEGENERATION

Fact. Smoking is a major risk factor for developing macular degeneration, a disease that gradually destroys sharp, central vision. Other risk factors include genetics, diet, exposure to bright sunlight, cardiovascular disease, and hypertension (high blood pressure).

Chapter 4 | **Vision Disorders: A Statistical Picture**

Chapter Contents

Section 4.1 | **Fast Facts about Vision Disorders**

This section includes text excerpted from "Vision Health Initiative (VHI)—Fast Facts," Centers for Disease Control and Prevention (CDC), July 25, 2017.

Approximately, 12 million people 40 years of age and over in the United States have vision impairment (VI), including 1 million who are blind, 3 million who have VI after correction, and 8 million who have VI due to uncorrected refractive error. As of 2012, 4.2 million Americans aged 40 years and older suffer from uncorrectable VI, out of which 1.02 million are blind; this number is predicted to become more than double by 2050 to 8.96 million due to the increasing epidemic of diabetes and other chronic diseases and the rapidly aging U.S. population.

Approximately, 6.8 percent of children younger than 18 years of age in the United States have a diagnosed eye and vision condition. Nearly 3 percent of children younger than 18 years of age are blind or visually impaired, defined as having difficulty in seeing even when wearing glasses or contact lenses. The National Institute for Occupational Safety and Health (NIOSH) reports that every day about 2,000 U.S. workers sustain job-related eye injuries that require medical treatment. However, safety experts and eye doctors believe the right eye protection can lessen the severity or even prevent 90 percent of these eye injuries. An estimated 61 million adults in the United States are at high risk for serious vision loss, but only half of them visited an eye doctor in the past 12 months.

The annual economic impact of major vision problems among the adult population 40 years of age and older is more than $145 billion. Vision disability is one of the top 10 disabilities among adults 18 years of age and older and one of the most prevalent disabling conditions among children. Early detection and timely treatment of eye conditions, such as diabetic retinopathy have been found to be efficacious and cost-effective. 90 percent of blindness caused by diabetes is preventable. Vision loss causes a substantial social and economic toll for millions of people including significant suffering, disability, loss of productivity, and diminished quality of life (QOL). The national and state data show that more than half of adult Americans who did not seek eye care are due to lack of awareness or costs; which often exacerbated by lack of adequate health insurance. More than 70 percent of survey respondents from the National Eye Health Education Program (NEHEP) 2005 Public Knowledge, Attitudes, and Practices survey consider that the loss of their eyesight would have the greatest impact on their day-to-day life; however, less than 11 percent knew that there are no early warning signs of glaucoma and diabetic retinopathy.

Section 4.2 | The Burden of Vision Loss

This section includes text excerpted from "The Burden of Vision Loss," Centers for Disease Control and Prevention (CDC), October 30, 2017.

POPULATION ESTIMATES

In 2015, a total of 1.02 million people were blind, and approximately 3.22 million people in the United States had vision impairment (VI), as defined by the best-corrected visual acuity in the better-seeing eye. In addition, 8.2 million people had VI due to uncorrected refractive error. By 2050, the numbers of these conditions are projected to double to approximately 2.01 million people who are blind, or having VI of 20/200 or worse, 6.95 million people with VI, and 16.4 million with VI due to uncorrected refractive error.

Through 2050, the number of people with VI are projected to continue to increase and remain higher among non-Hispanic White individuals compared with other racial/ethnic groups for both men and women. In 2050, the second highest number of VI cases is projected to shift from African American to Hispanic adults.

VISION LOSS AMONG TOP TEN DISABILITIES

An analysis of the 1999 Survey of Income and Program Participation (SIPP) (the Centers for Disease Control and Prevention (CDC), 2001) revealed blindness or vision problems to be among the top

10 disabilities among adults aged 18 years and older. Vision loss has serious consequences for the individual as well as those who care for and about people who have compromised vision because it impedes the ability to read, drive, prepare meals, watch television, and attend to personal affairs. Reduced vision among mature adults has been shown to result in social isolation, family stress, and ultimately a greater tendency to experience other health conditions or die prematurely.

ESTIMATED GROWTH IN POPULATION

During the next three decades, the population of adults with vision impairment and age-related eye diseases is estimated to double due to the rapidly aging U.S. population. In addition, the epidemic of diabetes, as well as other chronic diseases, will contribute to an increasing population of people who experience vision loss.

Chapter 5 | **Screening and Diagnostic Tests for Vision and Other Eye-Related Problems**

Chapter Contents

Section 5.1 | **Get Your Child's Vision Checked**

This section includes text excerpted from "Get Your Child's Vision Checked," Office of Disease Prevention and Health Promotion (ODPHP), U.S. Department of Health and Human Services (HHS), January 22, 2020.

WHY YOUR CHILD'S VISION NEEDS TO BE CHECKED

It is important for all children to have their vision checked at least once between three and five years of age. Even if children do not show signs of eye problems, they still need their vision checked. Finding and treating eye problems early on can save a child's sight.

Healthy eyes and vision are very important to a child's development. Growing children constantly use their eyes, both at play and in the classroom.

What Are the Common Eye Problems in Children?

These common eye problems can be treated if they are found early enough:

- Lazy eye (amblyopia)
- Crossed eyes (strabismus)
- Other conditions—such as being nearsighted or farsighted—can be corrected with glasses or contact lenses. Conditions such as these are called "refractive errors."

Is My Child at Risk for Vision Problems?

If your family has a history of childhood vision problems, your child may be more likely to have eye problems. Talk to the doctor about eye problems in your family.

EYE EXAMS

Eye exams are a part of regular checkups. The doctor will check your child's eyes during each checkup, beginning with your child's first well-baby visit.

Around the ages three or four, the doctor will do a more complete eye exam to make sure your child's vision is developing normally. If there are any problems, the doctor may send your child to an eye doctor.

SEE A DOCTOR

Follow these steps to protect your child's vision.

Talk to Your Child's Doctor

Ask the doctor or nurse if there are any problems with your child's vision.

If the doctor recommends a visit to an eye-care professional:

- Ask the doctor for the name of an eye doctor who is good with kids. You can also use these tips to find an eye doctor.
- Write down any information about your child's vision problem
- Plan your child's visit to the eye doctor

What about Cost

Under the Affordable Care Act (ACA), the healthcare reform law passed in 2010, health insurance plans must cover vision screening for kids.

If you have private insurance, your child may be able to get screened at no cost to you. Check with your insurance provider.

Medicaid and the Children's Health Insurance Program (CHIP) also cover vision care for kids.

EYE PROBLEMS

Schedule an eye exam for your child if you see signs of an eye problem, for instance, if your child's eyes:

- Look crossed
- Turn outwards
- Do not focus together
- Are red, crusted, or swollen around the eyelids

PREVENT EYE INJURIES

The following are tips for you to protect your child's eyes from injuries.

- Do not let your child play with toys that have sharp edges or points.
- Keep sharp or pointed objects, such as knives and scissors, away from your child.
- Protect your child's eyes from the sun with kids' sunglasses that block 100 percent of long wave ultraviolet A (UVA) and short wave ultraviolet B (UVB) rays.
- Keep chemicals and sprays (such as cleaners and bug spray) in places that kids cannot reach.
- Make sure your child wears the right eye protection for sports.

VISION DEVELOPMENT

Help develop your child's vision. It takes skill to match up what we see with what we want to do—such as when we want to bounce a ball or read a book.

Here are some activities that can help your child develop vision skills:

- Read to your child and let your child see what you are reading.
- Play with your child using a chalkboard, finger paints, or blocks.
- Take your child to the playground to climb the jungle gym and walk on the balance beam.
- Play catch with your child.

Section 5.2 | **Comprehensive Dilated Eye Exam**

This section includes text excerpted from "Get a Dilated Eye Exam," National Eye Institute (NEI), August 2, 2019.

WHAT IS A DILATED EYE EXAM?

A dilated eye exam is the best thing you can do for your eye health! It is the only way to check for eye diseases early on when they are easier to treat—and before they cause vision loss.

The exam is simple and painless. Your eye doctor will check for vision problems that make it difficult to see clearly, such as being nearsighted or farsighted. Then your doctor will give you some eye drops to dilate (widen) your pupil and check for eye diseases.

Since many eye diseases have no symptoms or warning signs, you could have a problem and not know it. Even if you think your eyes are healthy, getting a dilated eye exam is the only way to know for sure.

HOW OFTEN DO YOU NEED TO GET A DILATED EYE EXAM?

How often you need a dilated eye exam depends on your risk for eye disease. Talk to your doctor about what is right for you.

Get a dilated eye exam every one to two years if you:

- Are over 60 years of age
- Are African American and over 40 years of age
- Have a family history of glaucoma

If you have diabetes or high blood pressure, ask your doctor how often you need an exam. Most people with diabetes or high blood pressure need to get a dilated eye exam done at least once a year.

WHAT HAPPENS DURING A DILATED EYE EXAM

The exam includes:

- A **visual acuity test** to check how clearly you see. Your doctor will ask you to read letters that are up close and far away.

- A **visual field test** to check your peripheral (side) vision. Your doctor will test how well you can see objects off to the sides of your vision without moving your eyes.
- An **eye muscle function test** to check for problems with the muscles around your eyeballs. Your doctor will move an object around and ask you to follow it with your eyes.
- A **pupil response test** to check how light enters your eyes. Your doctor will shine a small flashlight into your eyes and check how your pupils react to the light.
- A **tonometry test** to measure the pressure in your eyes. Your doctor will use a machine to blow a quick puff of air onto your eye, or gently touch your eye with a special tool. Do not worry—it does not hurt!
- **Dilation** to check for problems with the inner parts of your eye. Your doctor will give you some eye drops to dilate (widen) your pupil. This helps the doctor see inside your eye.

Depending on your needs, your doctor may include other tests too. Ask your doctor if you have any questions.

HOW DOES DILATION WORK?

Dilating your pupil lets more light into your eye—just like opening a door lets light into a dark room. Dilation helps your eye doctor check for many common eye problems, including diabetic retinopathy, glaucoma, and age-related macular degeneration (AMD).

WHAT HAPPENS AFTER A DILATED EYE EXAM

For a few hours after a dilated eye exam, your vision may be blurry and you may be sensitive to light. Ask a friend or family member to drive you home from your appointment.

If your eye doctor finds refractive errors in your vision, you may get a prescription for eyeglasses or contact lenses to help you see more clearly.

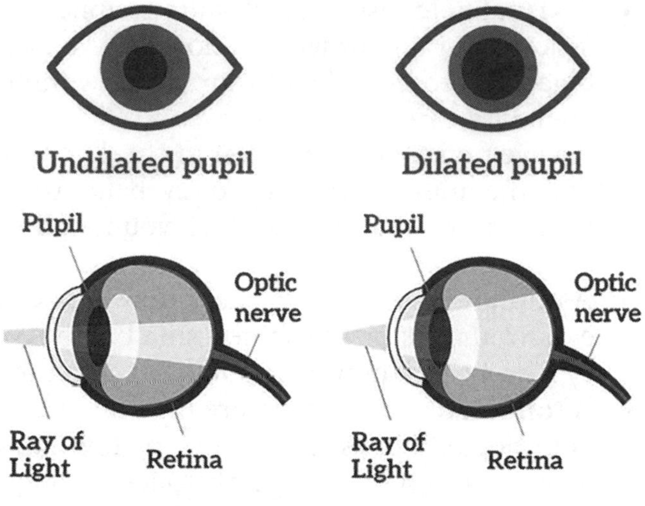

Figure 5.1. Undilated Pupil versus Dilated Pupil

If your eye doctor finds signs of an eye disease, you can talk about treatment options and decide what is right for you. Also, learn more about these common eye diseases:

- Diabetic retinopathy
- Age-related macular degeneration (AMD)
- Cataract
- Glaucoma

If you are seeing clearly and there are no signs of eye disease, you are all set until your next exam. Make an appointment for your next dilated eye exam before you leave the office—that way, you will not forget.

Section 5.3 | **Individualized Exam Schedule for Diabetic Eye Disease**

This section includes text excerpted from "Individualized Exam Schedule for Diabetic Eye Disease," National Institutes of Health (NIH), May 2, 2017.

People with diabetes have blood sugar (glucose) levels that are too high. Over time, high levels of blood glucose can cause health problems, such as eye damage. The part of the eye that is at risk for damage is the retina, the light-sensitive tissue that lines the back of the eye. Without treatment, retinal damage can lead to permanent blindness.

Signs of diabetic retinal disease (retinopathy) can be detected through a comprehensive dilated eye exam before symptoms occur and in time to take action to prevent vision loss. Pupil dilation, or widening, is an important part of the exam because it allows a much better view of the retina. To diagnose diabetic eye disease while it is treatable, experts currently suggest that people with type 1 diabetes get an eye exam at least once a year starting three to five years after diagnosis.

To find out whether the exam frequency could be tailored to individual risk, researchers analyzed 30 years of data from about 1,400 people with type 1 (insulin-dependent) diabetes. The study was funded mainly by the National Institutes of Health (NIH) and the National Institute of Diabetes and Digestive and Kidney Diseases (NIDDK). The NIH's National Eye Institute (NEI) and others also provided support. Results were published on April 20, 2017, in the *New England Journal of Medicine*.

The researchers analyzed data from about 24,000 eye exams with retinal photography. The results enabled them to develop a model to predict the likelihood of an individual progressing to significant, vision-threatening retinopathy based on their current retina exam and blood glucose level.

The analysis showed that, among people with type 1 diabetes and recent blood glucose level near the normal range (as measured by an A1C level of 6%), those with no detectable retinal damage could be screened every four years. Those with mild retinal damage could be examined every three years without increasing the risk of vision loss. People with moderate or severe retinal damage, the researchers found, should be examined more often than the current recommendation: every six or three months, respectively. On an average, this tailored schedule would result in fewer eye exams and earlier detection and treatment to save vision.

People who have type 1 diabetes and poorer blood glucose control (such as a current A1C of 8 to 10%) are at risk of developing retinal disease sooner. For that reason, the researchers recommended more frequent eye exams for these people.

"The results could save money and time while getting better health outcomes—a win all around," says Dr. Catherine Cowie, who oversaw the study at the NIDDK. "The findings from this landmark type 1 diabetes study will inform a precision medicine approach, where treatment is tailored to the individual."

The new evidence-based exam schedule could prove more efficient than the annual schedule at detecting vision-threatening retinal disease. The next step is for experts to consider these findings for modifying clinical guidelines for people with type 1 diabetes.

Chapter 6 | **Working with Your Eye-Care Doctor**

Chapter Contents

Section 6.1 | **Finding an Eye Doctor**

This section includes text excerpted from "Finding an Eye Doctor," National Eye Institute (NEI), October 24, 2019.

Seeing an eye doctor is the best way to stay on top of your eye health—and eye doctors are not just for people who need glasses or contacts. Many common eye diseases do not have any early warning signs, so getting an eye exam is the only way to be sure your eyes are healthy.

WHEN DO YOU NEED TO SEE AN EYE DOCTOR?

Your regular doctor may check your eyes quickly during an appointment. But that is not enough to keep your eyes healthy in the long run. It is time to see an eye doctor if:

- Your vision is blurry or your eyes are red, swollen, or painful
- You are not seeing in focus, even when you are wearing your glasses or contacts
- You think you may have a vision problem or eye disease
- Your doctor says you need a dilated eye exam

WHAT KIND OF EYE DOCTOR DO YOU NEED?

There are two basic types of eye doctors: optometrists and ophthalmologists. The best choice depends on your eye care needs.

For All-Around Eye Care

Either an optometrist or ophthalmologist is a good option. Both of these types of eye doctors can:

- Give you a comprehensive dilated eye exam
- Write a prescription for glasses or contacts
- Prescribe medicines

For Treating Serious Eye Problems

You may want to see an ophthalmologist. This type of eye doctor may offer treatments—such as surgery—that optometrists do not. Some ophthalmologists specialize in specific eye diseases, such as glaucoma or diabetic retinopathy.

HOW DO YOU FIND A DOCTOR WHO IS THE RIGHT FIT?

Ask for Recommendations

Start by asking your regular doctor to share the names of local eye doctors. Talk to your family and trusted friends, too. What do they like—or not like—about their eye doctors?

Look Online

Use these online tools to find an eye doctor near you:

- Find an Optometrist (www.aoa.org/doctor-locator-search?sso=y) (American Optometric Association (AOA))
- Find an Ophthalmologist (secure.aao.org/aao/find-ophthalmologist) (American Academy of Ophthalmology (AAO))
- Find a Retina Specialist (www.asrs.org/find-a-specialist) (American Society for Retina Specialists (ASRS))

If you have health insurance, you can also check your plan's website to find eye doctors in your area.

Find Out How Much You Will Need to Pay

If you have health insurance, call your insurance company and ask:

- What eye-care services does my plan cover?
- What will my out-of-pocket costs be?
- Can you give me a list of eye doctors who are in my plan's network?

Keep in mind that many plans—including some Medicare plans—do not cover routine eye exams or eyeglasses.

If you do not have health insurance, or if your plan does not cover eye care, call the eye doctor's office and ask how much the appointment will cost.

Schedule an Appointment

Before you meet with your eye doctor, it is a good idea to write down your questions to help you make the most of your visit.

Think about Whether It Is a Good Fit

After the appointment, ask yourself:

- Did the doctor and office staff explain things in a way you could understand?
- Did you get a chance to ask questions?
- Did you feel rushed during the appointment?
- Do you feel like you and the doctor could work together as a team?

Taking the time to find an eye doctor you trust is worth it. If you are not happy with how things are going, it is okay to look for a different eye doctor.

Note: The National Eye Institute (NEI) does not endorse or recommend specific eye-care professionals.

Section 6.2 | Talking to Your Eye-Care Doctor

This section includes text excerpted from "Talking with Your Eye Doctor," National Eye Institute (NEI), June 26, 2019.

Have you recently been diagnosed with an eye disease or a vision problem? Keep this in mind: when you and your eye doctor work together as a team and communicate well, you will feel more confident about your treatment plan, and you will get better care.

PLAN AHEAD TO MAKE THE MOST OF YOUR APPOINTMENTS

Working together is all about good communication. There is nothing wrong with asking lots of questions. Remember, it is your doctor's job to answer them.

But since it is easy to forget what you wanted to ask during an appointment, plan ahead and write down your questions before you meet.

ASK QUESTIONS—KEEP ASKING UNTIL YOU UNDERSTAND

Your doctor needs to listen carefully to your questions and concerns—and you need to make sure you understand exactly what your doctor tells you about your eye health, your treatment plan, and what you need to do next.

Here are some questions you may want to ask:

- What condition do I have?
- What does cause this condition?
- Will it affect my vision, now or in the future?
- Do I need to make any changes to my everyday life?
- Are there any symptoms I need to watch for? What do I need to do if I notice those symptoms?
- Can you give me some information about my condition to take home with me?

Questions about tests:

- Do I need any tests?
- What do you want to find out from the test?
- When will I get my test results?
- Does the test have any risks or side effects?
- Will I need more tests later?

Questions about treatment:

- What treatment do you recommend for me? Can you tell me why?
- When will I start treatment and how long will it last?
- What do I need to know about the medicine you are prescribing?

- What are the risks and benefits of this treatment?
- Are there other treatment options?

KEEP TRACK OF WHAT YOU LEARNED DURING YOUR APPOINTMENT

To help you remember everything your doctor tells you:

- Take notes during your appointment. You can write down your notes, or record your conversation with your cell phone so you can listen to it later.
- Ask a friend or family member to come with you to the appointment. They can take notes, help you ask questions, or just be there to listen and support you.
- Ask your doctor to write down the main points from the visit. They may also be able to print instructions or other important information for you.

Chapter 7 | Pediatric Vision Concerns

Children with unaddressed eye problems may face many barriers in life, academics, and athletics. Early detection can help eliminate these barriers and enable children to reach their maximum potential. Vision does not just happen. Just as with learning to walk or talk, a child's brain learns to use its eyes to see. For this reason, the longer a vision problem goes undiagnosed and untreated, the harder it will be for the child's brain to optimally adapt to the vision deficiency.

COMMON VISION PROBLEMS IN CHILDREN

According to the 2017 American Community Survey (ACS), almost 502,191 children below 18 years of age are visually impaired or described as having trouble seeing even when wearing glasses or contact lenses. Some of the common vision problems in children are:

- Lazy eye (Amblyopia)
- Crossed eyes (Strabismus)
- Refractive errors
    - Nearsightedness (myopia)
    - Farsightedness (hyperopia)
    - Astigmatism

Other common eye conditions that require immediate medical attention are retinopathy of prematurity (ROP), a disease that affects the eyes of premature babies and includes eye conditions associated with family history, including:

- **Retinoblastoma**—a tumor in the retina that can affect a child in their first three years, which may result in vision loss and whiteness in the pupil
- **Infantile cataracts**—a cataract (the clouding of the eye's lens) affecting newborns
- **Congenital glaucoma**—a rare condition in infants that can be inherited as a result of high intraocular pressure in the eye, due to incorrect or incomplete development of the eye's drainage system before birth. This can be corrected with medication and surgery.

To avoid irreversible harm from these conditions, children need to have routine eye checkups and screenings from an early age.

CAUSES OF VISION PROBLEMS IN CHILDREN

Children may have a vision problem from birth or it may occur later as a result of disease or injury. Some of the most common reasons for vision problems in children are:

- Any neurological condition that affects the part of the brain that controls vision
- Genetic conditions
- Any illnesses that occur in premature babies or newborns who had complications during birth
- Viral infections during pregnancy
- Any structural problem with the eye
- Damage or injury to the eye, the pathway that connects the eye to the brain, or the visual center of the brain

SYMPTOMS OF VISION DEFICIENCIES IN A CHILD

Some of the symptoms that can be spotted in a child with a vision problem are:

- Constant rubbing of the eyes
- Severe light sensitivity
- Poor focus

- Poor visual tracking (following an object)
- Unusual alignment or movement of the eyes
- Chronic redness or tearing of the eyes
- A white pupil
- Difficulty seeing distant objects
- Difficulty reading the blackboard
- Squinting
- Difficulty reading
- Sitting too close to the TV or holding a book too close to the eyes

Watch for these symptoms and have the child examined right away if you spot any of them so that the issue does not become permanent.

STATISTICS ON PEDIATRIC VISION CONCERNS

Eighty percent of what a child learns is acquired through visual processing. The risk of failing a grade is three times greater for a child with a vision deficiency. Statistics on pediatric vision concerns in the United States follow:

- 2 percent of children 6 to 72 months of age have been diagnosed with amblyopia (lazy eye), the most common cause of vision loss in children.
- 2 to 4 percent of children under the age of 6 have been diagnosed with strabismus (crossed eyes).
- 4 percent of children 6 to 72 months of age and 9 percent of children 5 to 17 years of age have been diagnosed with myopia (nearsightedness).
- The prevalence of hyperopia (farsightedness) has been seen in 21 percent of children between 6 to 72 months of age and 13 percent in children 5 to 17 years of age.
- 15 to 28 percent of children 5 to 17 years of age have astigmatism.
- A child's eye is 80 percent more prone to be damaged by ultraviolet (UV) rays.

EYE-EXAM ROUTINES FOR CHILDREN

It is necessary for children between three to five years of age to have their vision checked at least once even if the child does not show any symptoms of having an eye problem. Finding and treating an eye problem early can help save the child's sight. Some points to consider for routine eye checkups include:

- High-risk newborns (including premature infants), children with a family history of eye problems, and children with obvious eye irregularities should be examined by an eye doctor as early as possible.
- All infants need to be routinely screened for eye health during general checkups with their pediatrician or family doctor until they reach the age of one.
- Children must have an eye-health screening and visual sharpness tests between the ages of three and four.
- Children around the age of five should have their vision and eye alignment checked by their pediatrician or family doctor. If a child fails either of the tests, then she or he must be examined by an eye doctor as soon as possible.
- Routine screening should be done at school and the primary doctor's office when the child reaches the age of five or earlier if the teacher notices that a child is not seeing well in class or shows any symptoms of a visual deficiency, such as squinting or frequent headaches.
- Children who already wear prescribed glasses or contact lenses should have an annual checkup with an eye doctor to monitor any changes in their vision.

A child's development greatly depends on healthy eyes and vision. Their eyes need to be examined regularly because many vision problems, when detected early, can be treated more effectively.

References

1. "Vision Impairment," Raising Children Network, November 12, 2019.

2. "Shocking Vision Statistics," Essilor of America, September 23, 2014.
3. "Children's Vision and Eye Health: A Snapshot of Current National Issues," Prevent Blindness, National Center for Children's Vision & Eye Health, February 15, 2016.
4. "Your Child's Vision," Kids Health, June 27, 2014.

Chapter 8 | Adult Vision Concerns

Chapter Contents

Section 8.1 | **Common Vision Problems in Adults**

This section includes text excerpted from "Common Eye Disorders," Centers for Disease Control and Prevention (CDC), September 29, 2015. Reviewed March 2020.

Approximately 11 million Americans aged 12 years and older could improve their vision through proper refractive correction. More than 3.3 million Americans aged 40 years and older are either legally blind (having best-corrected visual acuity of 6/60 or worse (=20/200) in the better-seeing eye) or are with low vision (having best-corrected visual acuity less than 6/12 (<20/40) in the better-seeing eye, excluding those who were categorized as being blind). The leading causes of blindness and low vision in the United States are primarily age-related eye diseases, such as age-related macular degeneration (AMD), cataract, diabetic retinopathy, and glaucoma. Other common eye disorders include amblyopia and strabismus.

REFRACTIVE ERRORS

Refractive errors are the most frequent eye problems in the United States. Refractive errors include myopia (nearsightedness), hyperopia (farsightedness), astigmatism (distorted vision at all distances), and presbyopia that occurs between 40 to 50 years of age (loss of the ability to focus up close, inability to read letters of the phone book, need to hold newspaper farther away to see clearly) can be corrected by eyeglasses, contact lenses, or in some cases surgery. The studies conducted by the National Eye Institute (NEI) showed that proper refractive correction could improve vision among 11 million Americans aged 12 years and older.

AGE-RELATED MACULAR DEGENERATION

Macular degeneration often called "age-related macular degeneration" (AMD) is an eye disorder associated with aging and results in damaging sharp and central vision. Central vision is needed for seeing objects clearly and for common daily tasks such as reading and driving. AMD affects the macula, the central part of the retina that allows the eye to see fine details. There are two forms of AMD—wet and dry.

Wet AMD is when the abnormal blood vessels behind the retina start to grow under the macula, ultimately leading to blood and fluid leakage. Bleeding, leaking, and scarring from these blood vessels cause damage and lead to rapid central vision loss. An early symptom of wet AMD is that straight lines appear wavy.

Dry AMD is when the macula thins over time as part of the aging process, gradually blurring central vision. The dry form is more common and accounts for 70 to 90 percent of cases of AMD and it progresses more slowly than the wet form. Over time, as less of the macula functions, central vision is gradually lost in the affected eye. Dry AMD generally affects both eyes. One of the most common early signs of dry AMD is drusen.

Drusen are tiny yellow or white deposits under the retina. They often are found in people who are 60 years of age and above. The presence of small drusen is normal and does not cause vision loss. However, the presence of large and more numerous drusen raises the risk of developing advanced dry AMD or wet AMD.

It is estimated that 1.8 million Americans who are 40 years of age and above are affected by AMD and an additional 7.3 million with large drusen are at substantial risk of developing AMD. The number of people with AMD is estimated to reach 2.95 million in 2020. AMD is the leading cause of permanent impairment of reading and fine or close-up vision among people 65 years of age and above.

CATARACT

A cataract is a clouding of the eye's lens and is the leading cause of blindness worldwide, and the leading cause of vision loss in the United States. Cataracts can occur at any age because of a variety of causes and can be present at birth. Although treatment for the removal of a cataract is widely available, access barriers, such as insurance coverage, treatment costs, patient's choice, or lack of awareness prevents many people from receiving the proper treatment.

An estimated 20.5 million (17.2%) Americans who are of 40 years of age and older have a cataract in one or both eyes, and 6.1 million (5.1%) have had their lens removed operatively. The total number of people who have cataracts is estimated to increase to 30.1 million by 2020.

DIABETIC RETINOPATHY

Diabetic retinopathy (DR) is a common complication of diabetes. It is the leading cause of blindness in American adults. It is characterized by progressive damage to the blood vessels of the retina, the light-sensitive tissue at the back of the eye that is necessary for good vision. DR progresses through four stages, mild nonproliferative retinopathy (microaneurysms), moderate nonproliferative retinopathy (blockage in some retinal vessels), severe nonproliferative retinopathy (more vessels are blocked leading to the retina being deprived of blood supply, which leads to the abnormal growth of new blood vessels), and proliferative retinopathy (most advanced stage). DR usually affects both eyes.

The risks of DR are reduced through disease management that includes good control of blood sugar, blood pressure, and lipid abnormalities. Early diagnosis of DR and timely treatment reduces the risk of vision loss; however, as many as 50 percent of patients are not getting their eyes examined or are diagnosed too late for treatment to be effective.

It is the leading cause of blindness among working-age adults who are 20 to 74 years of age. An estimated 4.1 million and 899,000 Americans are affected by retinopathy and vision-threatening retinopathy, respectively.

GLAUCOMA

A glaucoma is a group of diseases that can damage the eye's optic nerve and result in vision loss and blindness. Glaucoma occurs when the normal fluid pressure inside the eyes slowly rises. However, the findings now show that glaucoma can occur with normal eye pressure. With early treatment, you can often protect your eyes against serious vision loss.

There are two major categories "open-angle" and "closed-angle" glaucoma. Open-angle is a chronic condition that progresses slowly over a long period of time without the person noticing vision loss until the disease is very advanced, that is why it is called "sneak thief of sight." Angle-closure can appear suddenly and is painful. Visual loss can progress quickly; however, the pain and discomfort lead patients to seek medical attention before permanent damage occurs.

AMBLYOPIA

Amblyopia, also referred to as "lazy eye," is the most common cause of vision impairment in children. Amblyopia is the medical term used when the vision in one of the eyes is reduced because the eye and the brain are not working together properly. The eye itself looks normal, but it is not being used normally because the brain is favoring the other eye. Conditions leading to amblyopia include strabismus, an imbalance in the positioning of the two eyes; more nearsighted, farsighted, or astigmatic in one eye than the other eye, and rarely other eye conditions such as cataract.

Unless it is successfully treated in early childhood, amblyopia usually persists into adulthood, and is the most common cause of permanent one-eye vision impairment among children and young and middle-aged adults. An estimated two to three percent of the population suffer from amblyopia.

STRABISMUS

Strabismus involves an imbalance in the positioning of the two eyes. Strabismus can cause the eyes to cross in (esotropia) or turn out (exotropia). Strabismus is caused by a lack of coordination between the eyes. As a result, the eyes look in different directions and do not focus simultaneously on a single point. In most cases of strabismus in children, the cause is unknown. In more than half of these cases, the problem is present at or shortly after birth (congenital strabismus). When the two eyes fail to focus on the same image, there is reduced or absent depth perception and the brain may learn to ignore the input from one eye, causing permanent vision loss in that eye (one type of amblyopia).

Section 8.2 | **Normal Changes in the Aging Eye and Their Symptoms**

This section includes text excerpted from "Aging and Your Eyes," National Institute on Aging (NIA), National Institutes of Health (NIH), January 31, 2017.

COMMON EYE PROBLEMS

The following common eye problems can be easily treated. But, sometimes they can be signs of more serious issues.

- **Presbyopia** is a slow loss of ability to see close objects or small print. It is normal to have this problem as you get older. People with presbyopia often have headaches or strained, tired eyes. Reading glasses usually fix the problem.
- **Floaters** are tiny specks or "cobwebs" that seem to float across your vision. You might see them in well-lit rooms or outdoors on a bright day. Floaters can be a normal part of aging. But, sometimes they are a sign of a more serious eye problem, such as retinal detachment. If you see many new floaters and/or flashes of light, see your eye-care professional right away.
- **Tearing** (or having too many tears) can come from being sensitive to light, wind, or temperature changes, or having a condition called "dry eye." Wearing sunglasses may help. So, might eye drops. Sometimes tearing is a sign of a more serious eye problem, such as an infection or a blocked tear duct. Your eye-care professional can treat these problems.
- **Eyelid problems** can result from different diseases or conditions. Common eyelid problems include red and swollen eyelids, itching, tearing, and crusting of eyelashes during sleep. These problems may be caused by a condition called "blepharitis" and are treated with warm compresses and gentle eyelid scrubs.

EYE DISEASES AND DISORDERS

The following eye conditions can lead to vision loss and blindness. They may have few or no early symptoms. Regular eye exams are your best protection. If your eye-care professional finds a problem early, there are certain things you can do to keep your eyesight.

- **Cataracts** are cloudy areas in the eye's lens that cause blurred or hazy vision. Some cataracts stay small and do not change your eyesight a lot. Others become large and reduce vision. Cataract surgery can restore good vision. It is a safe and common treatment. If you have a cataract, your eye-care professional will watch for changes over time to see if you would benefit from surgery.
- **Corneal diseases and conditions** can cause redness, watery eyes, pain, problems with vision, or a halo effect of the vision (things appear to have an aura of light around them). Infection and injury are some of the things that can hurt the cornea. Treatment may be simple—for example, changing your eyeglass prescription or using eye drops. In severe cases, surgery may be needed.
- **Dry eyes** happen when tear glands do not work well. You may feel stinging or burning, a sandy feeling as if something is in the eye, or other discomforts. Dry eye is more common as people get older, especially for women. Your eye-care professional may tell you to use a home humidifier or air cleaner, special eye drops (artificial tears), or ointments to treat dry eye.
- **Glaucoma** often comes from too much fluid pressure inside the eye. If not treated, it can lead to vision loss and blindness. People with glaucoma often have no early symptoms or pain. You can protect yourself by having dilated eye exams yearly. Glaucoma can be treated with prescription eye drops, lasers, or surgery.
- **Retinal disorders** are a leading cause of blindness in the United States. Retinal disorders that affect aging eyes include:
    - **Age-related macular degeneration (AMD).** AMD can harm the sharp, central vision needed to see objects clearly and to do common things such as driving and reading. During a dilated eye exam,

your eye-care professional will look for signs of AMD. There are treatments for AMD. If you have AMD, ask for special dietary supplements that could lower your chance of it getting worse.

- **Diabetic retinopathy (DR).** This problem may occur if you have diabetes. Diabetic retinopathy develops slowly and often has no early warning signs. If you have diabetes, be sure to have a dilated eye exam at least once a year. Keeping your blood sugar, blood pressure, and cholesterol under control can prevent diabetic retinopathy or slow its progress. Laser surgery can sometimes prevent it from getting worse.
- **Retinal detachment.** This is a medical emergency. When the retina separates from the back of the eye, it is called "retinal detachment." If you see new floaters or light flashes, or if it seems as if a curtain has been pulled over your eye, go to your eye-care professional right away. With treatment, doctors often can prevent loss of vision.

WHAT IS LOW VISION?

Low vision means you cannot fix your eyesight with glasses, contact lenses, medicine, or surgery. Low vision affects some people as they age.

You may have low vision if you:

- Cannot see well enough to do everyday tasks, such as reading, cooking, or sewing
- Have difficulty recognizing the faces of your friends or family
- Have trouble reading street signs
- Find that lights do not seem as bright

If you have any of these problems, ask your eye-care professional to test you for low vision. Special tools can help people with low vision to read, write, and manage daily tasks. These tools include large-print reading materials, magnifying aids, closed-circuit televisions, audio tapes, electronic reading machines, and computers with large print and a talking function.

Other tips that may help include:

- Brighten the lighting in your room.
- Write with bold, black felt-tip markers.
- Use paper with bold lines to help you write in a straight line.
- Put colored tape on the edge of your steps to help you see them and prevent you from falling.
- Install dark-colored light switches and electrical outlets that you can see easily against light-colored walls.
- Use motion lights that turn on when you enter a room. These may help you avoid accidents caused by poor lighting.
- Use telephones, clocks, and watches with large numbers; put large-print labels on the microwave and stove.

HOW CAN YOU PROTECT YOUR EYESIGHT?

Have your eyes checked regularly by an eye-care professional—either an ophthalmologist or optometrist. People over 60 years of age should get dilated eye exams yearly. During this exam, the eye-care professional will put drops in your eyes to widen (dilate) your pupils so that she or he can look at the back of each eye. This is the only way to find some common eye diseases that have no early signs or symptoms. If you wear glasses or contact lenses, your prescription should be checked, too. See your doctor regularly to check for diseases such as diabetes and high blood pressure. These diseases can cause eye problems if not controlled or treated.

See an eye-care professional right away if you:

- Suddenly cannot see or everything looks blurry
- See flashes of light
- Have eye pain
- Experience double vision
- Have redness or swelling of your eye or eyelid

TIPS FOR HEALTHY EYES

- Protect your eyes from too much sunlight by wearing sunglasses that block ultraviolet (UV) radiation and a hat with a wide brim when you are outside.
- Stop smoking.
- Make smart food choices.
- Be physically active and maintain a healthy weight.
- Maintain normal blood pressure.
- Control diabetes (if you have it).
- If you spend a lot of time at the computer or focusing on one thing, you may forget to blink. Every 20 minutes, look away about 20 feet for 20 seconds to prevent eyestrain.

Section 8.3 | **Vision Concerns during Pregnancy**

During pregnancy, a woman's body undergoes many physical changes in order to support a growing fetus. Natural fluctuations in hormone levels, metabolism, circulation, and fluid retention can affect the eyes just as they affect other organs. As a result, many pregnant women experience changes in their eyes or vision. Although most pregnancy-related eye issues are minor and disappear on their own after delivery, a few types of vision changes can indicate a health condition that requires medical attention. Experts recommend that expectant mothers check with their doctors if they experience any of the following symptoms:

- Double vision
- Temporary loss of vision
- Sensitivity to light
- Seeing spots, auras, or blinking lights

NORMAL VISION CHANGES DURING PREGNANCY

Most of the vision changes that occur during pregnancy are temporary. Although they can be annoying, they are usually not a cause for concern. They occur due to changing hormone levels and fluid retention, which are a normal part of pregnancy. Some of the common eye changes that occur during pregnancy include blurry vision, dry eyes, and puffy eyelids.

Blurry Vision

The fluid retention that most women experience during pregnancy can temporarily change the thickness and shape of the cornea, the transparent layer that helps focus light as it enters the eye. These changes can affect the power of corrective lenses the woman needs, resulting in blurry vision. Since the cornea will likely return to normal following delivery, experts generally recommend against getting a new prescription for corrective lenses during pregnancy. Many eye doctors can provide a temporary lens if the blurry vision makes it difficult to drive a car or perform other everyday tasks safely.

Dry Eyes

Many expectant mothers find that their eyes become dry and irritated during pregnancy and breastfeeding. This problem can be uncomfortable and make it difficult to wear contact lenses. Experts suggest using over-the-counter (OTC) lubricating or rewetting eye drops to soothe dry eyes and relieve discomfort. Pregnant women may switch to glasses temporarily and take frequent breaks while working at a computer to avoid eyestrain.

Puffy Eyelids

Many women experience swollen ankles during pregnancy as a result of water retention. A lesser-known effect of pregnancy hormones is swelling around the eyes and puffy eyelids, which can interfere with peripheral vision. To limit fluid retention, experts recommend drinking lots of water and eating a healthy diet low in sodium and caffeine.

VISION CHANGES OF CONCERN DURING PREGNANCY

A few vision changes that may occur during pregnancy can be symptoms of a serious medical condition, such as preeclampsia or gestational diabetes. Expectant mothers who experience sudden or severe vision disruptions should seek medical attention.

Preeclampsia

Preeclampsia is a complication that occurs in 5 percent to 8 percent of all pregnancies. The main symptoms are high blood pressure, swelling of the hands and feet, and protein in the urine. Many women who develop preeclampsia experience vision problems, such as double vision, temporary loss of vision, sensitivity to light, or seeing spots, auras, or blinking lights. Preeclampsia can progress quickly to cause bleeding, organ damage, and detachment of the retinas in the eyes. Expectant mothers who experience symptoms of preeclampsia should seek medical attention and have their blood pressure checked immediately.

Diabetes and Gestational Diabetes

Diabetes is a disease that affects the body's ability to metabolize carbohydrates, resulting in high levels of sugar in the blood. High blood sugar can damage the blood vessels in the retina, causing a serious eye condition called "diabetic retinopathy." Women who are diabetic need to monitor their blood sugar closely and get regular eye screenings to check for damage to the retina. This is especially important during pregnancy, which increases the risk of vision loss associated with diabetes.

Gestational diabetes is a form of diabetes that develops during pregnancy. Expectant mothers who develop the condition should be examined by an eye doctor for signs of retinopathy. Pregnant women with either form of diabetes should also seek medical attention if they experience blurry vision, which can be a sign of elevated blood sugar levels.

References

1. "Can Pregnancy Affect Your Eyes?" WebMD, 2017.
2. "How Pregnancy Affects Vision," Northwest Vision, August 30, 2015.
3. "Pregnancy and Your Vision," Prevent Blindness, 2017.
4. "Vision Changes during Pregnancy," BabyCenter, 2017.

Part 2 | Understanding and Treating Refractive, Eye Movement, and Alignment Disorders

Chapter 9 | Refractive Disorders

Chapter Contents

Section 9.1 | **An Overview of Refractive Errors**

This section includes text excerpted from "Refractive Errors," National Eye Institute (NEI), July 11, 2019.

WHAT ARE REFRACTIVE ERRORS?

Refractive errors are a type of vision problem that makes it hard to see clearly. They happen when the shape of your eye keeps light from focusing correctly on your retina (a light-sensitive layer of tissue in the back of your eye).

Refractive errors are the most common type of vision problem. More than 150 million Americans have a refractive error—but many do not know that they could be seeing better. That is why eye exams are so important.

If you have a refractive error, your eye doctor can prescribe eyeglasses or contact lenses to help you see clearly.

WHAT ARE THE TYPES OF REFRACTIVE ERRORS?

There are four common types of refractive errors:

- **Nearsightedness (myopia)** makes far-away objects look blurry.
- **Farsightedness (hyperopia)** makes nearby objects look blurry.
- **Astigmatism** can make far-away and nearby objects look blurry or distorted.
- **Presbyopia** makes it hard for middle-aged and older adults to see things up close.

WHAT CAUSES REFRACTIVE ERRORS

Refractive errors can be caused by:

- Eyeball length (when the eyeball grows too long or too short)
- Problems with the shape of the cornea (the clear outer layer of the eye)
- Aging of the lens (an inner part of the eye that is normally clear and helps the eye focus)

WHAT ARE THE SYMPTOMS OF REFRACTIVE ERRORS?

The most common symptom is blurry vision. Other symptoms include:

- Double vision
- Hazy vision
- Seeing a glare or halo around bright lights
- Squinting
- Headaches
- Eyestrain (when your eyes feel tired or sore)
- Trouble focusing when reading or looking at a computer

Some people may not notice the symptoms of refractive errors. It is important to get eye exams regularly—so your eye doctor can make sure you are seeing as clearly as possible.

If you wear glasses or contact lenses and still have these symptoms, you might need a new prescription. Talk to your eye doctor and get an eye exam if you are having trouble with your vision.

ARE YOU AT RISK FOR REFRACTIVE ERRORS?

Anyone can have refractive errors, but you are at higher risk if you have family members who wear glasses or contact lenses. Most types of refractive errors, such as nearsightedness, usually start in childhood. Presbyopia is common in adults aged 40 and older. Talk with your doctor about your risk for refractive errors, and ask how often you need to get checked.

HOW WILL YOUR EYE DOCTOR CHECK FOR REFRACTIVE ERRORS?

Eye doctors can check for refractive errors as part of a comprehensive eye exam. The exam is simple and painless. Your doctor will ask you to read letters that are up close and far away. Then, they may give you some eye drops to dilate (widen) your pupil and check for other eye problems.

WHAT IS THE TREATMENT FOR REFRACTIVE ERRORS?

Eye doctors can correct refractive errors with glasses or contact lenses, or fix the refractive error with surgery.

- **Glasses**. Eyeglasses are the simplest and safest way to correct refractive errors. Your eye doctor will prescribe the right eyeglass lenses to give you the clearest possible vision.
- **Contacts**. Contact lenses sit on the surface of your eyes and correct refractive errors. Your eye doctor will fit you for the right lenses and show you how to clean and wear them safely.
- **Surgery**. Some types of surgery, such as laser eye surgery, can change the shape of your cornea to fix refractive errors. Your eye doctor can help you decide if surgery is right for you.

Talk over your options with your eye doctor. Remember these tips:

- See your doctor for eye exams regularly.
- Tell your doctor if your vision gets worse or if you are having problems with your glasses or contact lenses.
- Encourage family members to get checked for refractive errors, since they can run in families.

Section 9.2 | **Astigmatism**

This section includes text from excerpted "Astigmatism," National Eye Institute (NEI), March 20, 2009. Reviewed March 2020.

WHAT IS ASTIGMATISM?

Astigmatism is a common type of refractive error. It is a condition in which the eye does not focus light evenly onto the retina, the light-sensitive tissue at the back of the eye.

WHAT IS REFRACTION?

Refraction is the bending of light as it passes through one object to another. Vision occurs when light rays are bent (refracted) as they pass through the cornea and the lens. The light is then focused on the retina. The retina converts the light rays into messages that are sent through the optic nerve to the brain.

HOW DOES ASTIGMATISM OCCUR?

Astigmatism occurs when light is bent differently depending on where it strikes the cornea and passes through the eyeball. The cornea of a normal eye is curved like a basketball, with the same degree of roundness in all areas. An eye with astigmatism has a cornea that is curved more similar to that of a football, with some areas that are steeper or more rounded than others. This can cause images to appear blurry and stretched out.

WHO IS AT RISK FOR ASTIGMATISM?

Astigmatism can affect both children and adults. Some patients with slight astigmatism will not notice much change in their vision. It is important to have eye examinations at regular intervals in order to detect any astigmatism early on for children.

WHAT ARE THE SIGNS AND SYMPTOMS OF ASTIGMATISM?

Signs and symptoms of astigmatism include the following:

- Headaches
- Eyestrain
- Squinting
- Distorted or blurred vision at all distances
- Difficulty driving at night

If you experience any of these symptoms, visit your eye-care professional.

If you wear glasses or contact lenses and still have these issues, a new prescription might be needed.

HOW IS ASTIGMATISM DIAGNOSED?

Astigmatism is usually found during a comprehensive dilated eye exam. Being aware of any changes in your vision is important. It can help in detecting any common vision problems. If you notice any changes in your vision, visit your eye-care professional for a comprehensive dilated eye examination.

CAN A PERSON HAVE ASTIGMATISM AND NOT KNOW IT?

It is possible to have mild astigmatism and not know about it. This is especially true for children, who are not aware of their vision being other than normal. Some adults may also have mild astigmatism without any symptoms. It is important to have comprehensive dilated eye exams to make sure you are seeing your best.

HOW IS ASTIGMATISM CORRECTED?

Astigmatism can be corrected with eyeglasses, contact lenses, or refractive surgery. Individual lifestyles affect the way astigmatism is treated.

Eyeglasses

Eyeglasses are the simplest and safest way to correct astigmatism. Your eye-care professional will prescribe appropriate lenses to help you see as clearly as possible.

Contact Lenses

Contact lenses work by becoming the first refractive surface for light rays entering the eye, causing more precise refraction or focus. In many cases, contact lenses provide clearer vision, a wider field of vision, and greater comfort. They are a safe and effective option if fitted and used properly. It is very important to wash your hands and clean your lenses as instructed in order to reduce the risk of infection. If you have certain eye conditions, you may not be able to wear contact lenses. Discuss this matter with your eye-care professional.

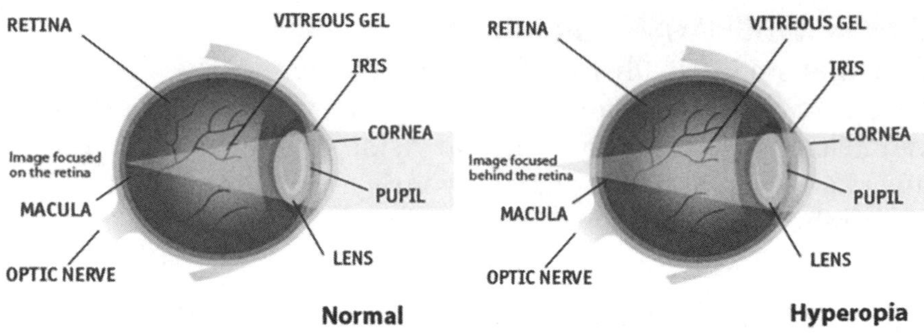

Figure 9.1. Normal Eye versus Hyperopia

Refractive Surgery

Refractive surgery aims to change the shape of the cornea permanently. This change in eye shape restores the focusing power of the eye by allowing the light rays to focus precisely on the retina for improved vision. There are many types of refractive surgeries. Your eye-care professional can help you decide if surgery is an option for you.

Section 9.3 | **Hyperopia**

This section includes text from excerpted "Hyperopia," National Eye Institute (NEI), March 20, 2009. Reviewed March 2020.

WHAT IS HYPEROPIA?

Hyperopia, also known as "farsightedness," is a common type of refractive error where distant objects may be seen more clearly than objects that are near. However, people experience farsightedness differently. Some people may not notice any problems with their vision, especially when they are young. For people with significant farsightedness, vision can be blurry for objects at any distance, near or far.

WHAT IS REFRACTION?

Refraction is the bending of light as it passes through one object to another. Vision occurs when light rays are bent (refracted) as they pass through the cornea and the lens. The light is then focused on the retina. The retina converts the light rays into messages that are sent through the optic nerve to the brain. The brain interprets these messages into the images we see.

WHAT ARE REFRACTIVE ERRORS?

In refractive errors, the shape of the eye prevents light from focusing on the retina. The length of the eyeball (longer or shorter), changes in the shape of the cornea, or aging of the lens can all cause refractive errors.

HOW DOES HYPEROPIA DEVELOP?

Hyperopia develops in eyes that focus images behind the retina instead of on the retina, which can result in blurred vision. This occurs when the eyeball is too short, which prevents incoming light from focusing directly on the retina. It may also be caused by an abnormal shape of the cornea or lens.

WHO IS AT RISK FOR HYPEROPIA?

Hyperopia can affect both children and adults. It affects about 5 to 10 percent of Americans. People whose parents are farsighted may also be more likely to get the condition.

WHAT ARE THE SIGNS AND SYMPTOMS OF HYPEROPIA?

The symptoms of hyperopia vary from person to person. Your eye-care professional can help you understand how the condition affects you. Common signs and symptoms of hyperopia include the following:

- Headaches
- Eyestrain
- Squinting
- Blurry vision, especially for close objects

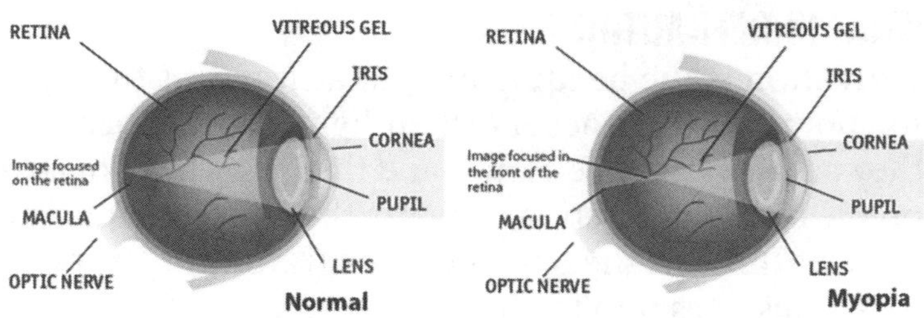

Figure 9.2. Normal Eye versus Myopia

HOW IS HYPEROPIA DIAGNOSED?

An eye-care professional can diagnose farsightedness and other refractive errors during a comprehensive dilated eye examination. People with this condition often visit their eye-care professionals with complaints of visual discomfort or blurred vision.

HOW IS HYPEROPIA CORRECTED?

Hyperopia can be corrected with eyeglasses, contact lenses, or refractive surgery.

Eyeglasses

Eyeglasses are the simplest and safest way to correct farsightedness. Your eye-care professional can prescribe lenses that will help correct the problem and help you see your best.

Contact Lenses

Contact lenses work by becoming the first refractive surface for light rays entering the eye, causing more precise refraction or focus. In many cases, contact lenses may provide a clearer vision, a wider field of vision, and greater comfort. They are a safe and effective option if fitted and used properly. However, contact lenses may not be the best option for everyone. If you have certain eye conditions, you may not be able to wear contact lenses. Discuss this matter with your eye-care professional.

Refractive Surgery

Refractive surgery aims to permanently change the shape of the cornea, which will improve refractive vision. Surgery can decrease or eliminate dependency on wearing eyeglasses and contact lenses. There are many types of refractive surgeries and surgical options should be discussed with an eye-care professional.

Section 9.4 | Myopia

This section includes text from excerpted "Myopia," National Eye Institute (NEI), March 20, 2009. Reviewed March 2020.

WHAT IS MYOPIA?

Myopia, also known as "nearsightedness," is a common type of refractive error where close objects appear clearly, but distant objects appear blurry.

WHAT IS REFRACTION?

Refraction is the bending of light as it passes through one object to another.

Vision occurs when light rays are bent (refracted) as they pass through the cornea and the lens. The light is then focused on the retina. The retina converts the light rays into messages that are sent through the optic nerve to the brain. The brain interprets these messages into the images we see.

WHAT ARE REFRACTIVE ERRORS?

In refractive errors, the shape of the eye prevents light from focusing on the retina. The length of the eyeball (longer or shorter), changes in the shape of the cornea, or aging of the lens can cause refractive errors.

HOW DOES MYOPIA DEVELOP?

Myopia develops in eyes that focus images in front of the retina instead of on the retina, which results in blurred vision. This occurs when the eyeball becomes too long and prevents incoming light from focusing directly on the retina. It may also be caused by an abnormal shape of the cornea or lens.

WHO IS AT RISK FOR MYOPIA?

Myopia can affect both children and adults. The condition affects about 25 percent of Americans. Myopia is often diagnosed in children between 8 and 12 years of age and may worsen during the teen years. Little change may occur between 20 to 40 years of age, but sometimes nearsightedness may worsen with age. People whose parents are nearsighted may be more likely to get the condition.

WHAT ARE THE SIGNS AND SYMPTOMS OF MYOPIA?

Some of the signs and symptoms of myopia include the following:

- Headaches
- Eyestrain
- Squinting
- Difficulty seeing distant objects, such as highway signs

HOW IS MYOPIA DIAGNOSED?

An eye-care professional can diagnose myopia and other refractive errors during a comprehensive dilated eye examination. People with this condition often visit their eye-care professionals with complaints of visual discomfort or blurred vision.

HOW IS MYOPIA CORRECTED?

Myopia can be corrected with eyeglasses, contact lenses, or refractive surgery.

Eyeglasses

Eyeglasses are the simplest and safest way to correct nearsightedness. Your eye-care professional can prescribe lenses that will correct the problem and help you to see your best.

Contact Lenses

Contact lenses work by becoming the first refractive surface for light rays entering the eye, causing more precise refraction or focus. In many cases, contact lenses may provide a clearer vision, a wider field of vision, and greater comfort. They are a safe and effective option if fitted and used properly. However, contact lenses may not be the best option for everyone. If you have certain eye conditions, you may not be able to wear contact lenses. Discuss this matter with your eye-care professional.

Refractive Surgery

Refractive surgery aims to permanently change the shape of the cornea, which will improve refractive vision. Surgery can decrease or eliminate dependency on wearing eyeglasses and contact lenses. There are many types of refractive surgeries and surgical options should be discussed with an eye-care professional.

Section 9.5 | **Presbyopia**

This section includes text from excerpted "Presbyopia," National Eye Institute (NEI), March 20, 2009. Reviewed March 2020.

WHAT IS PRESBYOPIA?

Presbyopia is a common type of vision disorder that occurs as you age. It is often referred to as the "aging eye condition." Presbyopia results in the inability to focus up close, a problem associated with refraction in the eye. The cornea and lens bend (refract) incoming light rays so they focus precisely on the retina at the back of the eye.

WHAT IS REFRACTION?

Refraction is the bending of light as it passes through one object to another. Vision occurs when light rays are bent (refracted) by the cornea and lens. The light is then focused directly on the retina, which is a light-sensitive tissue at the back of the eye. The retina

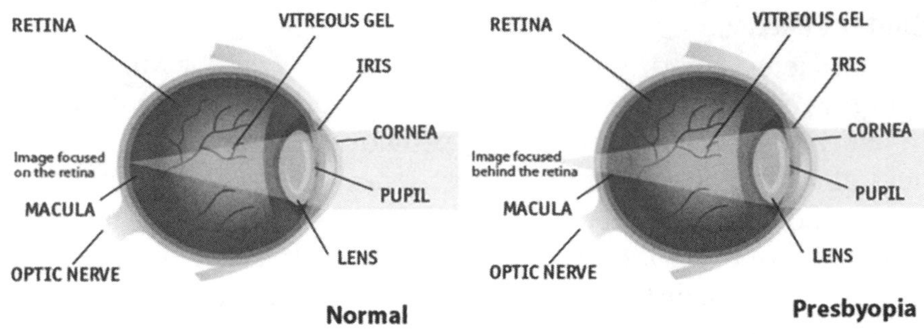

Figure 9.3. Normal Eye versus Presbyopia

converts the light rays into messages that are sent through the optic nerve to the brain. The brain interprets these messages into the images we see.

HOW DOES PRESBYOPIA OCCUR?

Presbyopia happens naturally in people as they age. The eye is not able to focus light directly onto the retina due to the hardening of the natural lens. Aging also affects muscle fibers around the lens, making it harder for the eye to focus on up close objects. The ineffective lens causes light to focus behind the retina, causing poor close-up vision.

When you are younger, the lens of the eye is soft and flexible, allowing the tiny muscles inside the eye to easily reshape the lens to focus on close and distant objects.

WHO IS AT RISK FOR PRESBYOPIA?

Anyone over the age of 35 is at risk for developing presbyopia. Everyone experiences some loss of focusing power for near objects as they age, but some will notice this more than others.

WHAT ARE THE SIGNS AND SYMPTOMS OF PRESBYOPIA?

Signs and symptoms of presbyopia include the following:

- Hard time reading small print

- The need to hold reading material farther than arm's distance
- Problems seeing objects that are close to you
- Headaches
- Eyestrain

If you experience any of these symptoms, you may want to visit an eye-care professional for a comprehensive dilated eye examination. If you wear glasses or contact lenses and still have these issues, a new prescription might be needed.

CAN A PERSON HAVE PRESBYOPIA AND ANOTHER TYPE OF REFRACTIVE ERROR AT THE SAME TIME?

Yes. It is common to have presbyopia and another type of refractive error at the same time. There are several other types of refractive errors: nearsightedness (myopia), farsightedness (hyperopia), and astigmatism. An individual may have one type of refractive error in one eye and a different type of refractive error in the other.

HOW IS PRESBYOPIA DIAGNOSED?

Presbyopia can be found during a comprehensive dilated eye exam. If you notice any changes in your vision, you should visit an eye-care professional. Eye exams are recommended more often after the age of 40 to check for age-related conditions.

HOW IS PRESBYOPIA CORRECTED?

Eyeglasses are the simplest and safest means of correcting presbyopia. Eyeglasses for presbyopia have higher focusing power in the lower portion of the lens. This allows you to read through the lower portion of the lens and clearly see distant objects through the upper portion of the lens. It is also possible to purchase reading eyeglasses. These types of glasses do not require a prescription and can help with reading vision.

Chapter 10 | **Eye Movement and Alignment Disorders**

Chapter Contents

Section 10.1 | **Amblyopia**

This section includes text excerpted from "Amblyopia (Lazy Eye)," National Eye Institute (NEI), July 2, 2019.

WHAT IS AMBLYOPIA?

Amblyopia (also called "lazy eye") is a type of poor vision that happens in just one eye. It develops when there is a breakdown in how the brain and the eye work together, and the brain cannot recognize the sight from one eye. Over time, the brain relies more and more on the other stronger eye—while vision in the weaker eye gets worse.

It is called a "lazy eye" because the stronger eye works better. But, people with amblyopia are not lazy, and they cannot control the way their eyes work.

Amblyopia starts in childhood, and it is the most common cause of vision loss in kids. Up to 3 out of 100 children have it. The good news is that early treatment works well and usually prevents long-term vision problems.

WHAT ARE THE SYMPTOMS OF AMBLYOPIA?

The symptoms of amblyopia can be hard to notice. Kids with amblyopia may have poor depth perception—they have trouble telling how near or far something is. Parents may also notice signs that their child is struggling to see clearly, such as:

- Squinting
- Shutting one eye
- Tilting their head

In many cases, parents do not know their child has amblyopia until a doctor diagnoses it during an eye exam. That is why it is important for all kids to get a vision screening at least once between three and five years of age.

IS YOUR CHILD AT RISK FOR AMBLYOPIA?

Some kids are born with amblyopia and others develop it later in childhood.

The chances of having amblyopia are higher in kids who:

- Were born early (premature)
- Were smaller than average at birth
- Have a family history of amblyopia, childhood cataracts, or other eye conditions
- Have developmental disabilities

WHAT CAUSES AMBLYOPIA

In many cases, doctors do not know the cause of amblyopia. But, sometimes, a different vision problem can lead to amblyopia.

Normally, the brain uses nerve signals from both eyes to see. But, if an eye condition makes vision in one eye worse, the brain may try to work around it. It starts to "turn off" signals from the weaker eye and rely only on the stronger eye.

Some eye conditions that can lead to amblyopia are:

- **Refractive errors.** These include common vision problems, such as nearsightedness (having trouble seeing far away), farsightedness (having trouble seeing things up close), and astigmatism (which can cause blurry vision). Normally, these problems are easy to fix with glasses or contacts. But, if they are not treated, the brain may start to rely more on the eye with a stronger vision.
- **Strabismus.** Usually, the eyes move together as a pair. But, in kids with strabismus, the eyes do not line up. One eye might drift in, out, up, or down.
- **Cataract.** This causes cloudiness in the lens of the eye, making things look blurry. While most cataracts happen in older people, babies and children can also develop cataracts.

HOW WILL YOUR CHILD'S DOCTOR CHECK FOR AMBLYOPIA?

As part of a normal vision screening, your child's doctor will look for signs of amblyopia. All kids three to five years of age need to have their vision checked at least once.

WHAT IS THE TREATMENT FOR AMBLYOPIA?

If there is a vision problem causing amblyopia, the doctor may treat that first. For example, doctors may recommend glasses or contacts (for kids who are nearsighted or farsighted) or surgery (for kids with cataract).

The next step is to retrain the brain and force it to use the weaker eye. The more the brain uses it, the stronger it gets. Treatments include:

- **Wearing an eye patch on the stronger eye.** By covering up this eye with a stick-on eye patch (similar to a Band-Aid), the brain has to use the weaker eye to see. Some kids only need to wear the patch for two hours a day, while others may need to wear it whenever they are awake.
- **Putting special eye drops in the stronger eye.** A once-a-day drop of the drug atropine can temporarily blur near vision, which forces the brain to use the other eye. For some kids, this treatment works as well as an eye patch, and some parents find it easier to use (for example, because young children may try to pull off eye patches).

After your child starts treatment, their vision may start to get better within a few weeks. But, it will probably take months to get the best results. After that, your child may still need to use these treatments from time to time to stop amblyopia from coming back.

It is important to start treating children with amblyopia early—the sooner the better. Kids who grow up without treatment may have lifelong vision problems. Amblyopia treatment is usually less effective in adults than in children.

Section 10.2 | **Brown Syndrome**

This section includes text excerpted from "Brown Syndrome," Genetic and Rare Diseases Information Center (GARD), National Center for Advancing Translational Sciences (NCATS), December 5, 2011. Reviewed March 2020.

Brown syndrome is an eye disorder characterized by abnormalities in the eye's ability to move. Specifically, the ability to look up and it is affected by a problem in the superior oblique muscle/tendon.

WHAT CAUSES BROWN SYNDROME

Brown syndrome may be present at birth (congenital) or it may develop following surgery or as a result of an inflammation or a problem with development. Some cases are constant while others are intermittent.

TREATMENT OF BROWN SYNDROME

Treatment recommendations vary depending on the cause and severity of the condition. In mild cases, a watch and wait approach may be sufficient. Visual acuity should be monitored. First-line therapy usually involves less invasive options, such as nonsteroidal anti-inflammatory medications such as Ibuprofen. Acquired causes of the inflammatory Brown syndrome may be successfully treated with corticosteroids. Surgery is considered in cases with double vision, compromised binocular vision, significant abnormalities in head position, or obvious eye misalignment when looking straight ahead.

Section 10.3 | Nystagmus

Nystagmus is a disorder that causes involuntary and uncontrollable movement of the eyes. This affects both the eyes of a person and results in three primary kinds of movement:

- Side to side (horizontal nystagmus)
- Up and down (vertical nystagmus)
- In a circle (rotary nystagmus)

These movements may vary between slow and fast, and the eyes may move rapidly when looking in certain directions, which may result in the person tilting or turning their head in an effort to see clearly and help slow the eye movements.

TYPES OF NYSTAGMUS

The different types of nystagmus include:

- **Congenital nystagmus**—a condition that is present from birth in which the eyes move together as they oscillate. Most of the other types of infantile nystagmus are classified as a form of strabismus, meaning the eyes do not necessarily work together all the time.
- **Latent nystagmus**—a conjugate jerk nystagmus that occurs when one eye is closed. The direction of this jerk depends on which eye is closed.
- **Manifest nystagmus**—a conjugate jerk nystagmus condition that is present at all times.
- **Manifest-latent nystagmus**—a conjugate jerk nystagmus condition that is present at all times but is worse when one eye is closed.
- **Acquired nystagmus**—a condition that can be caused by diseases and conditions such as multiple sclerosis, brain tumors, diabetic neuropathy, an accident, or any other neurological problem. In some rare cases, nystagmus can also be acquired through

hyperventilation, a flashing light in front of one eye, and nicotine. Some acquired nystagmus can be treated through medications or surgery.

CAUSES OF NYSTAGMUS

Some people are born with nystagmus, while others develop it later in their life. This might be caused by various factors that include:

- Other eye issues, such as cataracts or strabismus
- Diseases such as stroke or multiple sclerosis
- Head injuries
- Albinism (lack of melanin pigment)
- Inner-ear problems, such as Ménière disease
- Use of certain medications, such as lithium or other drugs used to treat seizures
- Use of alcohol or drugs

These are only a few of the reasons, however, and there can be instances in which the doctor may not know the exact cause of nystagmus.

SYMPTOMS OF NYSTAGMUS

The main symptom of nystagmus is rapid eye movement that cannot be controlled by the person. Other symptoms include:

- Extreme sensitivity to light
- Dizziness
- Difficulty seeing in the dark
- Vision problems
- Holding the head in a turned or tilted position, as this could help them reduce the eye movement

DIAGNOSIS OF NYSTAGMUS

If any symptoms of nystagmus are observed, then an immediate visit to an eye doctor is recommended. The eye doctor will check the insides of the eyes and test the vision. Other eye problems may also be checked.

Additional tests that may be included in the exam include:

- Ear exam
- Neurological exam
- Brain MRI
- Brain CT scan
- Recording of the eye movement

The doctor may ask the patient to spin around in a chair for 30 seconds, stop, and then try to stare at an object. If the person has nystagmus, their eyes will first move slowly in one direction, then move quickly the other way.

TREATMENT OF NYSTAGMUS

Those born with nystagmus cannot be completely cured of this condition. However, their eyesight can be improved with the help of glasses or contact lenses. Even though these assistive devices do not cure nystagmus, having clearer vision can help slow the eye movements.

In rare cases, a surgery to reposition the eye muscle may be performed. This may prevent the person from turning their head too far, and thereby reduce the jerking. This surgery does not cure nystagmus, but does allow the person to keep their head in a more comfortable position in order to limit eye movement.

There have been some instances when acquired nystagmus does go away when the condition causing the nystagmus is treated, however. These instances include treating a medical condition or stopping the use of alcohol or drugs.

If any symptoms of nystagmus are observed in a child or an adult, seek immediate medical attention, since early treatment can help control this disorder more effectively.

References

1. "Nystagmus: Causes and Treatment of the Involuntary Movement of the Eye," All About Vision, March 13, 2016.
2. "Nystagmus," WebMD, November 7, 2019.
3. "Nystagmus," Boyd, Kierstan, American Academy of Ophthalmology (AAO), December 20, 2019.

Section 10.4 | **Strabismus (Crossed Eyes)**

Crossed eyes, or strabismus, is a disorder in which the eyes are misaligned and point in different directions. One eye may point in a straight direction, while the other eye points in an inward, outward, upward, or downward direction. The eye that points straight and the one that is misaligned can differ.

Strabismus is common among children, and about four percent of children in the United States are affected by this disorder.

TYPES OF STRABISMUS

The types of strabismus are as follows:

Esotropia

Esotropia is further classified into infantile esotropia and accommodative esotropia. Infantile esotropia is when the eyes turn inward and it is a common type of strabismus in infants. Accommodative esotropia is a common form of strabismus that occurs in children who are two years of age or older. In this case, the eye turns inward when the child tries to focus on a thing. This crossing can happen when the child is trying to focus on something either at a distance or up close.

Exotropia

Exotropia is a condition in which the eye turns outward, which often occurs when a child is focusing on distant objects. This occurs usually when a child is daydreaming, ill, or tired. The child also may squint one eye to see more clearly in bright sunlight.

CAUSES OF STRABISMUS

Strabismus can be caused by issues with the eye muscles, the nerve that transmits information to the eye muscles, or the control center in the brain that directs eye movements. Stabismus can also develop due to other medical reasons or eye injuries. Some of the things that cause strabismus are:

- Family history
- Refractive error (farsightedness)

Strabismus has been found to be common among children with disorders that affect the brain, such as:

- Cerebral palsy
- Down syndrome
- Hydrocephalus
- Brain tumors
- Prematurity

SYMPTOMS OF STRABISMUS

The main symptom of strabismus is eyes that do not aim in the same direction, squinting one eye in bright sunlight, or tilting the head in an effort to use the eyes together. Some other symptoms include:

- Double vision
- Uncoordinated movement of the eyes
- Loss of vision or perception of depth

If any of these symptoms are noticed, immediately seek the help of an eye doctor.

DIAGNOSIS OF STRABISMUS

Strabismus can be diagnosed during an eye exam. It is recommended that children between three and four years of age have their vision checked by their pediatrician, a family doctor, or a person trained in vision assessment of children. Tests that will be carried out to determine how much the eyes are misaligned include:

- Corneal light reflex
- Cover/uncover test
- Retinal exam
- Standard ophthalmic exam
- Visual acuity

In addition to these, a brain and nervous system (neurological) exam will also be done to diagnose strabismus.

Note. If there is a family history of vision problems, then the child needs to be examined even earlier.

TREATMENT OF STRABISMUS

Those diagnosed with strabismus have various treatment options to help improve their vision, including:

- **Eyeglasses or contact lenses**—The first step in treating those affected with strabismus is prescribing glasses to them if required. For some, this may be the only treatment required for a permanent cure from the disorder.
- **Prism lenses**—These lenses are thicker on one side than the other. The lens alter the amount of light entering the eye and help reduce the act of turning in an effort to view an object. There have been instances in which prism lenses have eliminated eye turning altogether.
- **Vision therapy**—An ophthalmologist may prescribe a structured program of visual activities that will help improve eye coordination and focus. Vision therapy helps train the eyes and brain to work together more effectively. Eye exercises can help correct issues with the person's eye movement, focusing, and coordination, which will strengthen the eye–brain connection.
- **Eye muscle surgery**—This surgery usually changes the length and position of the muscles around the eyes so that they appear straight. However, those who undergo surgery may also require vision therapy to improve eye coordination so that the eye does not become misaligned again.

It is important to remember that, strabismus does not disappear with time—and, in fact, may get worse if not treated. It is necessary to seek early treatment if any of these symptoms are present, so that the vision is protected and there are no further problems.

References

1. "Strabismus (Crossed Eyes)," American Optometric Association (AOA), June 29, 2007.
2. "Strabismus," MedlinePlus, National Institutes of Health (NIH), August 28, 2018.
3. "What Is Strabismus?" MedlinePlus, American Academy of Ophthalmology (AAO), April 14, 2014.

Chapter 11 | Eyeglasses

Chapter Contents

Section 11.1 | **Eyeglasses for Refractive Errors**

This section includes text excerpted from "Eyeglasses for Refractive Errors," National Eye Institute (NEI), July 8, 2019.

Eyeglasses are the safest and simplest way to correct refractive errors.

WHAT ARE THE DIFFERENT TYPES OF EYEGLASSES?

People with different refractive errors need different types of eyeglass lenses to see clearly.

Reading Glasses

Reading glasses can help people with presbyopia read or see things up close. You can buy reading glasses at drug stores and convenience stores. Even though you can get reading glasses without a prescription, it is important to get regular eye exams to make sure you are seeing as clearly as possible.

Single Vision Prescription Lenses

Single vision prescription lenses correct near vision or distance vision, but not both. If you have nearsightedness, single vision lenses can help you see things far away. If you have farsightedness, they can help you see things up close.

Multifocal Prescription Lenses

Multifocal prescription lenses correct both near and distance vision. They can help people who have trouble seeing things up close and far away. For example, people who have both presbyopia and nearsightedness can use multifocal lenses for reading and driving.

- Bifocals correct near vision on the bottom and distance vision on the top.
- Trifocals correct middle-distance vision in between the near and distance vision areas.
- Progressive lenses are multifocal lenses that do not have a visible line between the near and distance vision areas.

HOW DO EYEGLASSES WORK?

Eyeglass lenses work by bending light—just like the lens and cornea in your eye. The eyeglass lens bends light to make it focus correctly on your retina (the light-sensitive layer of tissue at the back of the eye). Different eyeglass lenses can correct different errors caused by problems with the cornea, lens, or shape of the eye.

Glasses make your vision clearer while you are wearing them—but they do not change your eyes at all. Wearing glasses does not make your eyes weaker or your vision worse.

HOW DO YOU GET EYEGLASSES?

If you think you may need glasses, the first step is to see an eye doctor.

Eye doctors can prescribe eyeglasses as part of a regular eye exam. The vision test is simple and painless. Your doctor will ask you to read letters that are up close and far away. Then they may give you some eye drops to dilate (widen) your pupil and check the health of your eyes.

After your eye doctor gives you a written prescription for eyeglass lenses, go to an optician to pick out frames and buy your glasses. Your eye doctor may have an optician working in their office. You can also find opticians in stores that sell glasses and contacts.

If you wear eyeglasses, get an eye exam regularly—as often as your eye doctor recommends. That way, your doctor can make sure you are still seeing clearly.

Section 11.2 | **How to Read Your Eyeglass Prescription**

More than half of American adults—or around 150 million people—wear prescription eyeglasses to correct their vision. Yet few people understand the meaning behind the complicated series of letters, numbers, and symbols that appear on their eyeglass prescriptions. This shorthand code provides eyeglass manufacturers with specific information about a patient's vision, including the degree of nearsightedness, farsightedness, and astigmatism. This information enables the manufacturer to create custom eyeglasses to provide the patient with the best possible clarity of vision. Learning how to read an eyeglass prescription can provide patients with important knowledge about their eye health.

TERMINOLOGY USED IN EYEGLASS PRESCRIPTIONS

During an eye examination, the practitioner uses a process known as refraction to determine the exact amount of correction needed to give the patient clear vision. Refraction involves showing the patient a series of lenses using an instrument called a "phoropter." As the patient repeatedly chooses the lens option that provides greater clarity of vision, the lens power is fine-tuned until the practitioner determines the final prescription for corrective lenses. The prescription is similar to a formula or equation for the eyeglass manufacturer to follow in creating the lenses. A written eyeglass prescription typically includes the terminologies described below.

Oculus Dexter and Oculus Sinister

OD is an abbreviation for the Latin term "oculus dexter," which means "right eye." OS is an abbreviation for the Latin term "oculus sinister," which means "left eye." When both of the patient's eyes require the same amount of correction, the abbreviation OU—short for "oculus uterque," meaning "both eyes"—may appear instead. Although these Latin terms have traditionally been used, some eyecare practitioners have moved to the more modern abbreviations

RE for "right eye" and LE for "left eye." The information for the right eye is always listed before the information for the left eye because eye doctors work from left to right as they are facing a patient.

Sphere

The sphere or SPH on an eyeglass prescription indicates the lens power the patient requires to achieve a clear vision. The lens power is expressed in diopters (D), a unit of measurement used to describe the refractive or light-bending ability of a lens. Prescriptions are usually measured in quarter-diopter increments and expressed in decimal forms, such as 3.25D. If the sphere begins with a minus sign (–), it means the patient is myopic (nearsighted) and needs corrective lenses to see distant objects clearly. If the sphere begins with a plus sign (+) or has no sign, it means the patient is hyperopic (farsighted) and needs corrective lenses to see near objects clearly. A higher sphere number indicates that the patient needs a higher power lens, and thus more correction.

Cylinder

If CYL appears on an eyeglass prescription, it means that the patient has astigmatism. This common condition occurs when the eye, cornea, or lens has an irregular shape or curvature, rather than being perfectly round or spherical. Astigmatism can affect the way the eye focuses light, causing objects to appear blurry. The cylinder number indicates the amount of lens power required to correct astigmatism. If the number is preceded by a minus sign, it refers to nearsighted astigmatism, or if it is preceded by a plus sign or no sign, it refers to farsighted astigmatism. If there is no cylinder number, then the patient does not have astigmatism or has very mild astigmatism that does not require correction.

Axis

The axis (X) provides additional information to correct the vision of people with astigmatism. Due to the irregular shape of the eye, the cylinder lens power is not applied evenly to the entire eyeglass

Table 11.1. An Eyeglass Prescription

OD	-2.75 SPH	+1.50 add	0.5 PD BD
OS	-2.00 -0.50 x 180	+1.50 ad	0.5 PD BD

lens. Instead, the lens power is added to those meridians of the eye where it is needed to correct the imperfect curvature. The axis number describes the location on the eye where the astigmatism correction is needed. The axis number is expressed in whole numbers between 0 and 180 degrees. It is determined by placing an imaginary protractor through the middle of the eye, with the flat side running horizontally through the pupil and the curved side following the arch of the eyebrow. The 90-degree line runs vertically through the eye. The axis value on an eyeglass prescription indicates the meridian that contains no cylinder power to correct astigmatism, while the lens meridian that is 90 degrees away contains the cylinder power.

Add

"Add" refers to magnifying power that is added to bifocal, trifocal, or progressive lenses to correct presbyopia or blurry near vision. Many people develop presbyopia and need reading glasses as they reach middle age. The magnifying power is always positive. It usually ranges from +0.75 to +3.00 D and is the same for both eyes.

Prism and Base

Prism and base appear on a small percentage of eyeglass prescriptions. These terms provide the information needed to compensate for problems with eye alignment. The prismatic power is measured in prism diopters (PD) and may appear as a decimal or a fraction. The base (B) indicates the direction of the thickest part of the prism: BU (base up), BD (base down), BI (base in, toward the nose), or BO (base out, toward the ears).

SAMPLE EYEGLASS PRESCRIPTION

As an example, a patient might receive the following eyeglass prescription:

In the right eye (OD), the eye-care practitioner has prescribed -2.75 D sphere to correct nearsightedness. SPH indicates that the right eye is only being prescribed spherical power. Since there is no astigmatism in the right eye, no cylinder power or axis is noted.

In the left eye (OS), the practitioner has prescribed -2.00 D sphere to correct nearsightedness, plus -0.50 D cylinder to correct astigmatism. The axis for the cylinder power is 180, meaning the horizontal meridian of the eye has no added power for astigmatism, while the vertical (90-degree) meridian has -0.50 D applied.

In both eyes, the practitioner has added +1.50 D magnification to correct presbyopia. Finally, the practitioner has included a prismatic correction of 0.5 PD in each eye, with the prism orientation base down (BD) in the right eye and base in (BI) in the left eye.

EYEGLASS VERSUS CONTACT LENS PRESCRIPTIONS

It is important to note that separate prescriptions are needed for eyeglasses and contact lenses. Although both prescriptions may be provided at the same eye examination, they are not interchangeable. Eyeglass prescriptions only work for ordering eyeglasses, and contact lens prescriptions only work for ordering contact lenses.

The main reason the two types of prescriptions are different is that contact lenses are worn directly on the surface of the eyes, while glasses are positioned in frames at a distance from the eyes. The distance between the eye and the lens affects the power needed to provide a clear vision. In addition, contact lens prescriptions include additional information about the lens diameter, curvature, and manufacturer or brand that can only be determined through a special contact lens fitting.

THE PRESCRIPTION RELEASE RULE

Under a 1980 rule issued by the Federal Trade Commission (FTC), eye-care practitioners are required to provide patients with a copy of their eyeglass prescription. The rule is intended to protect consumers' right to shop around for the best deal when purchasing eyeglasses, rather than being compelled to purchase glasses from the practitioner who performed the eye examination.

Under the Prescription Release Rule, eye-care practitioners must provide a copy of the prescription whether the patient requests it or not. In addition, they cannot charge an extra fee or require the patient to meet any other conditions for the release of the prescription. Finally, practitioners cannot tell patients that the prescription may not be accurate if they purchase glasses from a different vendor. Practitioners who violate the rule face a $10,000 penalty from the FTC.

References

1. "Anatomy of an Eyeglass Prescription," FramesDirect, 2017.
2. Heiting, Gary. "How to Read Your Eyeglass Prescription," All About Vision, May 2016.

Section 11.3 | Prevent Eye Damage—Protect Yourself from UV Radiation

This section includes text excerpted from "Prevent Eye Damage—Protect Yourself from UV Radiation," U.S. Environmental Protection Agency (EPA), May 2013. Reviewed March 2020.

Most Americans understand the link between ultraviolet (UV) radiation and skin cancer. Many are less aware of the connection between UV radiation and eye damage. With increased levels of UV radiation reaching the Earth's surface, largely due to stratospheric ozone layer depletion, it is important to take the necessary precautions to protect your eyes.

POTENTIAL EFFECTS OF UV RADIATION ON EYES

Ultraviolet radiation, whether from natural sunlight or artificial UV rays, can damage the eye, affecting surface tissues and internal structures, such as the cornea and lens. Long-term exposure to UV radiation can lead to cataracts, skin cancer around the eyelids, and other eye disorders. In the short-term, excessive exposure to UV radiation from daily activities, including reflections off of snow, pavement, and other surfaces, can burn the front surface of the eye, similar to a sunburn on the skin. The cumulative effects of spending long hours in the sun without adequate eye protection can increase the likelihood of developing the following eye disorders:

- **Cataract,** clouding of the eye's lens that can blur vision
- **Snow blindness (photokeratitis),** a temporary but painful burn to the cornea caused by a day at the beach without sunglasses; reflections off of snow, water, or concrete; or exposure to artificial light sources such as tanning beds
- **Pterygium,** an abnormal, but usually noncancerous, growth in the corner of the eye. It can grow over the cornea, partially blocking vision, and may require surgery to be removed.
- **Skin cancer around the eyelids.** Basal cell carcinoma is the most common type of skin cancer to affect the eyelids. In most cases, lesions occur on the lower lid, but they can occur anywhere on the eyelids, in the corners of the eye, under the eyebrows, and on adjacent areas of the face.

EPA's SunWise Program

The SunWise Program is an environmental and health education program that teaches children and their caregivers how to protect themselves from overexposure to the sun. The program uses classroom, school, and community components to develop sustained sun-safe behaviors in children. When choosing sunglasses for children, SunWise, in partnership with Prevent Blindness America, recommends that you:

- Read the labels. Always look for labels that clearly state the sunglasses block 99 to 100 percent of UV-A and UV-B rays.

- Check often to make sure the sunglasses fit well and are not damaged
- Choose sunglasses that fit your child's face and lifestyle but that is large enough to shield the eyes from most angles
- Find a wide-brimmed hat to wear with sunglasses. Wide-brimmed hats greatly reduce the amount of UV radiation that reaches the eyes.

PROTECT YOUR EYES

The greatest amount of UV protection is achieved with a combination of sunglasses that block 99 to 100 percent of both UV-A and UV-B rays; a wide-brimmed hat; and for those who wear contact lenses, UV-blocking contacts. Wrap-around sunglasses and wide-brimmed hats add extra protection because they help block UV rays from entering the eyes from the sides and above.

Remember, exposure to UV radiation has cumulative effects on the eyes. Damage done by UV rays today leads to eye problems tomorrow.

FREQUENTLY ASKED QUESTIONS

Who Is at Risk for Eye Damage?

Every person in every ethnic group is susceptible to eye damage from UV radiation.

When Do I Need to Wear Sunglasses?

You need to wear sunglasses everyday, even on cloudy days. Snow, water, sand, and pavement reflect UV rays, increasing the amount reaching your eyes and skin.

What Should I Look for When Choosing a Pair of Sunglasses?

No matter what sunglass styles or options you choose, you should insist that your sunglasses block 99 to 100 percent of both UV-A and UV-B radiation.

Do I Have to Buy Expensive Sunglasses to Ensure That I Am Being Protected from UV Radiation?

No. As long as the label says that the glasses provide 99 to 100 percent UV-A and UV-B protection, price should not be a deciding factor.

Chapter 12 | **Contact Lenses**

Chapter Contents

Section 12.1 | About Contact Lenses

This section includes text excerpted from "Contact Lenses," National Eye Institute (NEI), July 8, 2019.

WHAT ARE CONTACT LENSES?

Contact lenses are thin lenses that sit on top of the cornea (the clear outer layer of the eye). They correct refractive errors to make your vision clearer—just like eyeglasses.

About 45 million Americans wear contact lenses. If you use them the right way, they can be a safe and effective alternative to eyeglasses. If you have a refractive error, such as being nearsighted or farsighted, your eye doctor can prescribe contact lenses to help you see clearly.

WHAT ARE THE DIFFERENT TYPES OF CONTACT LENSES?

When you are choosing contact lenses, there are three main things to know: whether they are soft or hard, how long you can wear them, and how often you need to replace them.

Soft or Hard Contact Lenses

Soft-contact lenses are much more common than hard lenses. Because they are soft and flexible, they can be more comfortable and easier to get used to.

Hard-contact lenses can make your vision crisper than soft lenses, and they are less likely to tear. But, they may take longer to get used to, and they can be harder to clean and take care of than soft lenses.

Daily-Wear or Extended-Wear Contact Lenses

You keep daily-wear contact lenses all day and take them out at night. You need to clean and disinfect daily-wear lenses every night. It is not safe to sleep in daily-wear lenses—it can put you at risk for serious eye infections.

You can leave extended-wear contact lenses overnight. Depending on the brand, you can wear them for as long as 30 days and nights before taking them out. Extended-wear lenses can be convenient—but they may also make it more likely that you will get a serious eye infection.

Single-Use or Reusable Contact Lenses

You wear single-use contact lenses for one day, then throw them away at night. The next day, you put in a brand new pair. You do not need to clean or disinfect single-use lenses.

You take reusable-contact lenses out at night, clean them, and wear them again the next day. Depending on the brand, you will need to replace them with a new pair after 7 to 30 days.

Some less common types of contact lenses fix specific vision problems or treat eye conditions.

WHAT ARE THE BENEFITS OF CONTACT LENSES?

Some people prefer to wear contacts instead of eyeglasses.

Contacts stay in place and improve peripheral (side) vision, so they can be easier to wear when being active or playing sports. They do not fog up the way glasses do, so they may also be more convenient for people who work or spend a lot of time outdoors in cold weather—or indoors in places that are very cold, such as a walk-in refrigerator or freezer.

If you wear contacts, you can wear nonprescription sunglasses to protect your eyes from ultraviolet (UV) rays. You can also wear contacts with UV protection built into the lenses.

WHAT ARE THE RISKS OF CONTACT LENSES?

Contact lenses are not risk-free. If you do not use them the right way, you can get serious eye conditions, including corneal ulcers (sores) and infections.

You can lower your risk by:

- Disinfecting and storing your contacts correctly—every time
- Only wearing your contacts for the amount of time your doctor recommends

- Taking out your contacts before you shower, swim, or go in for a bath or hot tub

The best way to prevent complications is to take good care of your contacts.

HOW DO YOU TAKE CARE OF YOUR CONTACT LENSES?

Most people use multipurpose contact lens solution to clean, disinfect, and store their contact lenses. Follow these steps to keep your contacts—and your eyes—clean and safe.

Every time you take out your lenses:

- Rub and rinse them with contact lens solution
- Store them in fresh solution in your contact lens storage case

Every time you put your lenses in your eyes:

- Rub and rinse the case with fresh solution
- Dump out the solution and dry the case with a clean tissue
- Store the case upside down on a clean tissue—leave the case open with the caps off

Some people use different systems to take care of their contacts. Talk to your eye doctor about which lens care system is right for you.

HOW DO YOU GET CONTACT LENSES?

Your eye doctor can prescribe eyeglasses or contact lenses as part of a dilated eye exam. The exam is simple and painless. Your doctor will ask you to read letters that are up close and far away. Then, they will give you some eye drops to dilate (widen) your pupil and check for other eye problems.

If you want to use contact lenses, your eye doctor will also put some trial lenses on your eyes to see how they fit and test your vision while wearing the lenses.

If you wear contacts, get an eye exam at least once a year—that way your eye doctor can make sure you are still seeing clearly.

Section 12.2 | **Contact Lens Care Systems and Solutions**

This section includes text excerpted from "Contact Lens Care Systems and Solutions," Centers for Disease Control and Prevention (CDC), March 21, 2016. Reviewed March 2020.

Lens care systems and solutions are products you use to clean, disinfect, and store your contact lenses. Proper contact lens care is important for keeping your eyes healthy and free from infection. Only your eye-care provider can determine which contact lens care system is best for you. Talk to your eye-care provider before using a new contact lens care system.

MULTIPURPOSE SOLUTION

Multipurpose solution is an all-in-one care system used to clean, rinse, disinfect, and store soft contact lenses. This solution is the most commonly used care system among soft contact lens wearers. Follow these steps for proper use of multipurpose solution:

- Rub and rinse your contact lenses and store them in fresh solution every time you take them out.
- Never mix fresh solution with old or used solution in the case—a practice called "topping off"—since it reduces the effectiveness of disinfection.
- Rub and rinse your contact lens storage case with fresh solution—never water—every day.
- Empty all excess solution out of the case, and dry it with a fresh, clean tissue.
- Store the clean case upside down on a fresh, clean tissue with the caps off after each use 8 in order to prevent germs from building up in the case.

HYDROGEN PEROXIDE-BASED SYSTEMS

Hydrogen peroxide-based systems clean, disinfect, and store contact lenses. An eye-care provider may prescribe this care system if you have an allergy to ingredients in a multipurpose solution that causes redness or irritation of the eye. Systems that use this type of solution require the use of a special case that comes with the solution when you buy it. The special case reacts with the hydrogen peroxide, converting it to the harmless saline solution over time. Never use another type of case with a hydrogen peroxide-based solution, as the solution will not convert to saline and will cause burning, stinging, and redness upon inserting the contact lenses.

- Carefully follow all instructions on the label for the proper use of hydrogen peroxide-based systems.
- Put the contact lenses in the special case with fresh solution. Never mix fresh solution with an old or used solution.
- Wait at least four to six hours—depending on the label's instructions—before inserting your contact lenses.
- Never rinse your contact lenses with hydrogen peroxide-based solutions and directly insert into your eyes, as this can cause burning, stinging, and redness.

SALINE

The saline solution does not disinfect contact lenses. Only use saline for rinsing contact lenses after cleaning and disinfecting with another care system. For example, some hydrogen peroxide-based systems suggest rinsing contact lenses with saline prior to insertion. Talk to your eye-care provider about whether or not you need to use saline with your lens-care system.

DAILY CLEANERS

The daily cleaner is intended for cleaning—not disinfecting—your contact lenses. The cleaner loosens and removes deposits and debris from the contact lens. Place a few drops in the palm of your hand and carefully rub the contact lens for as long as directed on both sides. You must use additional products, such as multipurpose solution, for rinsing the daily cleaner off, disinfecting, and storing the contact lenses.

ENZYMATIC PROTEIN REMOVERS

Enzymatic protein removers clean off material that your eyes deposit on the contact lenses over time. Depending on the type of contact lenses you wear and the amount of deposits that build upon the lens surface, your eye-care provider may recommend you use a product for removing the buildup. Enzymatic protein removers are available in liquid and tablet forms and are used on a daily or weekly basis depending on the product. Ask your eye-care provider before using this product.

RIGID GAS PERMEABLE CARE SYSTEMS

Care systems for rigid gas permeable, or hard contact lenses are different from care systems used for soft-contact lenses. Hard contact lenses typically require several different solutions for wetting, cleaning, and disinfecting. If you wear hard contact lenses, talk to your eye-care provider about which care system is best for you. Never use hard contact lens-care products on soft-contact lenses.

Your eye-care provider can help you determine which care system will work best for your eyes and your contact lens type.

Section 12.3 | **Things to Know about Decorative Contact Lenses**

This section includes text excerpted from "Decorative Contact Lenses for Halloween and More," U.S. Food and Drug Administration (FDA), October 28, 2019.

You may want to have the perfect look for Halloween or look similar to your favorite movie star or singer, but choosing to change the look of your eyes with contact lenses could cause a lot of damage to your eyesight if you get them without the input of your eye-care professional. Decorative contact lenses are sometimes called, among other names:

- Halloween contact lenses
- Fashion contact lenses
- Colored contact lenses
- Cosmetic contact lenses
- Theatre contact lenses

Decorative contact lenses change the look of your eyes. They may not correct your vision. They can temporarily change your brown eyes to blue or make your eyes look similar to that of cat eyes or vampire eyes for Halloween.

Did you know that these decorative contact lenses are actually medical devices? The U.S. Food and Drug Administration (FDA) oversees their safety and effectiveness, similar to contact lenses that correct your vision.

You should never buy contact lenses from a street vendor, beauty supply store, flea market, novelty store or Halloween store—and you should always have a prescription.

Before stepping out with your new look, here is what you need to know.

KNOW THE RISKS OF DECORATIVE- AND HALLOWEEN-CONTACT LENSES

Wearing decorative-contact lenses can be as risky as the contact lenses that correct your vision.

Wearing any kind of contact lenses, including decorative ones, can cause serious damage to your eyes if the lenses are obtained without a prescription or not used correctly.

These risks include:

- A cut or scratch on the top layer of your eyeball (corneal abrasion)
- Allergic reactions, such as itchy, watery red eyes
- Decreased vision
- Infection
- Blindness

When wearing any type of contact lenses, be aware of signs of possible eye infection, which include:

- Redness
- Pain in the eye(s) that does not go away after a short period of time
- Decreased vision

If you have any of these signs, you need to see a licensed eye doctor (optometrist or ophthalmologist) right away. An eye infection could become serious and cause you to become blind if it is not treated.

You can avoid some of these risks by getting any type of contact lenses from your doctor. Be sure to follow the directions for cleaning, disinfecting, and wearing the lenses that your doctor gives you. If your doctor does not give you any directions—ask for them.

DO'S AND DON'TS OF DECORATIVE AND HALLOWEEN LENSES

Do Get an Eye Exam

A licensed eye doctor will examine your eyes to make sure the contact lenses fit properly. The fit of your contact lenses is very important. A wrong fit can cause damage to your eyes. Be sure to always go for follow-up eye exams.

Do Get a Prescription

Your eye doctor will write you a prescription for all contact lenses, including decorative lenses. The prescription should include the brand name, correct lens measurements and expiration date.

Do Follow the Contact Lens-Care Instructions

Follow the instructions that come with contact lenses for wearing, cleaning, and disinfecting them. If you do not receive instructions, ask an eye doctor for them.

Seek Medical Attention

Do seek medical attention right away and remove your contact lenses if your eyes are red, have ongoing pain or discharge. Redness, pain, and discharge from the eyes are signs of an eye infection. If you think you have an eye infection from your contact lenses, remove them and see an eye doctor right away.

Do Not Share Your Contact Lenses with Anyone Else

You would not share your toothbrush, would you? All eyes are not the same size and shape and your contact lenses are fitted just for you.

Do Not Buy Any Contact Lenses without a Prescription

If you do not see an eye doctor and get a prescription, then the contact lenses you get may not fit properly and may not work well. They could even damage your eyes. Sometimes wearing contact lenses can damage the top layer of your eyeball (cornea). Even if you are not having any problems now, the lenses still could be causing damage to your eyes. By having regular checkups and buying contact lenses with a prescription, you will reduce the chances of any undetected damage to your eyes.

BUYING DECORATIVE- OR HALLOWEEN-CONTACT LENSES

You can buy contact lenses including decorative-contact lenses from your eye doctor, on the Internet, or from a mail-order company, which includes foreign manufacturers/distributors of decorative lenses. It is very important that you only buy contact lenses from a company that sells FDA-cleared or approved contact lenses and requires you to provide a prescription.

Anyone selling you contact lenses must get your prescription and verify it with your doctor. They should request not only the prescription but the name of your doctor and their phone number. If they do not ask for this information they are breaking federal law and could be selling you illegal-contact lenses.

Remember. Buying contact lenses without a prescription is dangerous.

Never buy contact lenses from a street vendor, a beauty supply store, flea market, novelty store or Halloween store, or from unknown online distributors as they may be contaminated and/or counterfeit and therefore not safe to use.

Even though there are a lot of products that you can buy without a prescription, contact lenses are not one of them. It is your job to make sure you protect your eyes by having an eye exam, getting a prescription, and buying contact lenses from a legal source.

REPORTING A PROBLEM

You can report:

- Adverse events including contact lens-related infections or potentially counterfeit products

    - FDA Medwatch (www.fda.gov/safety/medwatch-fda-safety-information-and-adverse-event-reporting-program)
- Unlawful Internet sales or contact lens vendors selling without a prescription
    - Report a Problem Web Form (www.fda.gov/safety/report-problem-fda/reporting-unlawful-sales-medical-products-internet)
    - Federal Trade Commission (FTC) Complaint Assistant (www.ftccomplaintassistant.gov/#crnt&panel1-1)
- E-mails promoting medical products that might be illegal
    - FDA Office of Regulatory Affairs (ORA) Web complaints (webcomplaints@ora.fda.org)
- Allegations that a medical device manufacturer or its product is in violation of the law
    - Allegations of Regulatory Misconduct Web Form (www.fda.gov/medical-devices/reporting-allegations-regulatory-misconduct/allegations-regulatory-misconduct-form)

Section 12.4 | What to Know If Your Child Wants Contact Lenses

This section includes text excerpted from "What to Know If Your Child Wants Contact Lenses," U.S. Food and Drug Administration (FDA), August 17, 2017.

These days, eyeglasses can look pretty cool. Still, the day may come when your son or daughter asks you for contact lenses.

There are pros to consider—and cons.

The U.S. Food and Drug Administration (FDA) regulates contact lenses and certain contact lens care products as medical devices. Contact lenses have benefits, says Bernard P. Lepri, O.D., M.S., M.Ed., an FDA optometrist in the agency's Contact Lens and Retinal Devices Branch.

"They can be better for sports activities because they do not break as frames and the lenses of glasses can. And they provide a better peripheral vision for sports or driving, if your teen is of driving age," Lepri explains. Moreover, in some cases, contact lenses improve the quality of vision in comparison to eyeglasses, especially when a child is very nearsighted, says Lepri.

"On the other hand, you have to remember that contact lenses are medical devices, not cosmetics," Lepri says. "Like any medical device, contact lenses should be used only if they can be used safely and responsibly. And only under the supervision of your eye-care professional." Serious injury to the eye can result, particularly if the contact lenses are not removed at the first hint of a problem.

CONTACT LENS RISKS AND SAFETY TIPS

Kids and contact lenses are not always the best fit.

"Eye-care professionals typically do not recommend contacts for kids until they are 12 or 13 years of age, because the risks are often greater than the benefits for younger children," Lepri says. "But age is not the only issue. It is also a question of maturity."

Lepri suggests that parents who are considering contacts for their kids take a look at how well they handle other responsibilities, especially personal hygiene. "It takes vigilance on the part of the parents," he says. "You need to constantly be looking over your child's shoulder to make sure they are properly caring for their lenses."

As many an eye-care professional can attest, kids find all sorts of ways to be less than hygienic. Common, dangerous behaviors include wearing another child's lens; using saliva to moisten a lens; and wearing decorative lenses purchased from flea markets, beauty supply stores, the Internet and other sources. These behaviors can result in injury.

In fact, according to a 2010 study published in Pediatrics, about 13,500 (or one-fourth) of the roughly more than 70,000 children who go to the emergency room each year for injuries and complications from medical devices are related to contact lenses. The problems from contact lenses include infections and eye abrasions—meaning that your eye can be bruised from contact lenses.

The reasons? Hygiene and responsibility. Or rather, Lepri says, the lack thereof. He adds that it is essential for all people who wear contact lenses to follow their eye-care professional's advice "to the letter." That means observing all hygienic precautions.

Even lenses without corrective power, such as decorative or so-called "colored" or "costume" contact lenses are still medical devices and have all the risks other contact lenses do, says Lepri.

"Never buy decorative/costume contact lenses without a prescription from your eye doctor," Lepri adds. And never buy contact lenses from any supplier that does not require a valid prescription. (Again, even zero-powered contact lenses require a prescription for correct and safe fitting.)

If considering contact lenses, your child should be able to follow the following safety tips.

- Always wash your hands before cleaning or inserting lenses, and carefully dry your hands with a clean, lint-free cloth.
- Rub, rinse, clean, and disinfect your contact lenses as directed and only with the products and solutions recommended by your eye-care professional.
- Never expose your contact lenses to any kind of water or saliva.
- Do not wear your lenses for longer than the prescribed wearing schedule. This means that you should not sleep in lenses that were not prescribed to be worn this way.
- Never wear someone else's lenses.
- Always have a prescription for any lenses you wear.
- When playing sports, wear safety goggles or glasses over your lenses.
- In general, always have a pair of back-up glasses handy.
- Never put a contact lens into an eye that is red.
- Do not ignore eye itching, burning, irritation or redness that could signal potentially dangerous infection. Remove the lenses and contact your eye-care professional. Apply cosmetics after inserting lenses, and remove your lenses before removing makeup.

Not taking the necessary safety precautions can result in ulcers (sores) of the cornea—which is the front of the eye that shields it from germs, dust, and other harmful material—and even blindness.

"Even an experienced lens wearer can scratch a cornea while putting in or taking out a lens," Lepri notes.

WHAT ELSE SHOULD YOU KNOW ABOUT CONTACT LENSES?

Eye-care professionals generally do not recommend extended wear lenses for kids and teens because they can increase the incidence of corneal ulcers, which can lead to permanent loss of vision.

Although they are a bit more expensive, daily disposable lenses can reduce some of the risks since the wearer is using a new pair of lenses every day.

In addition, children with seasonal allergies are usually not good candidates for wearing contact lenses. The lenses may only increase the itching and burning caused by their allergies.

You can talk with your child about the risks and responsibilities of wearing contact lenses and whether she or he is able to handle these responsibilities. Then talk with your eye-care provider to determine if your child is a good candidate for wearing contact lenses.

Section 12.5 | Risks of Contact Lens and How to Avoid Infection or Injury

This section contains text excerpted from the following sources: Text in this section begins with excerpts from "Contact Lens Risks," U.S. Food and Drug Administration (FDA), September 4, 2018; Text under the heading "How to Avoid Infection or Injury" is excerpted from "Focusing on Contact Lens Safety," U.S. Food and Drug Administration (FDA), October 16, 2019.

Wearing contact lenses puts you at risk of several serious conditions including eye infections and corneal ulcers. These conditions can develop very quickly and can be very serious. In rare cases, these conditions can cause blindness.

You cannot determine the seriousness of a problem that develops when you are wearing contact lenses. You have to get help from an eye-care professional to determine your problem.

If you experience any symptoms of eye irritation or infection:

- Remove your lenses immediately and do not put them back in your eyes.
- Contact your eye-care professional right way.
- Do not throw away your lenses. Store them in your case and take them to your eye-care professional. She or he may want to use them to determine the cause of your symptoms.
- Report serious eye problems associated with your lenses to the U.S. Food and Drug Administration's (FDA) MedWatch reporting program.

SYMPTOMS OF EYE IRRITATION OR INFECTION

- Discomfort
- Excess tearing or other discharge
- Unusual sensitivity to light
- Itching, burning, or gritty feelings
- Unusual redness
- Blurred vision
- Swelling
- Pain

SERIOUS HAZARDS OF CONTACT LENSES

Symptoms of eye irritation can indicate a more serious condition. Some of the possible serious hazards of wearing contact lenses are corneal ulcers, eye infections, and even blindness.

Corneal ulcers are open sores in the outer layer of the cornea. They are usually caused by infections. To reduce your chances of infection, you should:

- **Rub and rinse** your contact lenses as directed by your eye-care professional.
- **Clean and disinfect** your lenses properly according to the labeling instructions.
- **Do not "top-off" the solutions in your case.** Always discard all of the leftover contact lens solution after each use. Never reuse any lens solution.

- **Do not expose your contact lenses to any water**: tap, bottled, distilled, lake, or ocean water. Never use nonsterile water (distilled water, tap water or any homemade saline solution). Tap and distilled water have been associated with *Acanthamoeba* keratitis, a corneal infection that is resistant to treatment and cure.
- **Remove your contact lenses before swimming**. There is a risk of eye infection from bacteria in swimming pool water, hot tubs, lakes, and the ocean.
- **Replace your contact lens storage case** every three months or as directed by your eye-care professional.

OTHER RISKS OF CONTACT LENSES

Other risks of contact lenses include:

- Pink eye (conjunctivitis)
- Corneal abrasions
- Eye irritation

HOW TO AVOID INFECTION OR INJURY

Contact lens users run the risk of infections, such as the pink eye (conjunctivitis), corneal abrasions, and eye irritation. A common result of eye infection is corneal ulcers, which are open sores in the outer layer of the cornea. Many of these complications can be avoided through everyday care of the eye and contact lenses.

In general, if you are using a multipurpose contact lens solution, replace your contact- lens storage case at least every three months or as directed by your eye-care provider. If you are using a contact lens solution that contains hydrogen peroxide, always use the new contact lens case that comes with each box—and follow all directions that are included on or inside the packaging.

Clean and disinfect your lenses properly. When using contact lens solution, read and follow all instructions on the product label to avoid eye injury. This is particularly important if your eye-care professional has recommended a solution with hydrogen peroxide, as these solutions require special care.

Always remove contact lenses before swimming.

Never reuse any lens solution. Always discard all of the used solutions after each use, and add fresh solution to your lens case.

Do not expose your contacts to any water (which includes the lake, pond, and ocean water as well as distilled water, tap water, and homemade saline solution) because it can be a source of microorganisms that may cause serious eye infections. (Contact lens solution is sold in "sterile" containers, which means it is free from living germs or microorganisms.)

Never put your lenses in your mouth or put saliva on your lenses. The saliva is not sterile.

Never transfer contact lens solutions into smaller travel-size containers. These containers are not sterile, and unsterile solution can damage your eyes.

Do not wear contact lenses overnight unless your eye-care provider has prescribed them to be worn that way. Any lenses worn overnight can increase your risk of infection. Wearing contact lenses overnight can stress the cornea by reducing the amount of oxygen to the eye. They can also cause microscopic damage to the surface of the cornea, making it more susceptible to infection.

Never ignore symptoms of eye irritation or infection that may be associated with wearing contact lenses. These symptoms include discomfort, excess tearing or other discharge, unusual sensitivity to light, itching, burning, gritty feelings, unusual redness, blurred vision, swelling, or pain. If you experience any of these symptoms, remove your lenses immediately and keep them off. Contact your eye-care professional immediately. Keep the lenses, because they may help your eye-care professional determine the cause of your symptoms.

Section 12.6 | **The Danger of Using Tap Water with Contact Lenses**

This section includes text excerpted from "The Danger of Using Tap Water with Contact Lenses," U.S. Environmental Protection Agency (EPA), January 27, 2020.

More than 34 million people in the United States and 71 million people in the world wear contact lenses. Contact lens wearers include athletes, actors, musicians, and people in occupations where glasses get in the way. Some people wear contacts for cosmetic reasons.

WHAT IS *ACANTHAMOEBA*?

Acanthamoeba is a microbe that is very common in the environment, including tap water. It has two forms: the trophozoite and cyst. The infective form is the trophozoite, which can change into a cyst and survive a long time. These trophozoites and cysts can stick to the surface of your contact lenses and then infect your eye.

WHAT ARE THE SYMPTOMS OF *ACANTHAMOEBA* EYE INFECTION?

The symptoms of *Acanthamoeba* eye infection include severe pain in the eye, the sensation of a foreign body in the eye, and a whitish halo at the periphery of the eye. The infection can last weeks to months, and it never fully heals despite treatment. See your doctor immediately if you experience any of these symptoms.

HOW DO YOU GET *ACANTHAMOEBA* ON YOUR CONTACT LENSES?

Acanthamoeba gets on your lens when you use contaminated or homemade lens solutions to rinse or store your lenses. Eye infections often result when the microbe attaches to the surface of the lens and the contact case. You can also get infected when you swim while wearing your contact lenses.

WHO CAN GET INFECTED FROM *ACANTHAMOEBA* EYE INFECTION

- Anyone who wears contact lenses and does not use proper lens care
- Teens who share and swap their colored lenses
- People who use homemade saline solutions for contact lenses
- People who do not disinfect their contact lenses
- People who use saliva to wet their contacts
- People who buy contacts at beach shops and flea markets without going to the eye doctor for a prescription

CAN *ACANTHAMOEBA* EYE INFECTION BE TREATED?

The *Acanthamoeba* eye infection is difficult to treat. A doctor can successfully treat it with a combination of topical ointments, such as Brolene and Polyhexamethylene biguanide (PHMB). You can locate a contact lens doctor by visiting the website for the Contact Lens Association of Ophthalmologists (CLAO) (www.clao.org).

HOW CAN YOU PREVENT AN *ACANTHAMOEBA* EYE INFECTION?

- Practice good personal hygiene when handling your contact lenses.
- Remind young contact lens wearers about proper lens handling.
- Clean, rinse, and disinfect lenses with commercially made sterile solutions before placing them in the eyes.
- Clean lens cases with commercially made sterile solutions.
- Do not use tap water, homemade solutions, and other nonsterile solutions to disinfect and store contacts.
- Do not wet lenses with saliva.
- Follow manufacturer's instructions in rinsing and storing contact lenses.
- Do not swim while wearing your contacts.
- Do not trade, share, or borrow another person's lenses.
- Replace lenses and lens cases as often as possible.
- Only wear contact lenses prescribed by an eye-care professional.

WHAT IS ENVIRONMENTAL PROTECTION AGENCY DOING ABOUT *ACANTHAMOEBA*?

The U.S. Environmental Protection Agency (EPA) has issued guidance for vision care and healthcare providers on *Acanthamoeba* in contact lens wearers.

Chapter 13 | Laser-Assisted In Situ Keratomileusis (LASIK) Surgery

Chapter Contents

Section 13.1 | **LASIK: The Basics**

This section contains text excerpted from the following sources: Text in this section begins with excerpts from "What Is LASIK?" U.S. Food and Drug Administration (FDA), July 11, 2018; Text beginning with the heading "What Types of Surgery Can Fix Refractive Errors?" is excerpted from "Surgery for Refractive Errors," National Eye Institute (NEI), June 26, 2019.

The cornea is a part of the eye that helps focus light to create an image on the retina. It works in much the same way that the lens of a camera focuses light to create an image on film. The bending and focusing of light are also known as "refraction." Usually, the shape of the cornea and the eye are not perfect and the image on the retina is out-of-focus (blurred) or distorted.

These imperfections in the focusing power of the eye are called "refractive errors." There are three primary types of refractive errors: myopia, hyperopia, and astigmatism. People with myopia, or nearsightedness, have more difficulty seeing distant objects as clearly as near objects. People with hyperopia, or farsightedness, have more difficulty seeing near objects as clearly as distant objects. Astigmatism is a distortion of the image on the retina caused by irregularities in the cornea or lens of the eye.

Combinations of myopia and astigmatism or hyperopia and astigmatism are common. Glasses or contact lenses are designed to compensate for the eye's imperfections. Surgical procedures aimed at improving the focusing power of the eye are called "refractive surgery." In laser-assisted in situ keratomileusis (LASIK) surgery, precise and controlled removal of corneal tissue by a special laser reshapes the cornea changing its focusing power.

WHAT TYPES OF SURGERY CAN FIX REFRACTIVE ERRORS?

The most common type of refractive surgery is called "LASIK." Most types of refractive surgery, including LASIK, use lasers to change the shape of the cornea. Some use other tools, such as implants.

WHAT IS LASIK?

Laser-assisted in situ keratomileusis uses a laser (a strong beam of light) to change the shape of the cornea and help make vision clearer. It works best for adults with nearsightedness, farsightedness, or astigmatism. It cannot fix presbyopia. For LASIK to work correctly, your vision needs to be stable (meaning your eyeglass or contact lens prescription stays the same over time).

IS LASIK RIGHT FOR ME?

To find out if LASIK is right for you, you will need a comprehensive dilated eye exam. The exam is simple and painless. Your eye doctor will ask you to read letters that are up close and far away. Then they will give you some eye drops to dilate (widen) your pupil and check for other eye problems.

Laser-assisted in situ keratomileusis is not right for everyone. Some eye conditions can raise your risk for complications from LASIK, including:

- Keratoconus (a disease that makes the cornea thinner over time)
- Eye infections, such as keratitis or ocular herpes
- Dry eye
- Glaucoma
- Cataract
- Large pupils

Talk with your eye doctor to decide if LASIK or another type of refractive surgery is right for you.

WHAT ARE THE BENEFITS OF LASIK?

After LASIK, most people see well enough to stop wearing their eyeglasses or contact lenses for most of their daily activities. Since everyone gets presbyopia as they age, and LASIK cannot fix presbyopia, most people will still need single vision glasses or contact lenses at some point.

HOW LONG DOES IT TAKE TO RECOVER?

Right after surgery, your eyes might be irritated and your vision will be blurry, so you will need someone to give you a ride home from the doctor's office.

Your eye doctor may give you medicine or special eye drops to help with any pain after the surgery. You may also need to wear a special patch over your eye for several nights, to protect it while you are sleeping.

You will be able to see after surgery, but it takes two to three months for your eye to finish healing. Your vision will get clearer as your eye heals. Ask your doctor about when you can go back to your normal activities.

WILL YOU NEED MORE TREATMENT?
WHAT ARE THE OTHER TYPES OF REFRACTIVE SURGERY?

Alternatives to LASIK include:

- Laser epithelial keratomileusis (LASEK)
- EpiLasik
- Phakic intraocular lens (IOL) implantation
- Photorefractive keratectomy (PRK)

Section 13.2 | Wavefront LASIK

Custom wavefront laser-assisted in situ keratomileusis (LASIK) surgery is an advanced form of surgery that is also called "custom LASIK" or "wavefront LASIK." Introduction of this surgery in 1999 constituted a significant step forward in the field of refractive surgery, since the procedure uses a guided laser to reshape the cornea and improve a person's visual acuity.

Laser-assisted in-situ keratomileusis is a simple, fast, and effective procedure that is carried out to correct refractive errors such as nearsightedness (myopia), farsightedness (hyperopia and presbyopia), and astigmatism. Custom LASIK is a suitable option for reducing post-LASIK complications such as reduced night vision, halos, and glare, thereby improving visual acuity.

TYPES OF WAVEFRONT LASIK

There are two basic types of wavefront or custom LASIK procedures. They are:

1. **Wavefront-guided LASIK.** In this procedure, detailed wavefront-generated measurements are used to check how light waves travel through the eyes and fall upon the retina. In addition to treating nearsightedness, farsightedness, and astigmatism, wavefront-guided LASIK also reduces irregular higher-order aberrations that can reduce the quality of vision even after correcting all major refractive errors.
2. **Wavefront-optimized LASIK.** In this procedure, detailed measurements of the front curvature of the eye are taken to preserve the natural aspheric shape of the cornea. Preserving the natural shape of the cornea will help reduce the risk of a certain type of higher-order aberration called "spherical aberration," which often causes halos around light and other night-vision problems. This can naturally occur in an eye or can be caused by other types of laser-vision correction procedures.

ADVANTAGES AND DISADVANTAGES OF WAVEFRONT LASIK

Wavefront LASIK uses an individualized laser program to correct vision errors in the cornea. Customization is not done using the same methods used in conventional LASIK, however; instead, Wavefront LASIK uses the refractive error of the eyes to determine how to reshape the cornea. There can be advantages and disadvantages of custom LASIK.

Advantages

- A targeted approach to correcting the cornea
- More accurate correction of refractive errors
- Helps to correct other subtle distortions in the cornea
- Fewer cases of higher-order aberrations
- Side effects such as dry eye, itching, and night-vision problems as less frequent in wavefront LASIK

- Wavefront LASIK has shown higher rates of postsurgery 20/20 vision.
- Reduced problems of contrast sensitivity, or seeing black letters in a white background

Disadvantages

- The same amount of corneal aberrations occur in wavefront LASIK as in traditional LASIK.
- Changes required to adjust visual aberrations can leave the cornea too thin for any other LASIK procedure to be performed in the future.
- As with conventional LASIK, wavefront LASIK is not covered by most insurance plans, and wavefront LASIK is likely to cost more than traditional LASIK.
- The wavefront procedure may take longer than traditional LASIK surgery.

PROGNOSIS

Studies show that 90 to 94 percent of patients who received wavefront LASIK achieved visual acuity of 20/20 or better.

The postsurgery recovery period after wavefront LASIK is usually the same as the recovery time for traditional LASIK. There have been instances in which most patients have noticed a great improvement in their vision almost immediately after the procedure. Healing is quicker with wavefront LASIK, although patients are recommended to rest for the first 24 hours after the procedure. Most people return to their daily routine the following day.

An experienced refractive eye surgeon can determine if wavefront LASIK surgery is preferable for your eye-care needs by performing a preoperative examination and consultation. After analyzing all test results, the doctor will confirm whether wavefront LASIK surgery is suitable for you. It is important to work closely with the optometrist and/or ophthalmologist to determine the procedure that best suits your eyes.

References

1. "Custom Wavefront LASIK Surgery Is Safe and Effective," QualSight LASIK, July 4, 2017.
2. "Wavefront LASIK: Costs and Differences from Other Types," NVISION Eye Centers, December 23, 2018.
3. "Custom Wavefront LASIK: Personalized Vision Correction," All About Vision, June 2019.

Section 13.3 | Risks in LASIK

This section includes text excerpted from "What Are the Risks and How Can I Find the Right Doctor for Me?" U.S. Food and Drug Administration (FDA), August 8, 2018.

Most patients are very pleased with the results of their refractive surgery. However, like any other medical procedure, there are risks involved. That is why it is important for you to understand the limitations and possible complications of refractive surgery.

Before undergoing a refractive procedure, you should carefully weigh the risks and benefits based on your own personal value system, and try to avoid being influenced by friends who have had the procedure or doctors encouraging you to do so.

- **Some patients lose vision.** Some patients lose lines of vision on the vision chart that cannot be corrected with glasses, contact lenses, or surgery as a result of treatment.
- **Some patients develop debilitating visual symptoms.** Some patients develop glare, halos, and/or double vision that can seriously affect nighttime vision. Even with good vision on the vision chart, some patients do not see as well in situations of low contrast, such as at night or in fog, after treatment as compared to before treatment.
- **You may be undertreated or overtreated.** Only a certain percent of patients achieve 20/20 vision without glasses or contacts. You may require additional

treatment, but additional treatment may not be possible. You may still need glasses or contact lenses after surgery. This may be true even if you only required a very weak prescription before surgery. If you used reading glasses before surgery, you may still need reading glasses after surgery.

- **Some patients may develop severe dry eye syndrome.** As a result of surgery, your eye may not be able to produce enough tears to keep the eye moist and comfortable. Dry eye not only causes discomfort but can reduce visual quality due to intermittent blurring and other visual symptoms. This condition may be permanent. Intensive drop therapy and the use of plugs or other procedures may be required.
- **Results are generally not as good in patients with very large refractive errors of any type.** You should discuss your expectations with your doctor and realize that you may still require glasses or contacts after the surgery.
- **For some farsighted patients, results may diminish with age.** If you are farsighted, the level of improved vision you experience after surgery may decrease with age. This can occur if your manifest refraction (a vision exam with lenses before dilating drops) is very different from your cycloplegic refraction (a vision exam with lenses after dilating drops).
- **Long-term data is not available.** LASIK is a relatively new technology. The first laser was approved for LASIK eye surgery in 1998. Therefore, the long-term safety and effectiveness of LASIK surgery are not known.

ADDITIONAL RISKS

Monovision

Monovision is one clinical technique used to deal with the correction of presbyopia, the gradual loss of the ability of the eye to change focus for close-up tasks that progresses with age. The intent of monovision is for the presbyopic patient to use one eye for distance viewing and one eye for near viewing. This practice was first applied to fit contact lens wearers and more recently to LASIK and other refractive surgeries. With contact lenses, a presbyopic patient has one eye fit with a contact lens to correct distance vision, and the other eye fit with a contact lens to correct near vision. In the same way, with LASIK, a presbyopic patient has one eye operated on to correct the distance vision, and the other operated on to correct the near vision. In other words, the goal of the surgery is for one eye to have vision worse than 20/20, the commonly referred to goal for LASIK surgical correction of distance vision. Since one eye is corrected for distance viewing and the other eye is corrected for near viewing, the two eyes no longer work together. This results in poorer quality vision and a decrease in in-depth perception. These effects of monovision are most noticeable in low lighting conditions and when performing tasks requiring a very sharp vision. Therefore, you may need to wear glasses or contact lenses to fully correct both eyes for distance or near when performing visually demanding tasks, such as driving at night, operating dangerous equipment, or performing occupational tasks requiring very sharp close vision (e.g., reading small print for long periods of time).

Many patients cannot get used to having one eye blurred at all times. Therefore, if you are considering monovision with LASIK, make sure you go through a trial period with contact lenses to see if you can tolerate monovision, before having the surgery performed on your eyes. Find out if you pass your state's driver's license requirements with monovision.

In addition, you should consider how much your presbyopia is expected to increase in the future. Ask your doctor when you should expect the results of your monovision surgery to no longer be enough for you to see nearby objects clearly without the aid of glasses or contacts, or when a second surgery might be required to further correct your near vision.

Bilateral Simultaneous Treatment

You may choose to have LASIK surgery on both eyes at the same time or to have surgery on one eye at a time. Although the convenience of having surgery on both eyes on the same day is attractive, this practice is riskier than having two separate surgeries.

If you decide to have one eye done at a time, you and your doctor will decide how long to wait before having surgery on the other eye. If both eyes are treated at the same time or before one eye has a chance to fully heal, you and your doctor do not have the advantage of being able to see how the first eye responds to surgery before the second eye is treated.

Another disadvantage to having surgery on both eyes at the same time is that the vision in both eyes may be blurred after surgery until the initial healing process is over, rather than being able to rely on clear vision in at least one eye at all times.

THINGS TO CONSIDER BEFORE REFRACTIVE SURGERY

If you are considering refractive surgery, make sure you:

- **Compare.** The levels of risk and benefit vary slightly not only from procedure to procedure, but from device to device depending on the manufacturer, and from surgeon to surgeon depending on their level of experience with a particular procedure.
- **Do not base your decision simply on cost** and do not settle for the first eye center, doctor, or procedure you investigate. Remember that the decisions you make about your eyes and refractive surgery will affect you for the rest of your life.
- **Be wary of eye centers that advertise**, "20/20 vision or your money back" or "package deals." There are never any guarantees in medicine.
- **Read.** It is important for you to read the patient handbook provided to your doctor by the manufacturer of the device used to perform the refractive procedure. Your doctor should provide you with this handbook and be willing to discuss her/his outcomes (successes as well as complications) compared to the results of the studies outlined in the handbook.

Even the best screened patients under the care of most skilled surgeons can experience serious complications.

- **During surgery.** Malfunction of a device or other error, such as cutting a flap of cornea through instead of making a hinge during LASIK surgery, may lead to discontinuation of the procedure or irreversible damage to the eye.
- **After surgery.** Some complications, such as migration of the flap, inflammation or infection, may require another procedure and/or intensive treatment with drops. Even with aggressive therapy, such complications may lead to temporary loss of vision or even irreversible blindness.

Under the care of an experienced doctor, carefully screened candidates with reasonable expectations and a clear understanding of the risks and alternatives are likely to be happy with the results of their refractive procedure.

Section 13.4 | **LASIK Surgery Checklist**

This section includes text excerpted from "LASIK Surgery Checklist," U.S. Food and Drug Administration (FDA), July 11, 2018.

KNOW WHAT MAKES YOU A POOR CANDIDATE FOR LASIK

- **Career impact**—does your job prohibit refractive surgery?
- **Cost**—can you really afford this procedure?
- **Medical conditions**—e.g., do you have an autoimmune disease or other major illness? Do you have a chronic illness that might slow or alter healing?
- **Eye conditions**—do you have or have you ever had any problems with your eyes other than needing glasses or contacts?
- **Medications**—do you take steroids or other drugs that might prevent healing?

- **Stable refraction**—has your prescription changed in the last year?
- **High or Low refractive error**—do you use glasses/contacts only some of the time? Do you need an unusually strong prescription?
- **Pupil size**—are your pupils extra large in dim conditions?
- **Corneal thickness**—do you have thin corneas?
- **Tear production**—do you have dry eyes?

KNOW ALL THE RISKS AND PROCEDURE LIMITATIONS

- **Overtreatment or undertreatment**—are you willing and able to have more than one surgery to get the desired result?
- **May still need reading glasses**—do you have presbyopia?
- **Results may not be lasting**—do you think this is the last correction you will ever need? Do you realize that long-term results are not known?
- **May permanently lose vision**—do you know some patients may lose some vision or experience blindness?
- **Dry eyes**—do you know that if you have dry eyes they could become worse, or if you do not have dry eyes before you could develop chronic dry eyes as a result of surgery?
- **Development of visual symptoms**—do you know about glare, halos, starbursts, etc. and that night driving might be difficult?
- **Contrast sensitivity**—do you know your vision could be significantly reduced in dim light conditions?
- **Bilateral treatment**—do you know the additional risks of having both eyes treated at the same time?
- **Patient information**—have you read the patient information booklet about the laser being used for your procedure?

KNOW HOW TO FIND THE RIGHT DOCTOR FOR LASIK

- **Experienced**—how many eyes has your doctor performed LASIK surgery on with the same laser?

- **Equipment**—does your doctor use a U.S. Food and Drug Administration (FDA)-approved laser for the procedure you need? Does your doctor use each microkeratome blade only once?
- **Informative**—is your doctor willing to spend the time to answer all your questions?
- **Long-term care**—does your doctor encourage follow-up and management of you as a patient? Your preop and postop care may be provided by a doctor other than the surgeon.
- **Be comfortable**—do you feel you know your doctor and are comfortable with an equal exchange of information?

KNOW PREOPERATIVE, OPERATIVE, AND POSTOPERATIVE EXPECTATIONS

- **No contact lenses prior to evaluation and surgery**—can you go for an extended period of time without wearing contact lenses?
- **Have a thorough exam**—have you arranged not to drive or work after the exam?
- **Read and understand the informed consent**—has your doctor given you an informed consent form to take home and answered all your questions?
- **No makeup before surgery**—can you go 24 to 36 hours without makeup prior to surgery?
- **Arrange for transportation**—can someone drive you home after surgery?
- **Plan to take a few days to recover**—can you take time off to take it easy for a couple of days if necessary?
- **Expect not to see clearly for a few days**—do you know you will not see clearly immediately?
- **Know sights, smells, sounds of surgery**—has your doctor made you feel comfortable with the actual steps of the procedure?
- **Be prepared to take drops/medications**—are you willing and able to put drops in your eyes at regular intervals?

- **Be prepared to wear an eye shield**—do you know you need to protect the eye for a period of time after surgery to avoid injury?
- **Expect some pain/discomfort**—do you know how much pain to expect?
- **Know when to seek help**—do you understand what problems could occur and when to seek medical intervention?
- **Know when to expect your vision to stop changing**—are you aware that final results could take months?
- **Make sure your refraction is stable before any further surgery**—if you do not get the desired result, do you know not to have an enhancement until the prescription stops changing?

Section 13.5 | What to Expect before, during, and after LASIK Surgery

This section includes text excerpted from "What Should I Expect before, during, and after Surgery?" U.S. Food and Drug Administration (FDA), July 11, 2018.

What to expect before, during, and after surgery will vary from doctor to doctor and patient to patient. This section is a compilation of patient information developed by manufacturers and healthcare professionals, but cannot replace the dialogue you should have with your doctor.

BEFORE SURGERY

If you decide to go ahead with laser-assisted in situ keratomileuses (LASIK) surgery, you will need an initial or baseline evaluation by your eye doctor to determine if you are a good candidate. This is what you need to know to prepare for the exam and what you should expect:

If you wear contact lenses, it is a good idea to stop wearing them before your baseline evaluation and switch to wearing your glasses full-time. Contact lenses change the shape of your cornea for up to several weeks after you have stopped using them depending on the type of contact lenses you wear. Not leaving your contact lenses out long enough for your cornea to assume its natural shape before surgery can have negative consequences. These consequences include inaccurate measurements and a poor surgical plan, resulting in poor vision after surgery. These measurements, which determine how much corneal tissue to remove, may need to be repeated at least a week after your initial evaluation and before surgery to make sure they have not changed, especially if you wear rigid gas permeable (RGP) or hard lenses. If you wear:

- **Soft contact lenses**, you should stop wearing them for two weeks before your initial evaluation
- **Toric soft lenses** or **RGP lenses**, you should stop wearing them for at least three weeks before your initial evaluation
- **Hard lenses**, you should stop wearing them for at least four weeks before your initial evaluation

You should tell your doctor:

- About your past and present medical and eye conditions
- About all the medications you are taking, including over-the-counter (OTC) medications and any medications you may be allergic to

Your doctor should perform a thorough eye exam and discuss:

- Whether you are a good candidate
- What the risks, benefits, and alternatives of the surgery are
- What you should expect before, during, and after surgery
- What your responsibilities will be before, during, and after surgery

You should have the opportunity to ask your doctor questions during this discussion. Give yourself plenty of time to think about the risk/benefit discussion, to review any informational literature provided by your doctor, and to have any additional questions answered by your doctor before deciding to go through with surgery and before signing the informed consent form.

You should not feel pressured by your doctor, family, friends, or anyone else to make a decision about having surgery. Carefully consider the pros and cons.

The day before surgery, you should stop using:

- Creams
- Lotions
- Makeup
- Perfumes

These products as well as the debris along the eyelashes may increase the risk of infection during and after surgery. Your doctor may ask you to scrub your eyelashes for a period of time before surgery to get rid of residues and debris along the lashes.

Also before surgery, arrange for transportation to and from your surgery and your first follow-up visit. On the day of surgery, your doctor may give you some medicine to make you relax. Because this medicine impairs your ability to drive and because your vision may be blurry, even if you do not drive make sure someone can bring you home after surgery.

DURING SURGERY

The surgery should take less than 30 minutes. You will lie on your back in a reclining chair in an exam room containing the laser system. The laser system includes a large machine with a microscope attached to it and a computer screen.

A numbing drop will be placed in your eye, the area around your eye will be cleaned, and an instrument called a "lid speculum" will be used to hold your eyelids open.

Your doctor may use a mechanical microkeratome (a blade device) to cut a flap in the cornea.

If a mechanical microkeratome is used, a ring will be placed on your eye and very high pressures will be applied to create suction to the cornea. Your vision will dim while the suction ring is on and you may feel the pressure and experience some discomfort during this part of the procedure. The microkeratome, a cutting instrument, is attached to the suction ring. Your doctor will use the blade of the microkeratome to cut a flap in your cornea. Microkeratome blades are meant to be used only once and then thrown out. The microkeratome and the suction ring are then removed.

Your doctor may use a laser keratome (a laser device), instead of a mechanical microkeratome to cut a flap on the cornea.

If a laser keratome is used, the cornea is flattened with a clear plastic plate. Your vision will dim and you may feel the pressure and experience some discomfort during this part of the procedure. Laser energy is focused inside the cornea tissue, creating thousands of small bubbles of gas and water that expand and connect to separate the tissue underneath the corneal surface, creating a flap. The plate is then removed.

You will be able to see, but you will experience fluctuating degrees of blurred vision during the rest of the procedure. The doctor will then lift the flap and fold it back on its hinge, and dry the exposed tissue.

The laser will be positioned over your eye and you will be asked to stare at a light. This is not the laser used to remove tissue from the cornea. This light is to help you keep your eye fixed on one spot once the laser comes on.

Note: If you cannot stare at a fixed object for at least 60 seconds, you may not be a good candidate for this surgery.

When your eye is in the correct position, your doctor will start the laser. At this point in the surgery, you may become aware of new sounds and smells. The pulse of the laser makes a ticking sound. As the laser removes corneal tissue, some people have reported a smell similar to burning hair. A computer controls the amount of laser energy delivered to your eye. Before the start of surgery, your doctor will have programmed the computer to vaporize a particular amount of tissue based on the measurements taken at your initial evaluation. After the pulses of laser energy vaporize the corneal tissue, the flap is put back into position.

A shield should be placed over your eye at the end of the procedure as protection since no stitches are used to hold the flap in place. It is important for you to wear this shield to prevent you from rubbing your eye and putting pressure on your eye while you sleep, and to protect your eye from accidentally being hit or poked until the flap has healed.

AFTER SURGERY

Immediately after the procedure, your eye may burn, itch, or feel such as there is something in it. You may experience some discomfort, or in some cases, mild pain and your doctor may suggest you take a mild pain reliever. Both your eyes may tear or water. Your vision will probably be hazy or blurry. You will instinctively want to rub your eye, but do not! Rubbing your eye could dislodge the flap, requiring further treatment. In addition, you may experience sensitivity to light, glare, starbursts or halos around lights, or the whites of your eye may look red or bloodshot. These symptoms should improve considerably within the first few days after surgery. You should plan on taking a few days off from work until these symptoms subside. You should contact your doctor immediately and not wait for your scheduled visit, if you experience severe pain, or if your vision or other symptoms get worse instead of better.

You should see your doctor within the first 24 to 48 hours after surgery and at regular intervals after that for at least the first 6 months. At the first postoperative visit, your doctor will remove the eye shield, test your vision, and examine your eye. Your doctor may give you one or more types of eye drops to take at home to help prevent infection and/or inflammation. You may also be advised to use artificial tears to help lubricate the eye. Do not resume wearing contact lenses in the operated eye, even if your vision is blurry.

You should wait one to three days following surgery before beginning any noncontact sports, depending on the amount of activity required, how you feel, and your doctor's instructions.

To help prevent infection, you may need to wait for up to two weeks after surgery or until your doctor advises you otherwise before using lotions, creams, or makeup around the eye. Your doctor may advise you to continue scrubbing your eyelashes for a period of time after surgery. You should also avoid swimming and using hot tubs or whirlpools for one to two months.

Strenuous contact sports, such as boxing, football, karate, etc., should not be attempted for at least four weeks after surgery. It is important to protect your eyes from anything that might get into them and from being hit or bumped.

During the first few months after surgery, your vision may fluctuate.

- It may take up to three to six months for your vision to stabilize after surgery.
- Glare, haloes, difficulty driving at night, and other visual symptoms may also persist during this stabilization period. If further correction or enhancement is necessary, you should wait until your eye measurements are consistent for two consecutive visits at least three months apart before reoperation.
- It is important to realize that although distance vision may improve after reoperation, it is unlikely that other visual symptoms, such as glare or halos will improve.
- It is also important to note that no laser company has presented enough evidence for the U.S. Food and Drug Administration (FDA) to make conclusions about the safety or effectiveness of enhancement surgery.

Contact your eye doctor immediately if you develop any new, unusual or worsening symptoms at any point after surgery. Such symptoms could signal a problem that, if not treated early enough, may lead to a loss of vision.

Section 13.6 | **LASIK—FAQs**

This section includes text excerpted from "LASIK-FAQs (Frequently Asked Questions)," U.S. Food and Drug Administration (FDA), July 11, 2018.

WHERE CAN YOU FIND A GOOD LASIK SURGEON IN YOUR AREA?

You may want to go to your library and see if there is a local community services magazine that may provide comparison information on services for doctors in your area.

HOW DO YOU REPORT A BAD EXPERIENCE OR WHO DO YOU NOTIFY ABOUT A 'BAD' DOCTOR?

If you had a bad experience or sustained an injury, you should file a voluntary MedWatch report (800-FDA-1088 (800-332-1088)) to the FDA. Also, you could contact your state medical licensing board and file a complaint with them. In addition, you could contact your state health department or consumer complaint organization (e.g., Better Business Bureau (BBB)).

HOW MUCH DOES LASIK COST?

The FDA regulates the safety and effectiveness of medical devices for their intended use. The FDA does not regulate the marketing of or any fees associated with the use of that product. Again, you may want to go to your library and see if there is a local community services magazine that may provide comparison information on services for doctors in your area.

HOW CAN YOU FIND OUT IF A PARTICULAR LASER HAS BEEN APPROVED TO TREAT YOUR REFRACTIVE ERROR (NEARSIGHTEDNESS, FARSIGHTEDNESS, AND/OR ASTIGMATISM)?

You can find approved devices, their approval date, and a synopsis of the approved indications on the FDA-Approved Lasers page (www.accessdata.fda.gov/scripts/cdrh/devicesatfda/index.cfm?search_term=LZS%20or%20LASIK).

IF THE LASER YOU ARE INTERESTED IN HAS NOT YET BEEN APPROVED FOR A PARTICULAR INDICATION, HOW CAN YOU FIND OUT WHEN IT WILL BE APPROVED?

Confidentiality restrictions prohibit the FDA from commenting on the status of a device under regulatory review, but you can try asking the laser company for this information.

WHICH LASER IS THE BEST FOR TREATING YOUR REFRACTIVE ERROR?

The FDA does not provide comparisons between refractive lasers. It approves the safety and effectiveness of a device-independent of any other product. However, you are encouraged to review the approval documents to assess the capabilities of specific laser systems and make your own comparisons. Discuss any concerns you may have with your doctor.

HOW DOES WAVEFRONT LASIK COMPARE TO CONVENTIONAL LASIK?

Wavefront lasik adds an automatic measurement of more subtle distortions (called "higher-order aberrations") than just nearsightedness, farsightedness, and astigmatism corrected by conventional LASIK. However, these "higher-order aberrations" account for only a small amount (probably no more than 10%) of the total refractive error of the average person's eye. Conventional LASIK increases higher-order aberrations. Although wavefront-guided treatments attempt to eliminate higher-order aberrations, results from the clinical studies have shown that the average aberrations still increase, but less than they do after conventional LASIK. In a few studies comparing wavefront-guided LASIK to conventional LASIK, a slightly larger percentage of subjects treated with wavefront LASIK achieved 20/20 vision without glasses or contact lenses compared to subjects treated with conventional LASIK. Patient selection and the experience and competence of the surgeon are still the most important considerations.

WHAT IS "ALL-LASER LASIK" AND HOW DOES IT COMPARE TO TRADITIONAL LASIK SURGERY?

The difference between traditional LASIK and "all-laser LASIK" (also known as "bladeless LASIK") is the method by which the LASIK flap is created. In "all-laser LASIK," a laser device called a "laser keratome," is used to cut a corneal flap for LASIK surgery. This is a newer method to create a corneal flap than the traditional method of using a microkeratome, a mechanical device with a blade. There is no absolute agreement among eye surgeons on the better choice for flap creation. Some of the factors a surgeon considers when choosing a preferred method of flap creation during LASIK are as follows:

- Quality of vision
- Rate of complications
- Pain during and after surgery
- The precision of flap size and thickness
- Time taken to recover vision
- Expense

Discuss with your doctor any questions and concerns you have about how they chose their preferred method of flap creation.

WHAT PERCENTAGE OF PATIENTS ATTAIN 20/20 VISION OR BETTER WITHOUT GLASSES OR CONTACTS?

Data in the Approval Orders and related documents summarizes the outcomes from the clinical trials submitted to the FDA for each approved device. Links to these documents are included on the FDA-Approved Lasers (www.accessdata.fda.gov/scripts/cdrh/devicesatfda/index.cfm?search_term=LZS%20or%20LASIK) page.

Chapter 14 | **Photorefractive Keratectomy (PRK) Eye Surgery**

Photorefractive keratectomy (PRK) is a type of vision correction eye surgery in which a laser is used to reshape the cornea. The cornea is a clear layer in the front of the eye that helps to focus light images on the retina at the back of the eye. Errors in the way the cornea bends or refracts light through the eye create vision problems. PRK can be used to permanently correct refractive errors that cause nearsightedness (myopia), farsightedness (hyperopia), and astigmatism (irregularities in the shape of the eye).

In comparison to laser-assisted in situ keratomileusis (LASIK)—the most popular type of laser eye surgery—PRK is less invasive because the excimer laser is used on the surface of the cornea rather than deep within the cornea. Both types of surgery are highly effective in correcting mild to moderate vision problems, although PRK generally requires longer recovery time. PRK is often used for people who are ineligible for LASIK or whose corneas were previously treated with LASIK.

WHAT TO EXPECT

Before Photorefractive Keratectomy Eye Surgery

Before having PRK surgery, a patient must undergo a comprehensive eye examination to evaluate whether they are suitable

"Photorefractive Keratectomy (PRK) Eye Surgery," © 2017 Omnigraphics. Reviewed March 2020.

candidates for the procedure. The eye surgeon will ask questions about the patient's overall health, whether they have any medical conditions such as diabetes or arthritis, and what medications they are taking. The eye surgeon will also measure the thickness of the cornea, determine the amount of refractive error to be corrected in each eye, and use imaging technology to create a corneal map showing the precise curvature of the surface of each eye. Since contact lenses can affect the shape of the cornea, patients who wear rigid, gas permeable contact lenses may need to stop wearing them about three weeks before the initial eye examination, while those who wear soft contact lenses should avoid wearing them for three days before the initial visit.

Preparing for Photorefractive Keratectomy Eye Surgery

The PRK procedure is performed under local anesthesia, so patients are allowed to eat a light meal beforehand and take any prescribed medications. Patients should avoid wearing eye makeup and any hats or hair accessories that could interfere with the position of their head under the laser. The eyes are prepared for surgery by applying a topical anesthetic in the form of eye drops to numb the surface. A device called a "lid speculum" will be used to prevent the eyelids from closing during the procedure. The patient may also receive an oral sedative to promote relaxation.

During Photorefractive Keratectomy Eye Surgery

The PRK procedure itself only takes 10 to 15 minutes to treat both eyes. As the patient stares straight ahead, the surgeon begins by using an alcohol solution or a surgical instrument to carefully remove a layer of surface cells known as "epithelium" from the cornea. Next, the surgeon uses a computer-controlled excimer laser to direct pulses of ultraviolet (UV) light on the cornea. The laser energy removes microscopic amounts of tissue in a precise pattern to reshape the cornea to the specifications of the patient's prescription. In most cases, the procedure is completely painless, although some patients experience a feeling of pressure. Most patients elect to have both eyes treated on the same day, one immediately after the other, while some decide to have the second eye treated a few weeks after the first.

After Photorefractive Keratectomy Eye Surgery

Once the surgery is completed, the surgeon will place a bandage contact lens over the treated cornea to protect it while the epithelial cells grow back. The surgeon will also prescribe topical antibiotics, anti-inflammatory medications, and eye lubrication drops to reduce swelling and minimize discomfort. The patient can go home the same day with an escort to drive them, although they must return for several follow-up appointments over the next few weeks so the surgeon can monitor the healing process. The bandage contact lens is typically removed after four to six days.

Recovery from Photorefractive Keratectomy Eye Surgery

Recovery from PRK surgery can take a few weeks. Most patients experience some discomfort, irritation, and sensitivity to light for the first few days. Many patients find that their vision is blurry at first but gradually improves enough to drive a car within 1 to 3 weeks. It can take up to 6 months, however, for the patient's eyesight to be completely clear and stable. Around 90 percent of patients who undergo PRK have 20/20 vision without glasses or contact lenses one year after the surgery.

LONG-TERM RESULTS AND POSSIBLE COMPLICATIONS

Photorefractive keratectomy laser eye surgery has been performed millions of times around the world since the 1980s, and it is considered safe and effective. Nearly all patients who undergo PRK surgery experience significant improvements in the clarity of their vision. Although serious side effects and complications are rare, patients should be aware of the following potential side effects:

- Glare, starbursts, or halos around lights at night

- Abnormal corneal healing resulting in the formation of opaque cells that cause hazy vision
- Regression or partial loss of treatment effect in patients who have had PRK surgery to correct large amounts of farsightedness or astigmatism

In addition, most patients who undergo PRK surgery still require reading glasses with magnification to correct presbyopia (age-related loss of near vision) once they reach middle age. Some patients opt for a process called "monovision," in which one eye is corrected for distance vision and the other is corrected for near vision, either through contact lenses or laser surgery.

ADVANTAGES AND DISADVANTAGES OF PRK SURGERY

Photorefractive keratectomy is often compared to LASIK, the most popular form of laser eye surgery used to correct nearsightedness, farsightedness, and astigmatism. The two procedures use the same modern laser technologies and offer the same long-term results. The main difference between PRK and LASIK involves how much of the cornea is disturbed. In PRK procedures, only the epithelial layer or "skin" of the cornea is removed. This thin outer surface of the cornea grows back within a few days after the surgery, although patients may experience some discomfort and blurry vision during this time.

In LASIK procedures, the surgeon makes an incision with a microkeratome or a femtosecond laser to create a thin flap on the cornea. This flap is lifted so the underlying corneal tissue can be reshaped with an excimer laser. Although the flap is replaced at the end of the procedure, it can remain vulnerable to tearing or injury. The main reason LASIK is more popular is that patients experience little to no discomfort and achieve clear vision almost immediately.

PRK is often recommended for patients whose corneas are too thin for LASIK, or who have irregularities in the surface of their corneas that might complicate LASIK. In addition, PRK is often performed on patients who have already undergone LASIK but require additional correction to achieve clear vision.

References

1. Kozarsky, Alan. "Photorefractive Keratectomy Eye Surgery," WebMD, November 25, 2015.
2. "Photorefractive Keratectomy (PRK) Eye Surgery," Cleveland Clinic, 2015.
3. Wachler, Brian Boxer. "PRK Laser Eye Surgery," All About Vision, September 2016.

Chapter 15 | Laser Epithelial Keratomileusis (LASEK) Surgery

Laser epithelial keratomileusis (LASEK) is a type of vision correction eye surgery in which a laser is used to reshape the cornea. LASEK can be used to permanently correct vision problems such as nearsightedness (myopia), farsightedness (hyperopia), and astigmatism (irregularities in the shape of the eye). LASEK is a variation of two other laser eye surgery procedures, photorefractive keratectomy (PRK) and laser-assisted in situ keratomileusis (LASIK). The main difference between the procedures involves the way in which the eye is prepared for laser treatment:

- In PRK procedures, the eye surgeon removes and discards a very thin layer of epithelial cells from the surface of the cornea. This "skin" layer of the cornea regenerates within a few days after the surgery, but the healing process creates discomfort and occasionally results in a hazy vision.
- In LASIK procedures, the eye surgeon creates a thicker, circular flap of corneal tissue, performs the laser treatment underneath it, and then replaces it. Although this process allows for minimal discomfort and shorter recovery time than PRK, it can result in dry eyes, and the flap may be vulnerable to traumatic injury.
- LASEK procedures resemble PRK procedures because the eye surgeon removes a very thin surface layer

of cells from the cornea. Rather than discarding the epithelium, however, the surgeon replaces the flap following the laser treatment, as in LASIK procedures. LASEK is intended to reduce the discomfort and risk of corneal haze associated with PRK, as well as to avoid potential problems related to the thicker flap created in LASIK.

Laser epithelial keratomileusis, PRK, and LASIK all offer similar success rates and long-term vision outcomes. LASIK is the most popular type of laser eye surgery because it allows for minimal discomfort and provides clear vision almost immediately. Still, LASEK may be a good option for patients with thin corneas and who are not good candidates for LASIK, because they have thin corneas, or for patients who have already undergone LASIK but require additional correction to achieve clear vision. LASEK may be preferable to PRK for patients who have refractive errors greater than 6.00 diopters because it reduces the risk of corneal haze. A qualified eye surgeon can provide individualized advice about the best type of laser eye surgery for a patient's circumstances.

WHAT TO EXPECT

Before LASEK Surgery

Before having LASEK surgery, a patient must undergo a comprehensive eye examination to evaluate whether they are suitable candidates for the procedure. The eye surgeon will ask questions about the patient's overall health, whether they have any medical conditions such as diabetes or arthritis, and what medications they are taking. The eye surgeon will also measure the thickness of the cornea, determine the amount of refractive error to be corrected in each eye, and use imaging technology to create a corneal map showing the precise curvature of the surface of each eye. Since contact lenses can affect the shape of the cornea, patients who wear rigid, gas permeable contact lenses may need to stop wearing them about three weeks before the initial eye examination, while those who wear soft contact lenses should avoid wearing them for three days before the initial visit.

Preparing for LASEK Surgery

The LASEK procedure is performed under local anesthesia, so patients are allowed to eat a light meal beforehand and take any prescribed medications. Patients should avoid wearing eye makeup and any hats or hair accessories that could interfere with the position of their head under the laser. The eyes are prepared for surgery by applying a topical anesthetic in the form of eye drops to numb the surface. A device called a "lid speculum" will be used to prevent the eyelids from closing during the procedure. The patient may also receive an oral sedative to promote relaxation.

During LASEK Surgery

During the LASEK procedure, the eye surgeon uses a fine blade called a "trephine" to make a circular incision in the epithelium. Next, the surgeon places a diluted alcohol solution over the eye to loosen the edges of the epithelium flap so it can be moved gently to the side. The corneal tissue underneath the flap is then reshaped with an excimer laser to the patient's exact prescription. Following the laser treatment, the top layer of cells is returned to its original position on the eye, and a special contact lens bandage is put in place to protect the wound. In some cases, the thin flap of "skin" is too fragile and cannot be replaced on the eye. When the epithelial layer must be removed, the surgery technically becomes a PRK procedure rather than a LASEK procedure.

After LASEK Surgery

The main advantage of preserving the top layer of cells is that the patient experiences less discomfort following LASEK surgery than PRK surgery. However, the recovery process is similar for the two procedures and slower than for a LASIK procedure. The patient wears the protective contact lens bandage for four to six days while the epithelium heals. The surgeon will also prescribe topical antibiotics, anti-inflammatory medications, and eye lubrication drops to reduce swelling and minimize discomfort. The patient can go home the same day with an escort to drive them, although they must return for several follow-up appointments over the next few weeks so the surgeon can monitor the healing process.

Recovery from LASEK Surgery

Patients who undergo LASEK surgery usually regain clear vision within a week, although it may take several weeks for the eyesight to stabilize. Around 90 percent of patients who undergo LASEK have 20/20 vision without glasses or contact lenses one year after the surgery.

LONG-TERM RESULTS AND POSSIBLE COMPLICATIONS

Laser epithelial keratomileusis eye surgery is considered safe and effective. Nearly all patients who undergo LASEK experience significant improvements in the clarity of their vision. Although serious side effects and complications are rare, patients should be aware of the following side effects:

- Blurry vision, glare, or halos around lights at night
- Eye infection
- Dry eyes
- Regression or partial loss of treatment effect

In addition, most patients who have LASEK surgery still require reading glasses with magnification to correct presbyopia (age-related loss of near vision) once they reach middle age. Some patients opt for a process called "monovision," in which one eye is corrected for distance vision and the other is corrected for near vision, either through contact lenses or laser surgery.

ADVANTAGES AND DISADVANTAGES OF LASEK SURGERY

Although LASEK is considered a safe and effective alternative to LASIK or PRK, it is mainly used in patients who are not good candidates for the other procedures. LASEK is preferable to LASIK for people with thin corneas, dry eyes, or jobs and hobbies that put them at high risk of injury to the corneal flap. Many people opt for LASIK, however, because it offers minimal discomfort and a quick visual recovery.

Laser epithelial keratomileusis eye surgery is comparable to PRK in terms of visual recovery. Whereas eye surgeons once believed that replacing the epithelial level would lead to quicker healing, in practice, it takes the cornea less time to regrow a new layer of "skin." As a result, PRK is more popular than LASEK except for people with very strong prescriptions who face a higher risk of corneal hazing from PRK.

References

1. Hagele, Glenn. "LASEK—Laser-Assisted Sub-Epithelial Keratomileusis," USA Eyes, 2013.
2. "LASEK Eye Surgery," WebMD, 2016.
3. Wachler, Brian Boxer. "LASEK Eye Surgery: How It Works," All About Vision, April 2016.

Chapter 16 | **Phakic Intraocular Lenses**

Chapter Contents

Section 16.1 | **What Are Phakic Lenses?**

This section includes text excerpted from "What Are Phakic Lenses?" U.S. Food and Drug Administration (FDA), January 8, 2018.

Phakic intraocular lenses (pIOLs), or phakic lenses, are lenses made of plastic or silicone that are implanted into the eye permanently to reduce a person's need for glasses or contact lenses. "Phakic" refers to the fact that the lens is implanted into the eye without removing the eye's natural lens. During phakic lens implantation surgery, a small incision is made in the front of the eye. The phakic lens is inserted through the incision and placed just in front of or just behind the iris.

USES OF PHAKIC LENSES

Phakic lenses are used to correct refractive errors, errors in the eye's focusing power. All phakic lenses approved by the U.S. Food and Drug Administration (FDA) are for the correction of nearsightedness (myopia).

The cornea and natural lens of the eye focus light to create an image on the retina, much similar to the way the lens of a camera focuses light to create an image on film. The bending and focusing of light are also known as "refraction." Imperfections in the focusing power of the eye called "refractive errors," cause images on the retina to be out of focus or blurred.

People who are nearsighted have more difficulty seeing distant objects than near objects. For these people, the images of distant objects come to focus in front of the retina instead of on the retina.

Ideally, phakic lenses cause light entering the eye to be focused on the retina providing clear distance vision without the aid of glasses or contact lenses.

Surgery is not required to correct nearsightedness. You can wear glasses or contact lenses instead to correct your vision. Depending on how nearsighted you are, and other conditions of your eye, other refractive surgery (surgery to correct refractive errors) options may be available to you, including photorefractive keratectomy (PRK) and laser-assisted in situ keratomileusis (LASIK).

CAN PHAKIC LENSES BE REMOVED?

Phakic lenses are intended to be permanent. While the lenses can be surgically removed, returning to your previous level of vision or condition of your eye cannot be guaranteed.

WHAT IS THE DIFFERENCE BETWEEN PHAKIC INTRAOCULAR LENSES AND INTRAOCULAR LENSES FOLLOWING CATARACT SURGERY?

Phakic intraocular lenses are implanted in the eye without removing the natural lens. This is in contrast to intraocular lenses that are implanted into eyes after the eye's cloudy natural lens (cataract) has been removed during cataract surgery.

Section 16.2 | Are Phakic Lenses for You?

This section includes text excerpted from "Are Phakic Lenses for You?" U.S. Food and Drug Administration (FDA), January 8, 2018.

You are probably NOT a good candidate for phakic lenses if:

- **You are not an adult**. There are no phakic lenses approved by the U.S. Food and Drug Administration (FDA) for persons under 21 years of age.
- **You are not a risk-taker**. Certain complications are unavoidable in a percentage of patients, and there is no long-term data available for phakic lenses.
- **You required a change in your contact lens or glasses prescription in the last 6 to 12 months in order to obtain the best possible vision for you**. This is called "refractive instability." Patients who are:
  - In their early 20s or younger

- Whose hormones are fluctuating due to disease, such as diabetes
- Who are pregnant or breastfeeding
- Who are taking medications that may cause fluctuations in vision
- More likely to have refractive instability and should discuss the possible additional risks with their doctor

- **You may jeopardize your career.** Some jobs prohibit certain refractive procedures. Be sure to check with your employer/professional society/military service before undergoing any procedure.
- **Cost is an issue.** Most medical insurance will not pay for refractive surgery.
- **You have a disease or are on medications that may affect wound healing.** Certain conditions, such as autoimmune diseases (e.g., lupus, rheumatoid arthritis (RA), immunodeficiency states (e.g., human immunodeficiency viruses (HIV)) and diabetes, and some medications (e.g., retinoic acid and steroids) may prevent proper healing after intraocular surgery.
- **You have a low endothelial cell count or abnormal endothelial cells.** If, the endothelial cells, the cells that pump the fluid out of your cornea, are low in number relative to your age, or if your endothelial cells are abnormal, you have a higher risk of developing a cloudy cornea and requiring a corneal transplant.
- **You actively participate in sports with a high risk of eye trauma.** Your eye may be more susceptible to damage should you receive a blow to the face or eye, such as a blow to the head during boxing or hit in the eye by a ball during baseball. Your eye may be more susceptible to rupture or retinal detachment, and the phakic lens may dislocate.
- **You only have one eye with a potentially good vision.** If you only have one eye with good vision with glasses or contact lenses, due to disease, irreparable damage, or

amblyopia (eye with poor vision since childhood that cannot be corrected with glasses or contact lenses), you and your doctor should consider the risk of possible damage and/or loss of vision to your better eye, as a result, phakic lens implantation.

- **You have large pupils**. If your pupil dilates in low lighting conditions to a size that is larger than the size of the lens, you have a higher risk of experiencing visual disturbances after surgery that may affect your ability to function comfortably or normally under such conditions (e.g., while driving at night).
- **You have a shallow anterior chamber**. If the space between the cornea and the iris, the anterior chamber, is narrow, you have a higher risk of developing complications, such as greater endothelial cell loss, due to implantation of the phakic lens.
- **You have an abnormal iris**. If your pupil is irregularly shaped you have a higher risk of developing visual disturbances.
- **You have had uveitis**. If you have had inflammation in your eye, you may have a recurrence or worsening of your disease and/or may develop additional complications, such as glaucoma, as a result of surgery.
- **You have had problems with the posterior part of your eye**. If you have had any problems in the back part of your eye or are at risk for such problems, for example, proliferative diabetic retinopathy (growth of abnormal vessels in the back of the eye due to diabetes) or retinal detachment, you may not be a good candidate for phakic lens implantation. The phakic lens may not allow your eye doctor to get a clear view of the back part of your eye, preventing or delaying detection of a new or worsening problem, and/or the phakic lens may prevent or make treatment of a problem in the back of your eye more difficult.

The safety and effectiveness of phakic lenses have NOT been studied in patients with certain conditions. If any of the following conditions apply to you, make sure you discuss them with your doctor.

- **You have glaucoma** (damage to the nerve of the eye resulting in loss of peripheral and then central vision due to too high pressure inside the eye), ocular hypertension (high eye pressure), or glaucoma suspect (some indications, but not clear, that patient has glaucoma). You may have a higher risk of developing or worsening of glaucoma as a result of phakic lens implantation.
- **You have pseudoexfoliation syndrome** (abnormal deposits of material in the eye visible on the structures in the front part of the eye, such as on the front of the natural lens and the back of the cornea). This syndrome is associated with glaucoma and weakness of the structures holding the natural lens in place (the zonules). You may have a higher risk of surgical complications and/or complications after surgery if you have this syndrome.
- **You have had an eye injury or previous eye surgery**.
- **Your need for vision correction is outside the range for which the phakic lens has been approved**. Ask your eye doctor if the phakic lens that she or he recommends for you has been approved to treat your refractive error and/or check the FDA-Approved Phakic Lenses for the approved refractive range.
- **You are over the age of 45.** Some phakic lenses have not been studied in patients over the age of 45.

Section 16.3 | The Risks of Phakic Lenses

This section includes text excerpted from "What Are the Risks?" U.S. Food and Drug Administration (FDA), January 8, 2018.

Implanting a phakic lens involves a surgical procedure. As in any other medical procedure, there are risks involved. That is why it is important for you to understand the limitations and risks of phakic intraocular lens implant surgery.

Before undergoing surgery for implantation of a phakic intraocular lens, you should carefully weigh the risks and benefits and try to avoid being influenced by other people encouraging you to do it.

YOU MAY LOSE VISION

Some patients lose vision as a result of phakic lens implant surgery that cannot be corrected with glasses, contact lenses, or another surgery. The amount of vision loss may be severe.

YOU MAY DEVELOP DEBILITATING VISUAL SYMPTOMS

Some patients develop glare, halos, double vision, and/or decreased vision in situations of low-level lighting that can cause difficulty with performing tasks, such as driving, particularly at night or under foggy conditions.

YOU MAY NEED ADDITIONAL EYE SURGERY

You may need additional eye surgery to reposition, replace or remove the phakic lens implant. These surgeries may be necessary for your safety or to improve your visual function. If the lens power is not right, then a phakic lens exchange may be needed. You may also have to have the lens repositioned, removed, or replaced if the lens does not stay in the right place, is not the right size, and/or causes debilitating visual symptoms. Every additional surgical procedure has its own risks.

YOU MAY BE UNDERTREATED OR OVERTREATED

Many treated patients do not achieve 20/20 vision after surgery. The power of the implanted phakic lens may be too strong or too weak. This is because of the difficulties with determining exactly what power lens you need. This means that you will probably still need glasses or contact lenses to perform at least some tasks. For example, you may need glasses for reading, even if you did not need them before surgery. This also means that you may need a second surgery to replace the lens with another if the power of the originally implanted lens was too far from what you needed.

YOU MAY DEVELOP INCREASED INTRAOCULAR PRESSURE

You may experience increased pressure inside the eye after surgery, which may require surgery or medication to control. You may need long-term treatment with glaucoma medications. If the pressure is too high for too long, you may lose vision.

YOUR CORNEA MAY BECOME CLOUDY

The endothelial cells of your cornea are a thin layer of cells responsible for pumping fluid out of the cornea to keep it clear. If the endothelial cells become too few in number, the endothelial cell pump will fail and the cornea will become cloudy, resulting in loss of vision. You start with a certain number of cells at birth, and this number continuously decreases as you age, since these cells are not replenished. Normally, you die from old age before the number of endothelial cells becomes so low that your cornea becomes cloudy. Some lens designs have shown that their implantation causes endothelial cells to be lost at a faster rate than normal. If the number of endothelial cells drops too low and your cornea becomes cloudy, you will lose vision and you may require a corneal transplant in order to see more clearly.

YOU MAY DEVELOP A CATARACT

You may get a cataract, clouding of the natural lens. The amount of time for a cataract to develop can vary greatly. If your cataract develops and progresses enough to significantly decrease your vision, you may require cataract surgery and your doctor will have to remove both your natural and your phakic lenses.

YOU MAY DEVELOP A RETINAL DETACHMENT

The retina is the tissue that lines the inside of the back of your eyeball. It contains the light-sensing cells that collect and send images to your brain, much similar to the film in a camera. The risk of the retina becoming detached from the back of your eye increases after intraocular surgery. It is not known at this time by how much your risk of retinal detachment will increase as a result of phakic intraocular lens implantation surgery.

PAINFUL EXPERIENCE

You may experience infection, bleeding, or severe inflammation (pain, redness, and decreased vision). These are rare complications that can sometimes lead to permanent loss of vision or loss of the eye.

LACK OF LONG-TERM DATA

Long-term data is not available. Phakic lenses are a new technology and have only recently been approved by the U.S. Food and Drug Administration (FDA). Therefore, there may be other risks to having phakic lenses implanted that may not have been reported yet.

Section 16.4 | **Checklist of Questions for Your Doctor**

This section includes text excerpted from "Checklist of Questions for Your Doctor," U.S. Food and Drug Administration (FDA), January 8, 2018.

Use the following checklist to help you guide your discussion with your doctor about phakic lenses.

KNOW WHAT MAKES YOU A POOR CANDIDATE

- Do I have any conditions that would increase my risks?
- Are the size of my pupils under low lighting conditions bigger than the size of the lens? If so, what are my additional risks?
- Is my anterior chamber shallow? If so, what are my additional risks?

KNOW ALL THE BENEFITS, RISKS, AND ALTERNATIVES

- What are the benefits of the phakic lens for my amount of nearsightedness?
- What are the risks of having the phakic lens implanted?
- What is my risk of needing a corneal transplant in the future, if I have the phakic lens implanted, based on my age and my endothelial cell count?
- What could happen if I get hit in the eye or head after phakic lens implantation that might be different from what could happen if I did not have the lens implanted? Are my chances greater for a more severe injury after phakic lens implantation?
- Can the phakic lens be removed? What are the risks of removing the phakic lens?
- What other options are available for correcting my nearsightedness?

KNOW PREOPERATIVE, OPERATIVE, AND POSTOPERATIVE EXPECTATIONS

- Will I need to limit my activities after treatment? If so, for how long?
- What quality of vision can I expect in the first week, first few months, and a year after surgery?
- What is the possibility that the phakic lens will not completely correct my vision or that my prescription might be worse than before surgery? What options for additional treatment will be available to me if needed?

- How likely is it that I will need to wear glasses or contact lenses immediately after surgery and as I grow older?
- Should I have the phakic lens implanted in both eyes?
- What vision problems might I experience if I have the phakic lens implanted in only one eye?
- How long will I have to wait before having surgery on my other eye?

KNOW WHAT THE COSTS ARE

- How much will the surgery and follow-up cost? Will my health insurance cover this surgery?
- Will there be additional costs if I need additional procedures because the phakic lens implanted in my eye is too strong or too weak or because I have astigmatism? What is the likelihood of this happening?

Section 16.5 | **Phakic Lens Implantation Surgery—Before, during, and after Surgery**

This section includes text excerpted from "Before, during, and after Surgery," U.S. Food and Drug Administration (FDA), January 8, 2018.

This section gives you a general idea of what you might expect if you decide to have phakic intraocular lens implantation surgery. What to expect before, during, and after surgery will vary according to:

- The type of phakic lens implanted
- The practices of the medical facility where the surgery will be performed and of the doctor who will be providing your care
- Your unique health circumstances and body's response.

The information provided here may not apply to your particular situation and should not replace an in-depth discussion with your doctor.

WHAT SHOULD YOU EXPECT BEFORE PHAKIC LENS IMPLANTATION SURGERY?

Initial Visit

Before deciding to have phakic intraocular lens implantation surgery, you will need an initial examination to make sure your eye is healthy and suitable for surgery. Your doctor will take a complete history about your medical and eye health and perform a thorough examination of both eyes, which will include measurements of your pupils, anterior chamber depth (the distance between your cornea and iris), and endothelial cell counts (the number of cells on the back of your cornea).

If you wear contact lenses, your doctor may ask you to stop wearing them before your initial examination (from the day of, to a few weeks before), so that your refraction (a measure of how much your eye bends light) and central keratometry readings (a measure of how much the cornea curves) are more accurate.

At this time, you should tell your doctor if you:

- Take any medications, including over-the-counter (OTC) medications, vitamins, and other supplements
- Have any allergies
- Have had any eye conditions
- Have undergone any previous eye surgery
- Have had any medical conditions

Deciding to Have Surgery

To help you decide whether phakic lenses are right for you, talk to your doctor about your expectations and whether there are elements of your medical history, eye history, or eye examination that might increase your risk or prevent you from having the outcome you expect. Before you sign an informed consent document (a form giving permission to your doctor to operate on your eye), you should discuss with your doctor:

- Whether you are a good candidate
- What are the risks, benefits, and alternatives of the surgery
- What you should expect before, during, and after surgery

- What your responsibilities will be before, during, and after surgery

You should have the opportunity to ask questions to your doctor during this discussion. Ask your doctor for the patient labeling of the lens that she or he recommends for you. Give yourself plenty of time to think about the risk/benefit discussion, to review any informational literature provided by your doctor, and to have any additional questions answered by your doctor before deciding to go through surgery and before signing the informed consent document. You should not feel pressured by anyone to make a decision about having surgery. Carefully consider the pros and cons.

PREPARING FOR PHAKIC LENS IMPLANTATION SURGERY

Within Weeks of Surgery

About one to two weeks before surgery, your eye doctor may schedule you for a laser iridotomy to prepare your eye for implantation of the phakic lens. Before the procedure, your eye doctor may put drops in your eye to make the pupil small and to numb the eye. While you are seated, your doctor will rest a large lens on your eye. She or he will then make a small hole (or holes) in the extreme outer edge of the iris (the colored part of your eye) with a laser. This hole (holes) is to prevent fluid buildup and pressure in the back chamber of your eye after phakic lens implantation surgery. This procedure is usually performed in an office or clinic setting, not in an operating room, and usually only takes a few minutes.

After the iridotomy procedure, the doctor may have you wait around a while before checking your eye pressure and letting you go home. The procedure should not prevent you from driving home, but you should check with your eye doctor when you schedule your appointment. You will be given a prescription for steroid drops to put in your eye at home for several days to reduce inflammation from the iridotomy procedure. It is important that you follow all the instructions your doctor gives you after the iridotomy procedure.

Possible complications of laser iridotomy include:

- Iritis (inflammation in the front part of the eye)
- Increase in eye pressure (usually within one to four hours after the procedure)
- Cataract (clouding of the natural lens) from the laser
- Hyphema (bleeding into the anterior chamber of the eye, behind the cornea and in front of the iris, that can cause high pressure inside the eye)
- Injury to the cornea from the laser that can result in clouding of the cornea
- Incomplete opening of the hole all the way through the iris
- Closure of the new opening
- Rarely, retinal burns

Your doctor may ask you to stop wearing contact lenses before your surgery (anywhere from the day of the surgery to a few weeks before).

Before your surgery, your eye doctor may ask you to temporarily stop taking certain medications that increase the risk of bleeding during surgery. How long before surgery you may need to stop these medications depends upon which medications you are using and the conditions they are treating. You and your eye doctor may need to discuss stopping certain medications with the doctor who prescribed them, since you may need some of these medications to prevent life-threatening events. For example, you may need medications that stop blood clotting to keep from having a stroke.

Within Days of Surgery

Your doctor may give you prescriptions for antibiotic drops to prevent infection and/or anti-inflammatory drops to prevent inflammation to put in your eye for a few days before surgery.

Arrange for transportation to and from surgery and to your follow-up doctor's appointment the day after surgery, since you will be unable to drive. Your doctor will let you know when it is safe for you to drive again.

Your eye doctor will probably tell you not to eat or drink anything after midnight the night before your surgery.

WHAT YOU SHOULD EXPECT DURING PHAKIC LENS IMPLANTATION SURGERY

Just before surgery, drops will be put in your eye. You will have to lie down for the surgery and remain still. If you cannot lie down flat on your back, you may not be a good candidate for this surgery. Usually, patients are not put to sleep for this type of surgery, but you may be given a sedative or other medication to make you relax and an intravenous (IV) may be started. Your doctor may inject medication around the eye to make it numb. The doctor also may give you an injection around the eye to prevent you from being able to move your eye or see out of your eye. You will have to ask your doctor to find out exactly which type of anesthesia will be used in your case. Your eye and the surrounding area will be cleaned and an instrument called a "lid speculum" will be used to hold your eyelids open.

The doctor will make an incision in your cornea, sclera (the white part of your eye), or limbus (where the cornea meets the sclera). She or he will place a lubricant into your eye to help protect the back of the cornea (the endothelial cells) during the insertion of the phakic lens. The doctor will insert the phakic lens through the incision in the eye into the anterior chamber, behind the cornea and in front of the iris. Depending upon the type of phakic lens, the doctor will either attach the lens to the front of the iris in the anterior chamber of the eye or move it through the pupil into position behind the iris and in front of the lens in the posterior chamber of the eye. The doctor will remove the lubricant and may close the incision with tiny stitches, depending upon the type of incision. Your doctor will place some eye drops or ointment in your eye and cover your eye with a patch and/or a shield. The surgery will probably take around 30 minutes.

After the surgery is over, you may be brought to a recovery room for a couple of hours before you will be allowed to go home. You will be given prescriptions for antibiotics and anti-inflammatory drops to use at home as directed. You will be given an Implant Identification Card, which you should keep as a permanent record of the lens that was implanted in your eye. Make sure you show this card to anyone who takes care of your eyes in the future. You will be asked to go home and take it easy for the rest of the day.

WHAT YOU SHOULD EXPECT AFTER PHAKIC LENS IMPLANTATION SURGERY

Immediately after Surgery

After the surgical procedure, you may be sensitive to light and have a feeling that something is in your eye. You may experience minor discomfort after the procedure. Your doctor may prescribe pain medication to make you more comfortable during the first few days after the surgery. You should contact your eye doctor immediately if you have severe pain.

You should see your eye doctor the day after surgery. Your doctor will remove the patch and/or shield and will check your vision and the condition of your eye. Your doctor will instruct you on how to use the eye drops that you were prescribed for after the surgery. You will need to take these drops for up to a few weeks after surgery to decrease inflammation and help prevent infection. Your doctor may instruct you to continue wearing the shield all day and all night or just at night. You should wear the shield until your doctor tells you that you no longer have to do so. The shield is meant to prevent you from rubbing your eye or putting pressure on your eye while you sleep and to protect your eye from accidentally being hit or poked while it is healing.

As You Recover

Your vision will probably be somewhat hazy or blurry for the first several days after surgery. Your vision should start to improve after the first several days but may continue to fluctuate for the next several weeks. It usually takes about two to four weeks for the vision to stabilize. Do NOT rub your eyes, especially for the first three to five days. You may also experience sensitivity to light, glare, starbursts or halos around lights, or the whites of your eye may look red or bloodshot. These symptoms should decrease as your eye recovers over the next several weeks.

Remember to:

- Wash your hands before putting drops in your eye.
- Use the prescribed medications to help minimize the risk of infection and inflammation. Serious infection or inflammation can result in loss of vision.
- Try not to wet your eyes until your doctor says it is okay to do so.
- Try not to bend from the waist to pick up objects on the floor, as this can cause undue pressure to your eyes. Do not lift any heavy objects.
- Do not engage in any strenuous activity until your doctor says it is okay to do so. It will take about eight weeks for your eye to heal.

In the Long Term

Your doctor will instruct you to return for additional follow-up visits to monitor your progress. Initially, these visits will be closer together (a few days to a few weeks apart) and then they will be spread out (several weeks to several months apart). It is important to go to all these appointments, even if you think you are doing well so that the doctor can check for complications that you may not be aware of.

Because you will have a permanent implant in your eye with long-term risks, and especially since all these risks are not known at this time, you will need to be followed by an eye doctor on a regular basis for the rest of your life. Endothelial cell counts will have to be performed on a regular basis. You and/or your doctor should maintain records of these measurements, so as to be able to estimate the rate of cell loss. It is especially important for you to have your endothelial cells counted before you and your eye doctor consider any other intraocular procedures, such as cataract surgery, that will decrease the endothelial cell count even further.

Annual eye exams are usually recommended. However, if you have any problems with your vision or your eyes, such as flashing lights, floating spots, or blank spots in your vision (symptoms of a retinal detachment), you should see an eye doctor right away and inform her or him that you have a phakic lens implant. When participating in sports or other activities during which you might injure your eye, such as home improvement work, always wear protective eyewear, such as safety goggles.

Part 3 | **Understanding and Treating Disorders of the Cornea, Conjunctiva, Sclera, Lens, Iris, and Pupil**

Chapter 17 | The Cornea and Corneal Disease: An Overview

WHAT IS THE CORNEA?

The cornea is the clear outer layer at the front of the eye. The cornea helps your eye to focus light so you can see clearly.

WHAT ARE THE MAIN TYPES OF CORNEAL CONDITIONS?

There are several common conditions that affect the cornea.

- **Injuries.** Small abrasions (scratches) on the cornea usually heal on their own. Deeper scratches or other injuries can cause corneal scarring and vision problems.
- **Allergies.** Allergies to pollen can irritate the eyes and cause allergic conjunctivitis (pink eye). This can make your eyes red, itchy, and watery.
- **Keratitis.** Keratitis is inflammation (redness and swelling) of the cornea. Infections related to contact lenses are the most common cause of keratitis.
- **Dry eye.** Dry eye happens when your eyes do not make enough tears to stay wet. This can be uncomfortable and may cause vision problems.
- **Corneal dystrophies.** Corneal dystrophies cause cloudy vision when material builds up on the cornea. These diseases usually run in families.

This chapter includes text excerpted from "Corneal Conditions," National Eye Institute (NEI), August 3, 2019.

- There are also a number of less common diseases that can affect the cornea—including ocular herpes, Stevens-Johnson syndrome, iridocorneal endothelial syndrome, and pterygium.

WHEN TO GET HELP RIGHT AWAY

Go to the eye doctor or the emergency room if you have:

- Intense eye pain
- Change in vision
- Blurry vision
- Very red, watery eyes
- An object stuck in your eye
- A serious eye injury or trauma—like getting hit hard in the eye

AM I AT RISK FOR CORNEAL CONDITIONS?

Some corneal conditions, such as corneal dystrophies, run in families. But there are steps you can take to lower your risk of corneal injuries and infections.

To prevent corneal injuries, wear protective eyewear when you:

- Play sports that use a ball or puck, such as baseball or hockey
- Do yardwork, such as mowing the lawn or using a weedwhacker
- Make repairs, such as painting or hammering
- Use machines, such as sanders or drills
- Use chemicals, such as bleach or pesticides

If you wear contact lenses, always follow the instructions to clean, disinfect, and store your lenses. This can help prevent corneal infections, such as keratitis.

FEEL LIKE SOMETHING IS STUCK IN YOUR EYE?

- Try blinking several times
- Try rinsing your eye with clean water or saline (salt) solution

- Try pulling your upper eyelid down over your lower eyelid
- Do not rub your eye—you could scratch your cornea
- If an object is stuck in your eye, do not try to remove it yourself—go to your eye doctor or the emergency room

HOW WILL MY EYE DOCTOR CHECK FOR CORNEAL CONDITIONS?

Eye doctors can check for corneal conditions as part of a comprehensive eye exam. The exam is simple and painless.

To check for corneal abrasions (scratches), your eye doctor may use a special type of eye drops called "fluorescein dye." The dye makes corneal abrasions easier to see.

WHAT IS THE TREATMENT FOR CORNEAL CONDITIONS?

Many corneal conditions can be treated with prescription eye drops or pills. If you have advanced corneal disease, you may need a different treatment.

- **Laser treatment.** To treat some corneal dystrophies and other conditions, doctors can use a type of laser treatment called "phototherapeutic keratectomy" (PTK) to reshape the cornea, remove scar tissue, and make vision clearer.
- **Corneal transplant surgery.** If the damage to your cornea can't be repaired, doctors can remove the damaged part and replace it with healthy corneal tissue from a donor.
- **Artificial cornea.** As an alternative to corneal transplant, doctors can replace a damaged cornea with an artificial cornea, called a "keratoprosthesis" (KPro).

Chapter 18 | Corneal Injury

The cornea is a thin transparent layer that covers the eye's iris and pupil. A corneal injury, also called a "corneal abrasion," is a scratch or scrape on the surface of the cornea. An infected corneal injury can also develop into more serious eye conditions such as corneal ulcer or iritis.

CAUSES OF CORNEAL INJURY

Any object that comes in direct contact with the front surface of the eye can cause a potential corneal injury. Most of the corneal injuries are not only caused by trauma but can also be due to any of the following reasons:

- When the eye is poked with a fingernail, pen, or makeup brush
- When dirt, sand, sawdust, ash, chemicals, or any such foreign objects enter the eye
- When the eye is rubbed too hard
- Overwearing or wearing poor-fitted, damaged, or dirty contact lenses
- Certain eye infections
- Engaging in sports or any other activity without proper eye protection

Apart from the abovementioned reasons, dry eyes can also increase the chances of having a corneal injury that commonly occurs during sleep. While sleeping the eyes dry out making the eyelids stick to the cornea and while waking the eyelids can rub across the dry surface of the eye causing a corneal injury.

SYMPTOMS OF CORNEAL INJURY

The cornea is one of the most sensitive parts of the body as it has many nerve endings and even a minor injury to it can be very painful. It may feel as if there is a large rough object in the eye even though it may not be visible to others' naked eyes.

In addition to extreme pain and a scratchy feeling, other signs and symptoms of a corneal injury include:

- Redness of the eye
- Teary eyes
- Light sensitivity
- Headache
- Blurry vision
- Eye twitching

In some cases, the corneal injury can be so severe that it causes nausea. If there is a corneal injury and these symptoms are experienced, see an ophthalmologist immediately.

DIAGNOSIS OF CORNEAL INJURY

To diagnose a corneal injury, an ophthalmologist shall apply eye drops to relax the eye muscles and widen the pupil. A dye called "fluorescein" is then applied on the surface of the eye to highlight the affected areas. After giving a corneal anesthetic to temporarily ease the pain, the ophthalmologist shall examine the eye using a slit lamp.

TREATMENT FOR CORNEAL INJURY

Immediate First Aid When There Is a Corneal Injury

When there is a feeling that something is stuck in the eye, it is natural to rub the eyes, which might make the injury more serious. If something gets in the eye, try to flush it out with water or a saline solution. Also, it is not recommended to wear an eye patch since it can speed up bacterial growth leading to an infection.

If redness, pain, or a foreign body sensation continues even after flushing the eyes, seek immediate medical help—the corneal injury can cause serious harm if not attended to within 24 hours.

Medical Treatment

The treatment depends on the severity and cause of the wound. Minor injuries are treated with lubricating eye drops or ointments, which comfort the eye during the natural healing process. The ophthalmologist shall prescribe antibiotic eye drops as a precaution to avoid possible eye infection. However, in case of more serious corneal injuries, the antibiotic needs to stay longer in the eye.

Steroids are given to decrease the swelling and scarring along with pain-relieving medications. A minor corneal scratch is treated with bandage contact lenses that, when used along with prescribed eye drops, can help relieve pain and speed up the healing process.

A follow-up appointment within the next 24 hours of the treatment may be scheduled by the ophthalmologist depending on the severity. This is necessary since many corneal injuries may not heal properly and can cause recurrent corneal erosion and other complication that may affect the eyesight.

While the eyes are healing:

- Do not rub the eye
- Do not wear contact lenses until it is safe
- Wear sunglasses to reduce any discomfort while stepping out

Immediate treatment to most corneal injuries results in complete recovery with no permanent vision loss. But, some deeper abrasions that occur in the center of the cornea (directly in front of the pupil) can leave a scar and may result in permanent loss of visual acuity.

PREVENTION OF CORNEAL INJURY

It may be difficult to prevent most of the corneal injuries but some of them can be avoided by taking certain precautions. Some safety measures that can be taken are as follows:

- Wear safety goggles while working in environments with a risk of airborne debris such as construction or welding.

- Wear protective glasses while cleaning the yard, using machines or tools, and while playing sports.
- Clip the fingernails regularly.
- Be cautious while using a hairbrush or curling iron and while putting on eye makeup.
- Follow proper directions while using contact lenses.

A corneal injury, even if it is minor has to be immediately attended by a professional so that it may not develop into more serious conditions or get infected. If there are any unusual symptoms or recurring pain in the affected eye, visit the doctor again. Prompt treatment will reduce the risk of developing permanent vision loss.

References

1. "What Is a Corneal Abrasion?" WebMD, December 9, 2017.
2. "Corneal Abrasion: Treatment of a Scratched Eye," All About Vision, November 30, 2015.
3. "What Is Corneal Abrasion?" Boyd, Kierstan. American Academy of Ophthalmology (AAO), April 9, 2019.
4. "What Is a Corneal Abrasion?" Healthline Media, November 5, 2019.

Chapter 19 | **Keratitis**

Chapter Contents

Section 19.1 | **Microbial Keratitis: An Overview**

This section includes text excerpted from "Germs & Infections," Centers for Disease Control and Prevention (CDC), April 17, 2014. Reviewed March 2020.

GERMS AND INFECTIONS

Being able to see well is a vital aspect of performing daily activities for most people. Worldwide, many people rely on contact lenses (as well as glasses and eye surgery) to improve their sight. Contact lenses can provide many benefits, but they are not risk-free—especially if contact lens wearers do not practice healthy habits and take care of their contact lenses and supplies. If patients seek care quickly, most complications can be easily treated by an eye doctor. However, more serious infections can cause pain and even permanent vision loss, depending on the cause and how long the patient waits to seek treatment.

KERATITIS

Contact lens wear is linked to higher risk of keratitis, or inflammation of the cornea (the clear dome that covers the colored part of the eye). Many contact lens wearers do not care for their contact lenses and supplies as instructed, which increases their risk of eye problems like keratitis.

TYPES OF MICROBIAL KERATITIS

- Bacterial Keratitis
- Fungal Keratitis
- Parasitic/Amebic Keratitis
- Viral Keratitis

SYMPTOMS OF EYE INFECTION

- Irritated, red eyes
- Worsening pain in or around the eyes—even after contact lens removal
- Light sensitivity
- Sudden blurry vision
- Unusually watery eyes or discharge

PREVENTION

Microbial keratitis can usually be prevented through healthy habits and proper care of contact lenses and supplies. Keep your eyes healthy while wearing contact lenses by following these tips, and always be sure to carry a pair of glasses with you—just in case you have to take out your contact lenses.

Section 19.2 | Bacterial Keratitis

This section includes text excerpted from "Basics of Bacterial Keratitis," Centers for Disease Control and Prevention (CDC), April 7, 2014. Reviewed March 2020.

WHAT IS BACTERIAL KERATITIS?

Bacterial keratitis is an infection of the cornea (the clear dome covering the colored part of the eye) that is caused by bacteria. It can affect contact lens wearers, and also sometimes people who do not wear contact lenses. Types of bacteria that commonly cause bacterial keratitis include:

- *Pseudomonas aeruginosa*
- *Staphylococcus aureus*

WHAT ARE THE SYMPTOMS OF BACTERIAL KERATITIS?

Symptoms of bacterial keratitis include:

- Eye pain
- Eye redness
- Blurred vision
- Sensitivity to light
- Excessive tearing
- Eye discharge

If you experience any of these symptoms, remove your contact lenses (if you wear them) and call your eye doctor right away. If left untreated, bacterial keratitis can result in vision loss or blindness.

WHERE ARE THESE BACTERIA FOUND?

Bacteria are common in nature and found in the environment and on the human body. *Pseudomonas* bacteria can be found in soil and water. *Staphylococcus aureus* bacteria normally live on human skin and on the protective lining inside the body called the "mucous membrane." Bacterial keratitis cannot be spread from person to person.

WHAT PUTS PEOPLE AT RISK FOR BACTERIAL KERATITIS?

Risks for developing bacterial keratitis include:

- Wearing contact lenses, especially:
  - Overnight wear
  - Temporary reshaping of the cornea (to correct nearsightedness) by wearing a rigid contact lens overnight, otherwise known as "orthokeratology" (Ortho-K)
  - Not disinfecting contact lenses well
  - Not cleaning contact lens cases
  - Storing or rinsing contact lenses in water
  - Using visibly contaminated lens solution
  - "Topping off" lens solution rather than discarding used solution and replacing
  - Sharing noncorrective contact lenses used for cosmetic purposes
- Recent eye injury
- Eye disease
- Weakened immune system
- Problems with the eyelids or tearing

HOW IS BACTERIAL KERATITIS DIAGNOSED?

It is critical that when you first notice unusual eye irritation that you remove your contact lenses and not wear them again until instructed to do so by your eye doctor. Your eye doctor will examine your eye. She or he may take a tiny scraping of your cornea and send a sample to a laboratory to be analyzed.

Section 19.3 | **Fungal Keratitis**

This section includes text excerpted from "Basics of Fungal Keratitis," Centers for Disease Control and Prevention (CDC), October 10, 2014. Reviewed March 2020.

WHAT IS FUNGAL KERATITIS?

Fungal keratitis is an infection of the cornea (the clear dome covering the colored part of the eye) that is caused by a fungus. Some fungi that have been known to commonly cause fungal keratitis include:

- *Fusarium* species
- *Aspergillus* species
- *Candida* species

WHAT ARE SYMPTOMS OF FUNGAL KERATITIS?

Symptoms of fungal keratitis include:

- Eye pain
- Eye redness
- Blurred vision
- Sensitivity to light
- Excessive tearing
- Eye discharge

If you experience any of these symptoms, remove your contact lenses (if you wear them) and call your eye doctor right away. Fungal keratitis is a very rare condition, but if left untreated, it can become serious and result in vision loss or blindness.

WHERE ARE THESE FUNGI FOUND?

Fusarium and *Aspergillus* species live in the environment. *Candida* species normally live on human skin and on the protective lining inside the body called the "mucous membrane." Fungal keratitis is most common in tropical and subtropical regions of the world, but can also occur in areas of the world with milder temperatures. It cannot be spread from person to person.

WHAT PUTS PEOPLE AT RISK FOR FUNGAL KERATITIS?

The most common way that someone gets fungal keratitis is after experiencing trauma to the eye— especially trauma caused by a stick, thorn, or plant.

Risks for developing fungal keratitis include:

- Recent eye trauma, particularly involving plants (for example, thorns or sticks)
- Underlying eye disease
- Weakened immune system
- Contact lens use

In 2006, the Centers for Disease Control and Prevention (CDC) investigated an outbreak of *Fusarium* keratitis that was associated with a specific type of contact lens solution, which was withdrawn from the market.

HOW IS FUNGAL KERATITIS DIAGNOSED?

Your eye doctor will examine your eye and may possibly take a tiny scraping of your cornea. The sample will be sent to a laboratory to be analyzed.

HOW IS FUNGAL KERATITIS TREATED?

Fungal keratitis must be treated with prescription antifungal medicine for several months. Patients who do not get better after skin treatment and oral antifungal medications may require surgery, including corneal transplantation.

Section 19.4 | **Parasitic/Amebic Keratitis**

This section includes text excerpted from "Basics of Parasitic/Amebic Keratitis," Centers for Disease Control and Prevention (CDC), November 17, 2014. Reviewed March 2020.

WHAT IS *ACANTHAMOEBA* KERATITIS?

Acanthamoeba keratitis, or AK, is a rare but serious infection of the eye that can cause permanent vision loss or blindness. This infection is caused by a tiny ameba (single-celled living organism) called "*Acanthamoeba*." *Acanthamoeba* causes *Acanthamoeba* keratitis when it infects the cornea, the clear dome that covers the colored part of the eye.

WHAT ARE THE SYMPTOMS OF *ACANTHAMOEBA* KERATITIS?

Symptoms of AK include:

- Sensation of something in the eye
- Eye pain
- Eye redness
- Blurred vision
- Sensitivity to light
- Excessive tearing

If you experience any of these symptoms, remove your contact lenses (if you wear them) and call your eye doctor right away. AK is a rare condition, but if left untreated it can result in vision loss or blindness.

WHERE IS *ACANTHAMOEBA* FOUND?

Acanthamoeba is very common in nature and can be found in bodies of water (for example, lakes and oceans) and soil. It can also be found in tap water, heating, ventilating, and air conditioning units, and whirlpools. Infection of the eye occurs when the *Acanthamoeba* organisms contained in water or contact lens solution enter the eye through small scrapes that can be caused by contact lens wear or other minor eye injuries. The *Acanthamoeba* organism has to make contact directly with the eyes in order to cause AK, so this type of corneal infection cannot occur from drinking or inhaling water that has this ameba in it. AK cannot be spread from person to person.

WHO PUTS PEOPLE AT RISK FOR *ACANTHAMOEBA* KERATITIS?

In the United States, an estimated 85 percent of AK cases occur in contact lens wearers. For people who wear contact lenses, the risk of getting *Acanthamoeba* keratitis is higher if they:

- Do not store or handle contact lenses properly. This can include not washing hands before touching contact lenses, not rubbing and rinsing lenses after taking them out, and not storing them in the recommended contact lens solution.
- Do not disinfect contact lenses properly. This can include using tap water to clean the lenses or lens case, or adding fresh solution to existing used solution in the case instead of using only fresh solution when storing contact lenses.
- Swim, use a hot tub, or shower while wearing lenses.
- Have a history of trauma to the cornea, such as a previous eye injury.

In 2007, the Centers for Disease Control and Prevention (CDC) investigated a nationwide outbreak of *Acanthamoeba* keratitis which led to the recall of a specific type of contact lens solution from the market. Another nationwide outbreak in 2011 pointed to inadequate hygiene among contact lens wearers, in addition to water exposure and "topping off"—adding fresh solution to old solution—in the contact case.

HOW IS *ACANTHAMOEBA* KERATITIS DIAGNOSED?

Early diagnosis is important because early treatment can prevent AK infections from becoming more severe. The infection is usually diagnosed by an eye doctor based on symptoms, lab results from a scraping of the eye, and/or through a close-up eye exam that allows the eye doctor to see the ameba.

HOW IS *ACANTHAMOEBA* KERATITIS TREATED?

Acanthamoeba Keratitis can be difficult to treat, and the best treatment regimen for each patient should be determined by an eye doctor. AK usually requires aggressive medical and surgical treatment. If you think that your eye may be infected with *Acanthamoeba*, see an eye doctor immediately.

Section 19.5 | **Viral Keratitis**

This section includes text excerpted from "Basics of HSV (Herpes Simplex Virus) Keratitis," Centers for Disease Control and Prevention (CDC), April 7, 2014. Reviewed March 2020.

WHAT IS HERPES SIMPLEX VIRUS KERATITIS?

Herpes simplex virus (HSV) keratitis is an infection of the cornea—the clear dome that covers the colored part of the eye—that is caused by HSV. The infection usually heals without damaging the eye, but more severe infections can lead to scarring of the cornea or blindness. HSV keratitis is a major cause of blindness worldwide. HSV-1, which is the type of HSV that also causes cold sores on the mouth, is the most common cause of corneal infections.

WHERE IS HERPES SIMPLEX VIRUS FOUND?

Herpes simplex virus is only found in humans and is spread through direct contact with someone who is infected with the virus. Most HSV keratitis infections happen after another part of the body—most commonly the mouth—has already been infected by HSV. HSV keratitis is often the result of a "flare up" (reactivation) of the earlier infection.

WHAT ARE THE SYMPTOMS OF HERPES SIMPLEX VIRUS KERATITIS?

Symptoms of HSV keratitis include:

- Eye pain
- Eye redness

- Blurred vision
- Sensitivity to light
- Watery discharge

If you experience any of these symptoms, remove your contact lenses (if you wear them) and call your eye doctor right away. If left untreated, HSV keratitis can result in vision loss or blindness.

WHAT PUTS PEOPLE AT RISK FOR HERPES SIMPLEX VIRUS KERATITIS?

People who have had HSV keratitis are at risk for recurrences of the same infection. For these people, wearing contact lenses may further increase the risk.

People most at risk for HSV-1 (but not necessarily HSV keratitis) are:

- Female
- Non-Hispanic black or Mexican American
- Born outside the United States
- Sexually active, or have had three or more lifetime sex partners

HOW IS HERPES SIMPLEX VIRUS KERATITIS DIAGNOSED?

Herpes simplex virus keratitis is usually diagnosed based on a patient's health history and findings from an eye exam. Lab testing is not usually necessary, but certain lab tests may further help to confirm HSV-1.

HOW IS HERPES SIMPLEX VIRUS KERATITIS TREATED?

The treatment of HSV keratitis usually involves medicine, including eye drops or antiviral medications taken by mouth. Surgery is rarely necessary but may be considered if scarring on the eye from HSV keratitis causes vision problems. Each case of HSV keratitis is unique, and an eye doctor should determine the best treatment for each patient. While some treatments can greatly lower the severity and recurrence of symptoms, there is no cure for HSV.

HOW DO YOU PREVENT HERPES SIMPLEX VIRUS KERATITIS?

Currently, there are no proven methods for preventing HSV keratitis, but some steps available from the Mayo Clinic may help to control HSV keratitis recurrences:

- Avoid touching your eyes or the area around your eyes unless you have washed your hands properly—especially if you have a cold sore or herpes blister.
- Only use eye drops that have been prescribed or recommended by an eye doctor or healthcare provider.

Section 19.6 | Tips to Protect Eyes While Wearing Contact Lenses

This section includes text excerpted from "Protect Your Eyes," Centers for Disease Control and Prevention (CDC), February 28, 2020.

When cared for properly, contact lenses can provide a safe and effective way to correct your vision. In fact, more than 45 million Americans wear contact lenses. However, wearing contact lenses can increase your chance of getting an eye infection—especially if you do not care for them the right way.

CONTACT LENS HEALTH STARTS WITH YOU

Your habits, supplies, and eye-care provider are all essential to keeping your eyes healthy. Both contact lens wearers and eye-care providers play an important role in proper eye care. By following your eye-care provider's instructions on how to properly wear, clean, and store your lenses, you can enjoy the comfort and benefits of contact lenses while lowering your chances of an eye infection.

FOLLOW THESE HEALTHY HABITS TO WEAR YOUR CONTACT LENS SAFELY AND HELP PROTECT YOUR EYES

Do Not Sleep in Your Contact Lenses

- Do not sleep in your contact lenses unless prescribed by your eye-care provider. Sleeping while wearing contact lenses has been shown to increase the chance of an eye infection by six to eight times.

- Replace your contact lenses as often as recommended by your eye care provider.

Wash Your Hands

- Always wash your hands with soap and water before handling your lenses.
- Dry your hands well with a clean cloth before touching your contact lenses every time.

Keep Contact Lenses Away from All Water

- Water can introduce germs to the eyes through contact lenses. Remove contact lenses before swimming and avoid showering in them.

Properly Clean Your Lenses

- Rub and rinse your contact lenses with contact lens disinfecting solution—never water or saliva—to clean them each time you remove them.
- Do not "top off" solution. Use only fresh contact lens disinfecting solution in your case—never mix fresh solution with old or used solution.
- Use only the contact lens solution recommended by your eye-care provider.

Take Care of Your Contact Lens Case

- Clean your contact lens case by rubbing and rinsing it with contact lens solution—never water—and then empty and dry with a clean tissue. Store upside down with the caps off after each use.
- Replace your contact lens case at least once every three months.

Talk with Your Eye-Care Provider

- Have a conversation with your eye-care provider during your next appointment to discuss your contact lens wear and care habits and to help prevent eye infections.
- Visit your eye-care provider yearly or as often as she or he recommends.
- Remove your contact lenses immediately and call your eye-care provider if you have eye pain, discomfort, redness, or blurred vision.

Be Prepared

- Carry a backup pair of glasses with a current prescription—just in case you have to take out your contact lenses.

TIPS FOR HARD, OR RIGID GAS PERMEABLE, CONTACT LENS WEARERS

The wear and care recommendations for soft contact lenses also apply to hard, or rigid gas permeable (RGP or GP), contact lenses. Follow these extra tips:

- To clean hard contact lenses, rub and rinse them with contact lens cleaning or multipurpose solution—never water or saliva—each time you remove them. Rinse them well with the solution recommended by your eye-care provider.
- Hard contact lenses can last much longer than soft contact lenses if cared for properly. Replace your hard contact lenses when recommended to do so by your eye-care provider.

Chapter 20 | Corneal Dystrophies

Corneal dystrophies are eye diseases that involve changes in the cornea (the clear front layer of your eye). These diseases usually run in families.

Most corneal dystrophies are progressive—they get worse over time. Some cause vision loss or pain, but some have no symptoms. The only way to know for sure if you have a corneal dystrophy is to get a comprehensive dilated eye exam. Your eye doctor will use a microscope with a bright light attached (called a "slit lamp") to check your eyes for signs of corneal dystrophies.

KERATOCONUS

Keratoconus is usually diagnosed in teens and young adults. It causes the middle and lower parts of the cornea to get thinner over time. While a normal cornea has a rounded shape, a cornea with keratoconus can bulge outward and become a cone shape. This different cornea shape can cause vision problems.

Symptoms of keratoconus include:

- Itchy eyes
- Double vision
- Blurry vision
- Nearsightedness (when far-away objects look blurry)
- Astigmatism (when things look blurry or distorted)
- Sensitivity to light

As keratoconus gets worse, it may cause eye pain and more serious vision problems.

This chapter includes text excerpted from "Corneal Dystrophies," National Eye Institute (NEI), June 26, 2019.

Most people with keratoconus can correct their vision problems by wearing glasses, soft contact lenses, or special hard contact lenses that change the shape of the cornea. Your doctor may also recommend a procedure called "corneal cross-linking" to strengthen your cornea. If your keratoconus causes severe corneal scarring or you have trouble wearing contact lenses, you may need a corneal transplant.

FUCHS' DYSTROPHY

Most people with Fuchs' dystrophy start to have symptoms around 50 to 60 years of age. This disease makes a type of cornea cells (called "endothelial cells") stop working. When these cells stop working, the cornea swells and gets thicker. These cornea changes can cause vision problems.

Symptoms of Fuchs' dystrophy include:

- Blurry vision that is worse in the morning and gets better later in the day
- Glare and halos in your vision that makes it hard to see things at night or in low light
- Cloudy corneas
- Sensitivity to light

As Fuchs' dystrophy gets worse, it may cause eye pain and more serious vision problems.

Treatments for Fuchs' dystrophy include eye drops, ointments, and special contact lenses to help reduce corneal swelling. If your disease is more severe, you may need a corneal transplant.

LATTICE DYSTROPHY AND MAP-DOT-FINGERPRINT DYSTROPHY

Lattice dystrophy usually begins in childhood. It causes material to build up on the cornea in a lattice (grid) pattern. As the material builds up, it can cause vision problems.

Map-dot-fingerprint dystrophy (also called "epithelial basement membrane dystrophy") is most common in adults 40 to 70 years of age. It causes a layer of the cornea to develop folds that can look like continents on a map, clusters of dots, or small fingerprints.

Sometimes these folds cause vision problems, which may come and go over time.

Lattice dystrophy and map-dot-fingerprint dystrophy can both cause corneal erosion, when the outer layer of the cornea is not attached to the eye correctly and starts to erode (wear away).

Symptoms of corneal erosion include:

- Eye pain that is worse in the morning and gets better later in the day
- Feeling like there is something in your eye
- Blurry vision
- Sensitivity to light
- Watery eyes

Treatments include eye drops, ointments, and special eye patches or contact lenses that stop your eyelid from rubbing against your cornea. If you have severe corneal erosions or corneal scarring, you may need a surgical treatment, like laser eye surgery or a corneal transplant.

Chapter 21 | Other Types of Corneal Disease

Several types of diseases can affect the cornea (the clear front layer of the eye). Your eye doctor can check for corneal diseases as part of a comprehensive dilated eye exam.

SHINGLES

If you have had chickenpox, you are at risk for shingles (also called "herpes zoster"). Shingles happen when the chickenpox virus gets reactivated in your nerve cells, usually many years after you had the chickenpox. When shingles affect the cornea, it can cause inflammation (swelling) and scarring.

Your eye doctor can prescribe antiviral medicine to help shingles go away faster and prevent damage to your cornea. If you get shingles on your face or in your nose or eyes, it is important to get a comprehensive eye exam to check for cornea problems.

OCULAR HERPES

When a herpes virus (the type of virus that causes cold sores and genital herpes) infects the eye, it can cause sores on the eyelid or the outer layer of the cornea. This is called "ocular (eye) herpes."

If an ocular herpes infection spreads deeper into the cornea or the other layers of the eye, it can become a serious eye infection called "keratitis." Keratitis can cause corneal scarring and vision loss.

This chapter includes text excerpted from "Other Types of Corneal Disease," National Eye Institute (NEI), June 26, 2019.

If you have ocular herpes, your eye doctor can prescribe an antiviral medicine to help control the virus and prevent damage to your cornea.

IRIDOCORNEAL ENDOTHELIAL SYNDROME

Iridocorneal endothelial syndrome (ICE) is most common in women 30 to 50 years of age. It happens when a type of corneal cells called "endothelial cells" move from the cornea into the iris (the colored part of the eye). When these cells move, they can block eye fluid from draining and raise eye pressure.

Iridocorneal endothelial syndrome has three main symptoms:

- Changes in the shape of the iris or pupil
- Swelling in the cornea
- Glaucoma

Your eye doctor can prescribe medicine to treat the corneal swelling and glaucoma. If the damage to the cornea is severe, you may need a corneal transplant.

PTERYGIUM

A pterygium is a pink-colored growth on the cornea shaped like a wing or triangle. It is most common in adults 20 to 40 years of age who spend a lot of time outdoors in the sun.

A pterygium may cause redness or irritate your eye. Eye drops can help with these symptoms. If a pterygium is large enough to cause vision problems, you may need surgery to remove it.

To protect your eyes and lower your risk of a pterygium, wear sunglasses or a wide-brimmed hat when you are in the sun.

STEVENS-JOHNSON SYNDROME

Stevens-Johnson syndrome (SJS), also called "erythema multiforme major," is a rare skin disorder that also affects the eyes. SJS can cause serious eye problems that may lead to vision loss, including:

- Severe pink eye (conjunctivitis)
- Iritis (inflammation inside the eye)
- Serious corneal damage

Stevens-Johnson syndrome can happen as an allergic reaction to a drug or medication, or as part of a viral infection. Anyone can get it, but it is more common in men and in children and young adults under 30 years of age.

If you have SJS, your eye doctor may prescribe medicines, such as antibiotics or a corticosteroid, as well as a type of eye drops called "artificial tears." With treatment, SJS usually goes away over time, but people who have had SJS before are more likely to get it again.

Chapter 22 | Corneal Transplant

If you have severe damage to your cornea (the clear front layer of your eye), doctors can replace the damaged part with healthy corneal tissue from a donor.

If you have scarring or other damage that affects the whole cornea, doctors can do a full-thickness corneal transplant (called a "penetrating keratoplasty"). If only part of your cornea is damaged, doctors can do a partial-thickness transplant (called a "lamellar keratoplasty").

WHAT HAPPENS DURING A CORNEAL TRANSPLANT

You may get general anesthesia to put you to sleep during the transplant surgery, or you may be awake. If you are awake, your doctor will put medicine in your eye to make it numb and give you another medicine to help you relax.

Your doctor will use a special tool to keep your eye open during surgery. They will remove the damaged part of your cornea and replace it with healthy donor tissue.

HOW LONG DOES IT TAKE TO RECOVER?

Corneal transplant is an outpatient surgery, so you can go home the same day. You will not be able to drive, so you will need someone to give you a ride home after surgery.

You will need a follow-up appointment the day after surgery to check how your eye is healing.

This chapter includes text excerpted from "Corneal Transplants," National Eye Institute (NEI), July 5, 2019.

After surgery, you will need to take steps to help your eye recover:

- Use special eye drops prescribed by your doctor.
- Avoid rubbing or pressing on your eye.
- Wear eyeglasses or a special shield to protect your eye.

Depending on the type of transplant, it can take up to a year to fully recover. Talk with your doctor about when you can get back to your normal activities.

When to Get Help Right Away

Cornea rejection can cause:

- Eye pain
- Sensitivity to light
- Red eyes
- Cloudy or hazy vision

If you have these symptoms after a corneal transplant, tell your eye doctor right away.

ARE THERE ANY SIDE EFFECTS?

Like any surgery, corneal transplant surgery has risks. One major risk is tissue rejection when your body sees the new cornea as a foreign object and tries to get rid of it. Your doctor can give you medicine to help stop the rejection and save your cornea.

A corneal transplant can also cause other eye problems, including:

- Infection
- Bleeding from the eye
- Retinal detachment
- Glaucoma

If you have tissue rejection or other severe problems with your new cornea, you may need another transplant. Talk with your doctor about the risks of a corneal transplant and whether this treatment is right for you.

Chapter 23 | Cataracts

Chapter Contents

Section 23.1 | **About Cataracts**

This section includes text excerpted from "Cataracts," National Eye Institute (NEI), August 3, 2019.

WHAT ARE CATARACTS?

A cataract is a cloudy area in the lens of your eye. Cataracts are very common as you get older. In fact, more than half of all Americans 80 years of age or older either have cataracts or have had surgery to get rid of cataracts.

At first, you may not notice that you have a cataract. But, over time, cataracts can make your vision blurry, hazy, or less colorful. You may have trouble reading or doing other everyday activities.

The good news is that surgery can get rid of cataracts. Cataract surgery is safe and corrects vision problems caused by cataracts.

TYPES OF CATARACTS

Most cataracts are age-related—they happen because of normal changes in your eyes as you get older. But, you can get cataracts for other reasons—for example, after an eye injury or after surgery for another eye problem (such as glaucoma).

No matter what type of cataracts you have, the treatment is always surgery.

SYMPTOMS OF CATARACTS

You might not have any symptoms at first when cataracts are mild. But, as cataracts grow, they can cause changes in your vision. For example, you may notice that:

- Your vision is cloudy or blurry
- Colors look faded
- You cannot see well at night
- Lamps, sunlight, or headlights seem too bright
- You see a halo around lights
- You see double (this sometimes goes away as the cataract gets bigger)
- You have to change the prescription for your glasses often

These symptoms can be a sign of other eye problems, too. Be sure to talk to your eye doctor if you have any of these problems.

Over time, cataracts can lead to vision loss.

ARE YOU AT RISK FOR CATARACTS?

Your risk for cataracts goes up as you get older. You are also at higher risk if you:

- Have certain health problems, such as diabetes
- Smoke
- Drink too much alcohol
- Have a family history of cataracts
- Have had an eye injury, eye surgery, or radiation treatment on your upper body
- Have spent a lot of time in the sun
- Take steroids (medicines used to treat a variety of health problems, such as arthritis and rashes)

If you are worried you might be at risk for cataracts, talk with your doctor. Ask if there is anything you can do to lower your risk.

WHAT CAUSES CATARACTS

Most cataracts are caused by degenerative changes in your eyes as you get older.

When you are young, the lens in your eye is clear. Around the age of 40, the proteins in the lens of your eye start to break down and clump together. This clump makes a cloudy area on your lens—or a cataract. Over time, the cataract gets more severe and clouds more of the lens.

HOW YOU CAN PREVENT CATARACTS

You can take steps to protect your eyes and delay cataracts.

- **Protect your eyes from the sun.** Wear sunglasses and a hat with a brim to block the sun.
- **Quit smoking.** If you are ready to quit, call 800-QUIT-NOW (800-784-8669) for free support.

- **Eat healthy.** Eat plenty of fruits and vegetables—especially dark, leafy greens such as spinach, kale, and collard greens.
- **Get a dilated eye exam.** If you are 60 years of age or above, get a dilated eye exam at least once every 2 years.

HOW DOES THE EYE DOCTOR CHECK FOR CATARACTS?

An eye doctor can check for cataracts as part of a dilated eye exam. The exam is simple and painless—your doctor will give you some eye drops to dilate (widen) your pupil and then check your eyes for cataracts and other eye problems.

TREATMENT FOR CATARACTS

Surgery is the only way to get rid of a cataract, but you may not need to get surgery right away.

- **Home treatment.** Early on, you may be able to make small changes to manage your cataracts. You can do things such as:
    - Use brighter lights at home or work
    - Wear antiglare sunglasses
    - Use magnifying lenses for reading and other activities
- **New glasses or contacts.** A prescription for eyeglasses or contact lenses can help you see better with cataracts early on.
- **Surgery.** Your doctor might suggest surgery if your cataracts start getting in the way of everyday activities such as reading, driving, or watching TV. During cataract surgery, the doctor removes the clouded lens and replaces it with a new, artificial lens (also called an "intraocular lens," or "IOL"). This surgery is very safe, and 9 out of 10 people who get it can see better afterward.

Talk about your options with your doctor. Most people do not need to rush into surgery. Waiting to have surgery usually would not harm your eyes or make surgery more difficult later. Remember these tips:

- Tell your doctor if cataracts are getting in the way of your everyday activities.
- See your doctor for regular check-ups.
- Ask your doctor about the benefits and risks of cataract surgery.
- Encourage family members to get checked for cataracts, since they can run in families.

Section 23.2 | **UV Rays May Contribute to Cataract**

This section includes text excerpted from "New Research Sheds Light on How UV Rays May Contribute to Cataract," National Eye Institute (NEI), June 3, 2014. Reviewed March 2020.

A study offers an explanation for how years of chronic sunlight exposure can increase the risk of cataract, a clouding of the eye lens that typically occurs with aging. The study firms up a link between the sun's damaging rays and a process called "oxidative stress." It was funded in part by the National Eye Institute (NEI).

It is well-known that exposure to ultraviolet (UV) light from the sun can cause skin damage. But, many studies show that UV light can also increase the risk of cataract and other eye conditions.

"Oxidative stress" refers to harmful chemical reactions that can occur when our cells consume oxygen and other fuels to produce energy. It is an unfortunate consequence of living, but it is also considered a major contributor to normal aging and age-related diseases-including cataract formation in the lens. The cells within the lens contain mostly water and proteins and lack the organelles (literally "tiny organs") typically found in other cells. This unusual makeup of lens cells renders the lens transparent, uniquely capable of transmitting light and focusing it on the retina at the back of the eye. When a cataract forms, the proteins inside lens cells show signs of oxidative damage, and they ultimately become clumped together, scattering light rather than transmitting it. So, the theory goes, oxidative stress (or something similar to it) is responsible for destroying the neatly ordered proteins inside the lens and producing a cataract.

The theory might sound simple, but there is a puzzling fact that does not fit. The oldest cells in the lens are not only devoid of the organelles that keep most other cells alive and functioning, but they also get little to no oxygen. So, how can they suffer from oxidative stress?

The study, led by researchers at Case Western Reserve University in Cleveland, Ohio, suggests that UV light may provide an answer. The study shows that UV light can damage lens proteins in a distinct way (called "glycation") that is typically seen in cataract and in cells damaged by oxidative stress. In other words, UV light can substitute for oxygen to trigger harmful oxidative reactions in the lens.

Prior studies have supported this theory. But, the Case Western team has unveiled a detailed play-by-play of the chemical changes induced in the lens by UV light.

Many clinical studies, including an NEI-funded study of fishermen in the Chesapeake Bay, have pointed to UV light exposure as a risk factor for age-related cataract. UV light rays are invisible and have shorter wavelengths than visible light. In the earth's atmosphere, UV light comes in two varieties: long wave ultraviolet A (UVA) and short wave ultraviolet B (UVB). Their relative contributions to cataract remain unclear, but UVA penetrates more deeply into the body and may be more likely to reach the lens. The NEI's National Eye Health Education Partnership (NEHEP) recommends wearing sunglasses with both UVA and UVB protection to shield your eyes from the sun. A hat can help, too.

"UV light has long been suspected to have a role in cataract formation, but the mechanism has not been clear," said Ram Nagaraj, Ph.D., the study's senior author and a professor of ophthalmology and visual sciences at Case Western.

Dr. Nagaraj and his colleagues tested the effects of UVA light on proteins and chemicals found in lens cells. They found that in the absence of oxygen, UVA light can trigger a chain reaction that begins with amino acid derivatives called "kynurenines," and ends with protein glycation in the lens. In earlier work, they also showed that mice genetically engineered to overproduce kynurenines developed a cataract by three months of age. In the current study, when lenses from these mice were exposed to two hours of intense UVA light, they accumulated damaged (glycated) proteins.

"Our study shows how UV light could promote cataract development, and reiterates the importance of wearing sunglasses to protect your eyes from the sun's harmful rays," Dr. Nagaraj said.

Unfortunately, the researchers found that a natural antioxidant in the eye and other tissues, called "glutathione," offered little protection against the damaging effects of UV light. Several clinical studies with mixed results have tested the potential for antioxidant supplements to prevent or slow age-related cataract.

"Overall, there is a need to better understand the extent to which natural antioxidants or other mechanisms within the lens might offer some protection against the sun," said Houmam Araj, Ph.D., who oversees programs on the lens, cataract and oculomotor systems at NEI. One such mechanism includes proteins called "chaperones," which can help prevent damaged proteins from clumping together.

"When do these mechanisms work in the lens and when do they fail? Answering those questions might lead to drug treatments for preventing cataracts, and perhaps even skin cancer," Dr. Araj said. "The eye and lens provide a useful, accessible system to study general countermeasures the body might have for defending itself against UV radiation."

Section 23.3 | **Cataract Surgery**

This section includes text excerpted from "Cataract Surgery," National Eye Institute (NEI), May 29, 2019.

A cataract is a cloudy area in the lens of your eye that can make it hard to see clearly. Surgery is the only way to get rid of cataracts.

WHO NEEDS CATARACT SURGERY

Your doctor will probably suggest cataract surgery if you have vision loss that gets in the way of everyday activities such as reading, driving, or watching TV.

Sometimes, your doctor might recommend cataract surgery even if your cataracts are not the main cause of your vision problems. For example, cataracts might need to be removed so that your doctor can see the back of your eye. If you have another eye condition, such as diabetic retinopathy or age-related macular degeneration (AMD), your doctor will need to see the back of your eye to help you manage it.

Cataracts are not a medical emergency, and you do not need to rush to have surgery to remove them. Ask your doctor about the risks and benefits of cataract surgery to decide if it is right for you.

HOW YOU CAN PREPARE FOR CATARACT SURGERY

At your doctor's office before the day of the surgery, your doctor will do some tests to measure the size and shape of your eye. You may need to use some special eye drops before the surgery, and your doctor may tell you not to eat anything the night before your surgery.

You would not be able to drive yourself home after the surgery, and you will need a friend or family member to make sure you get home safely—so be sure to bring someone with you.

If you have cataracts in both eyes, you will need to have surgery on each eye at a separate time, usually about four weeks apart.

WHAT HAPPENS DURING CATARACT SURGERY

During surgery, the doctor will remove the cloudy lens from your eye and replace it with an artificial lens (called an "intraocular lens"). The surgery lasts about an hour and is almost painless.

Usually, you will be awake during cataract surgery. You might notice lights or motion, but you would not be able to see what your doctor is doing.

When you get this surgery, your doctor will:

- Put numbing drops into your eye to keep you from feeling anything
- Use tiny tools to cut into your eye, break up the lens, and take it out
- Place the new artificial lens in your eye

Right after surgery, you will need to rest in a recovery area outside the operating room for a little while. Before you go home, the medical team will check to make sure you do not have any problems with your eye.

WHAT HAPPENS AFTER CATARACT SURGERY

Your doctor will explain how to protect your eye after cataract surgery. They will give you eye drops to help your eye heal and you may need to wear a special eye shield or glasses. You may need to avoid some activities for a few weeks, such as touching your eye, bending over, or lifting heavy things.

Your eye may feel a bit itchy or uncomfortable and sensitive to light and touch. After one or two days, your eye should feel better.

Call your doctor right away if you notice any of these problems after surgery:

- Vision loss
- Bad pain that would not go away even if you take medicine for it
- Eye redness
- Flashes of light or a lot of floaters (specks) in your vision

Most people get completely healed eight weeks after their surgery. Your doctor will schedule checkups to make sure your eye is healing correctly.

WILL YOUR VISION BE NORMAL AFTER CATARACT SURGERY?

About 9 out of 10 people who get cataract surgery see better afterward, but your vision might be blurry at first while your eye recovers.

Some people notice that colors seem brighter after cataract surgery. This is because the artificial lens is clear, while your natural lens had a yellow or brown tint from the cataract.

Once your eye is completely healed, you might need a new prescription for glasses or contact lenses to see clearly.

WHAT ARE THE RISKS OF CATARACT SURGERY?

Cataract surgery is one of the most common, safe, and effective types of surgery done in the United States. But, as in the case with any surgery, there are risks, including:

- Swelling, bleeding, or infections
- Vision loss or double vision
- Unusual changes in eye pressure
- Retinal detachment
- Secondary cataract (posterior capsule opacity)

Your doctor can treat these problems if they are detected early. Be sure to go to all of your checkups, and call your doctor if you notice anything wrong with your eyes or your vision.

WHAT IS SECONDARY CATARACT?

After cataract surgery, some people may develop a condition called "secondary cataract," or posterior capsule opacification. Secondary cataracts are not actually cataracts, because they are caused by cloudiness on the outside of your lens, not the inside—but they make your vision cloudy. Secondary cataracts can appear weeks, months, or even years after cataract surgery—but they are easy to fix with a laser treatment in the doctor's office.

Section 23.4 | New Early Detection Technique for Cataract

This section includes text excerpted from "From Outer Space to the Eye Clinic: New Cataract Early Detection Technique," National Institutes of Health (NIH), January 8, 2009.

A compact fiber-optic probe developed for the space program has now proven valuable for patients in the clinic as the first noninvasive early detection device for cataracts, the leading cause of vision loss worldwide.

Researchers from the National Eye Institute (NEI), part of the National Institutes of Health (NIH), and the National Aeronautics and Space Administration (NASA) collaborated to develop a simple, safe eye test for measuring a protein related to cataract formation. If subtle protein changes can be detected before a cataract develops, people may be able to reduce their cataract risk by making simple lifestyle changes, such as decreasing sun exposure, quitting smoking, stopping certain medications and controlling diabetes.

"By the time the eye's lens appears cloudy from a cataract, it is too late to reverse or medically treat this process," said Manuel B. Datiles III, M.D., NEI medical officer and lead author of the clinical study. "This technology can detect the earliest damage to lens proteins, triggering an early warning for cataract formation and blindness."

The new device is based on a laser light technique called "dynamic light scattering" (DLS). It was initially developed to analyze the growth of protein crystals in a zero-gravity space environment. NASA's Rafat R. Ansari, Ph.D., senior scientist at the John H. Glenn Research Center and coauthor of the study, brought the technology's possible clinical applications to the attention of NEI vision researchers when he learned that his father's cataracts were caused by changes in lens proteins.

Several proteins are involved in cataract formation, but one known as "alpha-crystallin" serves as the eye's own anticataract molecule. Alpha-crystallin binds to other proteins when they become damaged, thus preventing them from bunching together to form a cataract. However, humans are born with a fixed amount of alpha-crystallin, so if the supply becomes depleted due to radiation exposure, smoking, diabetes or other causes, a cataract can result.

"We have shown that this noninvasive technology that was developed for the space program can now be used to look at the early signs of protein damage due to oxidative stress, a key process involved in many medical conditions, including age-related cataract and diabetes, as well as neurodegenerative diseases such as Alzheimer and Parkinson," said NASA's Dr. Ansari. "By understanding the role of protein changes in cataract formation, we can use the lens not just to look at eye disease, but also as a window into the whole body."

The NEI-NASA clinical trial, reported in the December 2008 *Archives of Ophthalmology*, looked at 380 eyes of people 7 to 86 years of age who had lenses ranging from clear to severe cloudiness from cataract. Researchers used the DLS device to shine low-power laser light through the lenses. They had previously determined alpha-crystallin's light-scattering ability, which was then used to detect and measure the amount of alpha-crystallin in the lenses.

They found that as cloudiness increased, alpha-crystallin in the lenses decreased. Alpha-crystallin amounts also decreased as the participants' ages increased, even when the lenses were still transparent. These age-related, precataract changes would remain undetected by currently available imaging tools.

"This research is a prime example of two government agencies sharing scientific information for the benefit of the American people," said NEI director Paul A. Sieving, M.D., Ph.D. "At an individual level, this device could be used to study the effectiveness of anticataract therapies or the tendency of certain medications to cause cataract formation."

The DLS technique will now assist vision scientists in looking at long-term lens changes due to aging, smoking, diabetes, laser-assisted in situ keratomileusis (LASIK) surgery, eye drops for treating glaucoma, and surgical removal of the vitreous gel within the eye, a procedure known to cause cataracts within six months to one year. It may also help in the early diagnosis of Alzheimer disease (AD), in which an abnormal protein may be found in the lens. In addition, the NASA researchers will continue to use the device to look at the impact of long-term space travel on the visual system.

"During a three-year mission to Mars, astronauts will experience increased exposure to space radiation that can cause cataracts and other problems," Dr. Ansari explained. "In the absence of proper countermeasures, this may pose a risk for NASA. This technology could help us understand the mechanism for cataract formation so we can work to develop effective countermeasures to mitigate the risk and prevent it in astronauts."

The NASA John H. Glenn Research Center is one of NASA's 10 field centers, empowered with the resources for developing cutting-edge technologies and advancing scientific research that addresses NASA's mission to pioneer the future in space exploration, scientific discovery and aeronautics research. Working in partnership with government, industry, and academia, the Center serves to maintain the U.S. economy's global leadership while benefiting the lives of people around the world.

Section 23.5 | **Implanted Lens to Improve Vision after Cataract Surgery**

This section includes text excerpted from "FDA Approves First Implanted Lens That Can Be Adjusted after Cataract Surgery to Improve Vision without Eyeglasses in Some Patients," U.S. Food and Drug Administration (FDA), November 22, 2017.

The U.S. Food and Drug Administration (FDA) approved RxSight Inc., Light Adjustable Lens (LAL) and Light Delivery Device (LDD), the first medical device system that can make small adjustments to the artificial lens' power after cataract surgery so that the patient will have better vision when not using glasses.

Cataracts are a common eye condition where the natural lens becomes clouded, impairing a patient's vision. Following cataract surgery, during which the natural lens of the eye that has become cloudy is removed and replaced with an artificial lens (intraocular lens, or IOL), many patients have some minor residual refractive error requiring the use of glasses or contact lenses. Refractive error, which is caused when the artificial lens does not focus properly, causes blurred vision.

"Until now, refractive errors that are common following cataract surgery could only be corrected with glasses, contact lenses or refractive surgery," said Malvina Eydelman, M.D., director of the Division of Ophthalmic, and Ear, Nose and Throat at the FDA's Center for Devices and Radiological Health. "This system provides a new option for certain patients that allows the physician to make small adjustments to the implanted lens during several in-office procedures after the initial surgery to improve visual acuity without glasses."

The RxSight IOL is made of a unique material that reacts to UV light, which is delivered by the Light Delivery Device, 17 to 21 days after surgery. Patients receive three or four light treatments over a period of 1 to 2 weeks, each lasting about 40 to 150 seconds, depending upon the amount of adjustment needed. The patient must wear special eyeglasses for UV protection from the time of the cataract surgery to the end of the light treatments to protect the new lens from UV light in the environment.

A clinical study of 600 patients was conducted to evaluate the safety and effectiveness of the RxSight Light Adjustable Lens and Light Delivery Device. Six months after the procedure, patients on average saw an improvement of about one additional line down the vision chart, for distance vision without glasses, compared to a conventional IOL. Six months after surgery, 75 percent of the patients also had a reduction in astigmatism.

The device is intended for patients who have astigmatism (in the cornea) before surgery and who do not have macular diseases.

The device should not be used in patients taking systemic medication that may increase sensitivity to UV light, such as tetracycline, doxycycline, psoralens, amiodarone, phenothiazines, chloroquine, hydrochlorothiazide, hypericin, ketoprofen, piroxicam, lomefloxacin, and methoxsalen. Treatment in patients taking such medications may lead to irreversible eye damage. The device is also contraindicated in cases where patients have a history of ocular herpes simplex virus.

The FDA approved the Vision Light Adjustable Lens and the Light Delivery Device to RxSight Inc.

Chapter 24 | Disorders of the Conjunctiva, Sclera, and Pupil

Chapter Contents

Section 24.1 | **Conjunctivitis (Pink Eye)**

This section contains text excerpted from the following sources: Text in this section begins with excerpts from "Pinkeye," MedlinePlus, National Institutes of Health (NIH), October 30, 2017; Text beginning with the heading "Causes of Conjunctivitis" is excerpted from "Conjunctivitis (Pink Eye)," Centers for Disease Control and Prevention (CDC), January 4, 2019.

Conjunctivitis is the medical name for pink eye. It involves inflammation of the outer layer of the eye and inside of the eyelid. It can cause swelling, itching, burning, discharge, and redness. Causes include:

- Bacterial or viral infection
- Allergies
- Substances that cause irritation
- Contact lens products, eye drops, or eye ointments

Pink eye usually does not affect vision. Infectious pink eye can easily spread from one person to another. The infection will clear in most cases without medical care, but bacterial pink eye needs treatment with antibiotic eye drops or ointment.

CAUSES OF CONJUNCTIVITIS

The most common causes of conjunctivitis (pink eye) are:

- Viruses
- Bacteria
- Allergens

Other causes include:

- Chemicals
- Contact lens wear
- Foreign bodies in the eye (such as a loose eyelash)
- Indoor and outdoor air pollution caused, for example, by smoke, dust, fumes, or chemical vapors
- Fungi
- Ameba and parasites

It can be difficult to determine the exact cause of conjunctivitis because some symptoms may be the same no matter the cause.

Viral Conjunctivitis

- Infection of the eye caused by a virus
- Can be caused by a number of different viruses, such as adenoviruses
- Very contagious
- Sometimes can result in large outbreaks depending on the virus

Bacterial Conjunctivitis

- Infection of the eye caused by certain bacteria
- Can be caused by Staphylococcus aureus, *Streptococcus pneumoniae*, *Haemophilus influenzae*, *Moraxella catarrhalis*, or, less commonly, *Chlamydia trachomatis* and *Neisseria gonorrhoeae*
- Can be spread easily, especially with certain bacteria and in certain settings
- Children with conjunctivitis without fever or behavioral changes can usually continue going to school
- More common in kids than adults
- Observed more frequently December through April

Allergic Conjunctivitis

- The result of the body's reaction to allergens, such as pollen from trees, plants, grasses, and weeds; dust mites; molds; dander from pets; medicines; or cosmetics
- Not contagious
- Occurs more frequently among people with other allergic conditions, such as hay fever, asthma, and eczema
- Can occur seasonally, when allergens such as pollen counts, are high
- Can also occur year-round due to indoor allergens, such as dust mites and animal dander

Conjunctivitis Caused by Irritants

- Caused by irritation from a foreign body in the eye or contact with smoke, dust, fumes, or chemicals
- Not contagious
- Can occur when contact lenses are worn longer than recommended or not cleaned properly

SYMPTOMS OF CONJUNCTIVITIS

- Pink or red color in the white of the eye(s)
- Swelling of the conjunctiva (the thin layer that lines the white part of the eye and the inside of the eyelid) and/or eyelids
- Increased tear production
- Feeling like a foreign body is in the eye(s) or an urge to rub the eye(s)
- Itching, irritation, and/or burning
- Discharge (pus or mucus)
- Crusting of eyelids or lashes, especially in the morning
- Contact lenses that feel uncomfortable and/or do not stay in place on the eye

Depending on the cause, other symptoms may occur.

Viral Conjunctivitis

- Can occur with symptoms of a cold, flu, or other respiratory infection
- Usually begins in one eye and may spread to the other eye within days
- Discharge from the eye is usually watery rather than thick

Bacterial Conjunctivitis

- More commonly associated with discharge (pus), which can lead to eyelids sticking together
- Sometimes occurs with an ear infection

Allergic Conjunctivitis

- Usually occurs in both eyes

- Can produce intense itching, tearing, and swelling in the eyes
- May occur with symptoms of allergies, such as an itchy nose, sneezing, a scratchy throat, or asthma

Conjunctivitis caused by irritants can produce watery eyes and mucus discharge.

TRANSMISSION OF CONJUNCTIVITIS

How It Spreads

Several viruses and bacteria can cause conjunctivitis (pink eye), some of which are very contagious. Each of these types of germs can spread from person to person in different ways. They usually spread from an infected person to others through:

- Close personal contact, such as touching or shaking hands
- The air by coughing and sneezing
- Touching an object or surface with germs on it, then touching your eyes before washing your hands

When to Go Back to Work or School

If you have conjunctivitis but do not have fever or other symptoms, you may be allowed to remain at work or school with your doctor's approval. However, if you still have symptoms, and your activities at work or school include close contact with other people, you should not attend.

DIAGNOSIS OF CONJUNCTIVITIS

A doctor can often determine whether a virus, bacterium, or allergen is causing the conjunctivitis (pink eye) based on patient history, symptoms, and an examination of the eye. Conjunctivitis always involves eye redness or swelling, but it also has other symptoms that can vary depending on the cause. These symptoms can help a healthcare professional diagnose the cause of conjunctivitis. However, it can sometimes be difficult to make a firm diagnosis because some symptoms are the same no matter the cause.

It can also sometimes be difficult to determine the cause without doing laboratory testing. Although not routinely done, your healthcare provider may collect a sample of eye discharge from the infected eye and send it to the laboratory to help them determine which form of infection you have and how best to treat it.

Viral Conjunctivitis

The cause is likely a virus if:

- Conjunctivitis accompanies a common cold or respiratory tract infection, and
- Discharge from the eye is watery rather than thick

Bacterial Conjunctivitis

The cause may be bacterial if:

- Conjunctivitis occurs at the same time as an ear infection
- Occurs shortly after birth
- Discharge from the eye is thick rather than watery

Allergic Conjunctivitis

The cause is likely allergic if:

- Conjunctivitis occurs seasonally when pollen counts are high
- The patient's eyes itch intensely
- It occurs with other signs of allergic disease such as hay fever, asthma, or eczema

TREATMENT OF CONJUNCTIVITIS

There are times when it is important to seek medical care for conjunctivitis (pink eye). However, this is not always necessary. To help relieve some of the inflammation and dryness caused by conjunctivitis, you can use cold compresses and artificial tears, which you can purchase over the counter without a prescription. You should also stop wearing contact lenses until your eye doctor says it is okay to start wearing them again. If you did not need to see a doctor, do not wear your contacts until you no longer have symptoms of pink eye.

When to Seek Medical Care

You should see a healthcare provider if you have conjunctivitis along with any of the following:

- Pain in the eye(s)
- Sensitivity to light or blurred vision that does not improve when discharge is wiped from the eye(s)
- Intense redness in the eye(s)
- Symptoms that get worse or do not improve, including pink eye thought to be caused by bacteria which does not improve after 24 hours of antibiotic use
- A weakened immune system, for example from HIV infection, cancer treatment, or other medical conditions or treatments

Newborns with symptoms of conjunctivitis should see a doctor right away.

Viral Conjunctivitis

Most cases of viral conjunctivitis are mild. The infection will usually clear up in 7 to 14 days without treatment and without any long-term consequences. However, in some cases, viral conjunctivitis can take 2 to 3 weeks or more to clear up.

A doctor can prescribe antiviral medication to treat more serious forms of conjunctivitis. For example, conjunctivitis caused by herpes simplex virus or varicella-zoster virus. Antibiotics will not improve viral conjunctivitis; these drugs are not effective against viruses.

Bacterial Conjunctivitis

Your doctor may prescribe an antibiotic, usually given topically as eye drops or ointment, for bacterial conjunctivitis. Antibiotics may help shorten the length of infection, reduce complications, and reduce the spread to others.

Antibiotics may be necessary in the following cases:

- With discharge (pus)
- When conjunctivitis occurs in people whose immune system is compromised
- When certain bacteria are suspected

Mild bacterial conjunctivitis may get better without antibiotic treatment and without causing any complications. It often improves in two to five days without treatment but can take two weeks to go away completely.

Talk with your doctor about the best treatment options for your infection.

Allergic Conjunctivitis

Conjunctivitis caused by an allergen (such as pollen or animal dander) usually improves by removing the allergen from the person's environment. Allergy medications and certain eye drops (topical antihistamine and vasoconstrictors), including some prescription eye drops, can also provide relief from allergic conjunctivitis. In some cases, your doctor may recommend a combination of drugs to improve symptoms. Your doctor can help if you have conjunctivitis caused by an allergy.

Section 24.2 | **Dry Eye**

This section includes text excerpted from "Dry Eye," National Eye Institute (NEI), July 5, 2019.

WHAT IS DRY EYE?

Dry eye happens when your eyes do not make enough tears to stay wet, or when your tears do not work correctly. This can make your eyes feel uncomfortable, and in some cases it can also cause vision problems.

Dry eye is common—it affects millions of Americans every year. The good news is that if you have dry eye, there are lots of things you can do to keep your eyes healthy and stay comfortable.

WHAT ARE THE SYMPTOMS OF DRY EYE?

Dry eye can cause:

- A scratchy feeling, such as there is something in your eye

- Stinging or burning feelings in your eye
- Red eyes
- Sensitivity to light
- Blurry vision

ARE YOU AT RISK FOR DRY EYE?

Anyone can get dry eye, but you might be more likely to have a dry eye if you:

- Are 50 years of age or older
- Are female
- Wear contact lenses
- Do not get enough vitamin A (found in foods, such as carrots, broccoli, and liver) or omega-3 fatty acids (found in fish, walnuts, and vegetable oils)
- Have certain autoimmune conditions, such as lupus or Sjögren syndrome

WHAT CAUSES DRY EYE

Normally, glands above your eyes make tears that keep your eyes wet. Dry eye happens when your tears do not do their job. This could mean:

- Your glands do not make enough tears to keep your eyes wet
- Your tears dry up too fast
- Your tears just do not work well to keep your eyes wet

HOW WILL MY EYE DOCTOR CHECK FOR DRY EYE?

Your doctor can check for dry eye as part of a comprehensive dilated eye exam.

Be sure to tell your doctor if you think you might have a dry eye. To find out if you have dry eye, your doctor might check:

- The amount of tears your eyes make
- How long it takes for your tears to dry up
- The structure of your eyelids

Did You Know?

- Dry eye is common—nearly five million Americans have dry eye
- Dry eye can happen if you spend a lot of time looking at your computer, tablet, or smartphone
- If severe dry eye is not treated, it can sometimes damage your cornea, the clear outer layer of your eye

WHAT IS THE TREATMENT FOR DRY EYE?

Treatment for dry eye usually depends on what is causing your symptoms. There are a few different types of treatment that can ease your symptoms and help keep your eyes healthy.

- **Over-the-counter (OTC) eye drops.** The most common treatment for mild dry eye is a type of eye drops called "artificial tears." You can get these eye drops without a prescription. There are also over-the-counter (OTC) moisturizing gels and ointments that may help your eyes feel better.
- **Prescription medicines.** If your dry eye is more serious, your eye doctor may give you a prescription for medicines called "cyclosporine" (Restasis) or "lifitegrast" (Xiidra). These medicines are both types of eye drops that can help your eyes make more tears.
- **Lifestyle changes.** If something in your life or your environment is causing your dry eye, or making it worse, your doctor may suggest changes to help protect your eyes. For example, if a medicine you take for another health condition is causing dry eye, your doctor may also suggest that you try a different medicine. Your eyes may also feel better if you:
  - Try to avoid smoke, wind, and air conditioning
  - Use a humidifier to keep the air in your home from getting too dry
  - Limit screen time and take breaks from staring at screens
  - Wear wraparound sunglasses when you are outside

    - Drink plenty of water—try for 8 to 10 glasses every day
    - Get enough sleep—about 7 to 8 hours a night
- **Tear duct plugs.** If tears are draining too quickly from your eyes, your doctor may suggest putting special plugs (called "punctal plugs") in your tear ducts (small holes in the inner corners of your eyes). These plugs can help keep your tears in your eyes.
- **Surgery**. In some cases, dry eye can happen because your lower eyelids are too loose, causing tears to drain too quickly out of your eye. If this is the cause of your dry eye, your eye doctor may suggest surgery to fix your eyelids and help your tears stay on your eyes. This treatment is not very common.

Talk over your options with your doctor. If another health condition is causing your dry eye, treating that condition may improve your dry eye symptoms. Even if you have dry eye, there are lots of things you can do to help keep your eyes healthy. Remember these tips:

- Follow your doctor's instructions for using your eye drops (OTC or prescription).
- Tell your doctor if dry eye is getting in the way of everyday activities.

Section 24.3 | **Episcleritis**

Episcleritis is an inflammation of the episclera, a clear layer of tissue that covers the white of the eye (the sclera). Another clear layer outside the episclera is the conjunctiva. Episcleritis inflammation causes the eye to look red and irritated. Episcleritis often looks similar to pink eye, however, it does not cause discharge. Normally, episcleritis resolves without requiring medical attention.

TYPES OF EPISCLERITIS

There are two types of episcleritis:

Simple Episcleritis

Simple episcleritis is the most common type of episcleritis. It causes recurring inflammation that can last for around 7 to 10 days. Longer episodes may occur when the disease is associated with another systemic medical condition in addition to episcleritis. Simple episcleritis has two subtypes:

- **Sectoral**. The redness appears over a part of the episclera.
- **Diffuse**. The redness appears over all of the episclera.

Nodular Episcleritis

Nodular episcleritis is when a tiny nodule (bump) forms in the episcleral tissues of the eye. It is a more painful form of inflammation that causes people discomfort.

CAUSES AND RISK FACTORS OF EPISCLERITIS

Experts have yet to discover a specific reason why episcleritis occurs. However, they have found that about one-third of those affected by this condition have other systemic medical conditions such as rheumatoid arthritis, inflammatory bowel disease, lupus, Crohn disease, gout, rosacea, and collagen vascular diseases, as well.

Other causes include medications such as topiramate and pamidronate, or an injury.

Some people are more likely to be affected by episcleritis than others.

- **Gender**—Researchers have found that women are slightly more prone to be affected by episcleritis than men.
- **Age**— Episcleritis can affect children. However, it is more common in adults, especially those between the ages of 40 and 50.

- **Infection**—Sometimes, certain types of bacteria, fungi, or viruses can cause an infection, which may lead to episcleritis. In some cases, researchers have found that varicella virus, which is known to cause shingles, can be a cause for episcleritis disease as well.
- **Cancer**—Episcleritis has been linked to T-cell leukemia and Hodgkin lymphoma. However, these occur in extremely rare scenarios.

SYMPTOMS OF EPISCLERITIS

The symptoms for simple and nodular episcleritis are the same. Usually, redness of the eye is the only symptom of this disease. Some of the other symptoms include:

- Irritation or burning of the eye
- Light sensitivity
- Tearing

Episcleritis does not usually hurt, affect a person's vision, or cause permanent damage to the eyes. If the eyes are sore or painful, then this may be due to another medical condition, so immediate medical attention is required.

If a person has been diagnosed with episcleritis, then chances are it will recur. It may affect the other eye, but mostly occurs in the same eye. If episcleritis previously affected both the eyes, then it tends to recur in the same way.

DIAGNOSING EPISCLERITIS

To diagnose episcleritis, the ophthalmologist (eye doctor) will perform a thorough eye exam, starting with observation of the color of the eyes. If the discoloration is bluish-purple rather than red, then the doctor may diagnose the condition as scleritis instead of episcleritis.

The doctor will also complete a slit-lamp exam, which provides a 3D-view of the front of the eyes. The doctor may use eye drops to determine which layer of the eye is red.

TREATMENT OPTIONS

Episcleritis often goes away on its own within three weeks' time, even if left untreated. However, if you experience too much discomfort, or the condition recurs, then the doctor may suggest treatment options that can speed up the recovery process. Treatment of episcleritis includes:

- Corticosteroid eye drops to be used several times a day
- Lubricant eye drops, such as artificial tear eye drops
- Nonsteroidal anti-inflammatory medications such as ibuprofen (Advil, Motrin), for a severe forms of episcleritis
- Treatment to address any underlying inflammatory conditions

Some home remedies may also relieve the discomforts of episcleritis:

- Applying a cold pack over the eyes, at least three to four times daily
- Applying artificial-tear eye drops
- Wearing good quality sunglasses outdoors

Although episcleritis may look alarming, it is a common condition that does not usually cause any long-term damage. It typically goes away without treatment, but treatments are available to help speed up the recovery process. Pain is not associated with episcleritis, so immediate medical consultation is recommended should pain occur along with these symptoms.

References

1. "Episcleritis Symptoms and Treatments," Bedinghaus, Troy, Verywell Health, November 10, 2019.
2. "What Is Episcleritis?" WebMD, December 27, 2018.

Section 24.4 | Leukocoria

Leukocoria, commonly known as "white pupil" or "white pupillary reflex," is a condition in which the pupil of the eye is white, rather than its usual black. The pupil is always white in more obvious cases of leukocoria but, with other conditions, the pupil turns white when it enlarges in the dark.

RED REFLEX

When a bright light is shone on the eye, the eye normally appears red (red reflex). However, in the case of leukocoria, the eye appears white. Although a "white eye" is one of the primary signs of retinoblastoma, several other eye conditions may occur with leukocoria. Hence, it is important to differentiate retinoblastoma (a potentially life-threatening cancer) from pseudoretinoblastomas in order to determine proper diagnosis and treatment.

CAUSES OF LEUKOCORIA

Many conditions may cause leukocoria. Given the long list of possible causes, some of the most common causes are listed below:

- Astrocytic hamartoma (retinal lesions), anisometropia (eyes with differing refractive power)
- Cataract (restricted lens opacity), Coats disease (leaking retinal vessels), coloboma (hole in the eye)
- Endophthalmitis (inflammation of eye fluids)
- Familial exudative vitreoretinopathy (FEVR), a hereditary disorder that leads to vision loss
- Granuloma (a tissue mass that usually forms in response to allergens, infectious organisms, or a foreign body present in the eye)
- Incontinentia pigmenti (a rare genetic condition that causes skin lesions), inflammation (uveitis)
- Myelinated retinal nerve fiber layers (MRNF), frayed patches on the retinal nerve

- Norrie disease (a rare genetic disorder)
- Persistence of the fetal vasculature (PFV), a congenital developmental disorder
- Retinal dysplasia (disease characterized by retinal folds), retinoma (a benign tumor), retinopathy of prematurity (ROP, or Terry syndrome), a disease of the eye affecting some infants born prematurely
- Trauma (corneal scarring), toxocariasis (illness caused by roundworms)

In some cases, a diagnosis of abnormal red reflex can turn out to be nothing, or something minor. However, a dilated eye exam is always recommended in order to rule out the more serious conditions mentioned above.

SYMPTOMS OF LEUKOCORIA

In most cases, an obvious white pupil can be detected by casual observation. In other instances, the pupil only becomes larger in a darkened room or when the person looks in a particular direction.

Sometimes, leukocoria can be detected through flash photography, in which one of the pupils may reflect as having an abnormal white reflex, while the other eye has a typical red reflex.

Early diagnosis, achieved by checking for red reflex, can stop this disease from becoming more serious.

DIAGNOSIS OF LEUKOCORIA

Apart from the obvious detection of difference in the pupils, the ophthalmologist will use an ophthalmoscope to view the interior of the eye. Generally, dilating eye drops are used to enlarge the pupil, which can help with a more precise and thorough examination. However, some additional differential diagnoses of leukocoria may be diagnosed:

- Abnormalities of the anterior chamber or lens
- Choroidal hemangioma
- Congenital anomalies
- Corneal opacity

- Endophthalmitis
- Foreign body
- Glaucoma
- Hypopyon
- Neoplasia
- Ocular trauma
- Retinal detachment
- Retinal fibrosis
- Vascular abnormalities

TREATMENT OF LEUKOCORIA

Treatment for leukocoria may vary depending on the patient's conditions and the severity of the disease. Usually, the underlying condition responsible for the leukocoria is treated. Some recommended treatment options are surgery, chemotherapy, medications, and radiation.

People who desire a second opinion after diagnosis can consult with a doctor who specializes in diseases of the retina (a retina specialist). This would ensure that the patient sees a specialist who is most likely to have all the latest information on the diagnosis and treatment of this condition.

When treated early, leukocoria can often be stopped from developing into retinoblastoma.

If any of these symptoms are apparent, it is important to contact your doctor or ophthalmologist as soon as possible for a thorough examination of your eyes.

References

1. "What Is the Differential Diagnosis of Leukocoria?" PediatricEducation.org, January 2, 2007.
2. "Leukocoria," American Association for Pediatric Ophthalmology and Strabismus (AAPOS), March 2019.
3. "Leukocoria—White Pupil: Symptoms, Causes, Diagnosis and Treatment," Dr. Troup, Cameron, MD. Scope Heal (AAO), October 19, 2018.

Section 24.5 | Pinguecula

Pinguecula is a yellowish raised growth that is caused by the deposit of calcium, fat, or protein in the conjunctiva—a thin tissue that covers the white part of the eye (sclera). This growth usually occurs on the side of the eye closest to the nose, although it can occur on the other side as well. The growth happens in the part of the conjunctiva that is exposed when the eye is open.

CAUSES OF PINGUECULA

The exact cause of pinguecula is unknown. However, long-term exposure to the sun (ultraviolet (UV) light) and eye irritants such as dust may play a role in acquiring pinguecula. Arc-welding, farming, and construction are some of the major job-related risks that can increase a person's chances of acquiring pinguecula.

SYMPTOMS OF PINGUECULA

The symptoms of pinguecula can vary from mild to severe and include:

- Swelling and redness of the conjunctiva
- A yellow spot or bump in the white of the eye
- A dry, itchy, and burning sensation in the eye
- Discomfort such as a feeling of sand or grit being stuck in the eye
- Blurry eyesight

Pinguecula can usually be diagnosed by an eye exam.

TREATMENT FOR PINGUECULA

Treatment for pinguecula includes lubricating the eyes with drops which can help relieve the irritation caused by pinguecula. They also help relieve the feeling of having sand or grit stuck in the eye. If there is redness in the eyes, the doctor may recommend mild steroid eye drops to be used temporarily.

Since eye drops can help relieve any irritation or discomfort, surgery is rarely recommended for pinguecula. However, they might be done to remove the extra growth for more comfort or for cosmetic reasons.

Scleral contact lenses are another treatment option for pinguecula. These lenses cover both, the cornea, and a large part of the sclera (the white part of the eye), which helps to protect the eyes from further exposure to ultraviolet (UV) light. They will break up the protein, fat, or calcium deposit in the eyes causing the pinguecula to dissolve. This can be an easier option for those who face a problem where the pinguecula interferes with the application of their normal contact lenses since scleral contact lenses completely shield the cornea, overcoming the issues faced by an irregular corneal surface.

PINGUECULA VERSUS PTERYGIA

Sometimes, pinguecula is confused with another form of eye growth called the "pterygia." Though both are occasionally mentioned together, they are distinct conditions.

Pterygia, a fleshy tissue that grows in the sclera, can start off as pinguecula but can grow large enough to cover the cornea, affecting a person's vision. Pinguecula does not typically grow or cover the cornea, nor does it typically affect a person's vision. For these reasons, the two are considered to be separate conditions.

The suspected causes for both pinguecula and pterygia are the same: exposure to sunlight (UV rays) or exposure to dust. However, their development and prognosis are different.

PROGNOSIS

Even though a person may experience discomfort and distress upon seeing an unusual growth in the eye, pinguecula is noncancerous and is generally not a cause for concern. Pinguecula can be easily treated and minor lifestyle changes can return the eye to its normal appearance.

Long-term consequences of pinguecula are rare. However, there have been instances in which it grew back even after treatment, especially when the patient continued to expose their eyes to dust, sand, or ultraviolet (UV) rays.

PREVENTING PINGUECULA

Some practices that a person can adapt to help prevent a pinguecula or to keep an existing pinguecula from becoming worse include:

- Lubricating the eye with artificial tears
- Wearing good quality sunglasses
- Avoiding eye irritants such as dust or sand

Pinguecula is harmless, but if the growths change in size, shape, or color—or if you experience significant itching or burning of the eye (beyond what is to be expected from this disease)—then consult with a doctor immediately.

References

1. "Guide to Pinguecula (& How to Treat It)," NVISION Eye Centers, February 12, 2019.
2. "Pinguecula," MedlinePlus, National Institutes of Health (NIH), September 30, 2018.
3. "What Is a Pinguecula and a Pterygium (Surfer's Eye)?" Boyd, Kierstan. American Academy of Ophthalmology (AAO), August 29, 2019.

Section 24.6 | **Peters Anomaly**

This section includes text excerpted from "Peters Anomaly," Genetics Home Reference (GHR), National Institutes of Health (NIH), January 2014. Reviewed March 2020.

Peters anomaly is characterized by eye problems that occur in an area at the front part of the eye known as the "anterior segment." The anterior segment consists of structures including the lens, the colored part (iris) of the eye, and the clear covering of the eye (cornea). During the development of the eye, the elements of the anterior segment form separate structures. However, in Peters anomaly, the development of the anterior segment is abnormal, leading to incomplete separation of the cornea from the iris or the lens. As a result, the cornea is cloudy (opaque), which causes blurred vision. The opaque area (opacity) of the cornea varies in size and intensity from a small, faint streak to a large, white cloudy area that covers the front surface of the eye. Additionally, the location of the opacity varies; the cloudiness may be at the center of the cornea or off-center. Large, centrally located opacities tend to cause poorer vision than smaller, off-center ones.

Nearly half of the individuals affected with Peters anomaly have low vision early in life and about a quarter are legally blind. Due to a lack of visual stimulation, some individuals develop "lazy eye" (amblyopia). Peters anomaly is often associated with other eye problems, such as increased pressure within the eye (glaucoma), clouding of the lens (cataract), and unusually small eyeballs (microphthalmia). In most cases, Peters anomaly is bilateral, which means that it affects both eyes, although the level of vision impairment may be different in each eye. These individuals may have eyes that do not point in the same direction (strabismus). In some people with Peters anomaly, corneal clouding improves over time leading to improved vision.

There are two types of Peters anomaly, which are distinguished by their signs and symptoms. Peters anomaly type I is characterized by an incomplete separation of the cornea and iris and mild to moderate corneal opacity. Type II is characterized by an incomplete separation of the cornea and lens and severe corneal opacity that may involve the entire cornea.

FREQUENCY OF PETERS ANOMALY

The exact prevalence of Peters anomaly is unknown. This condition is one of a group of disorders known as "congenital corneal opacities," which affect 3 to 6 individuals per 100,000.

CAUSES OF PETERS ANOMALY

Mutations in the *FOXC1*, *PAX6*, *PITX2*, or *CYP1B1* gene can cause Peters anomaly. The *FOXC1*, *PAX6*, and *PITX2* genes are all members of a family called "homeobox genes" that direct the formation of many parts of the body. These three genes are involved in the development of the anterior segment of the eye. The *CYP1B1* gene provides instructions for making an enzyme that is active in many tissues, including the eye. The enzyme's role in these tissues is unclear; it is likely involved in the development of the anterior segment.

Mutations in any of these four genes disrupt the development of the anterior segment of the eye. These mutations can lead to severe developmental problems, such as incomplete separation of eye structures and complete corneal opacity, or they can result in minor eye abnormalities including small, faint opacities. It is likely that mutations that cause a complete absence of protein function result in the most severe eye problems. It is unknown why both eyes are affected in some cases and in others only one eye is abnormal.

In many cases of Peters anomaly, there is no mutation identified in any of these four genes. The cause of the condition in these cases is unknown.

Part 4 | Understanding and Treating Disorders of the Macula, Optic Nerve, Retina, Vitreous, and Uvea

Chapter 25 | Age-Related Macular Degeneration

WHAT IS AGE-RELATED MACULAR DEGENERATION?

Age-related macular degeneration (AMD) is an eye disease that can blur the sharp, central vision you need for activities, such as reading and driving. "Age-related" means that it often happens in older people. "Macular" means it affects a part of your eye called the "macula."

Age-related macular degeneration is a common condition—it is a leading cause of vision loss for people 50 years of age and older. AMD does not cause complete blindness, but losing your central vision can make it harder to see faces, drive, or do close-up work, such as cooking or fixing things around the house.

Age-related macular degeneration happens very slowly in some people. Even if you have early AMD, you may not experience vision loss for a long time. For other people, AMD progresses faster and can lead to central vision loss in one eye or both eyes.

WHAT ARE THE SYMPTOMS OF AGE-RELATED MACULAR DEGENERATION?

As AMD progresses, many people see a blurry area near the center of their vision. Over time, this blurry area may get bigger or you may see blank spots. Things may also seem less bright than before.

Some people may also notice that straight lines start to look wavy. This can be a warning sign for late AMD. If you notice these symptoms, see your eye doctor right away.

This chapter includes text excerpted from "Age-Related Macular Degeneration," National Eye Institute (NEI), August 2, 2019.

ARE YOU AT RISK FOR AGE-RELATED MACULAR DEGENERATION?

Your risk for AMD increases as you get older. People over 60 years of age are more likely to have AMD. The risk for AMD is also higher for people who:

- Have a family history of AMD
- Are Caucasian
- Smoke

If you are at risk for AMD because of your age, family history, or other factors, it is important to get regular eye exams. Early AMD does not have any symptoms, so do not wait for your vision to change.

HOW YOU CAN LOWER YOUR RISK FOR AGE-RELATED MACULAR DEGENERATION

Research shows that you may be able to lower your risk of AMD (or slow its progression) by making these healthy choices:

- Quit smoking—or do not start
- Get regular physical activity
- Maintain a healthy blood pressure and cholesterol levels
- Eat healthy foods, including leafy green vegetables and fish

Did You Know?

- Late AMD can happen in one eye or both eyes.
- If you have late AMD in only one eye, you may not notice any changes in your vision—but it is still important to get your eyes checked.
- Having late AMD in one eye puts you at a higher risk of developing late AMD in your other eye.

HOW DOES THE EYE DOCTOR CHECK FOR AGE-RELATED MACULAR DEGENERATION?

Eye doctors can check for AMD as part of a comprehensive dilated eye exam. The exam is simple and painless—your doctor will give you some eye drops to dilate (widen) your pupil and then check your eyes for AMD and other eye problems.

If your doctor dilates your pupils, your vision may be blurry and sensitive to light for a few hours after the exam. It is a good idea to ask a friend or family member to drive you home—especially if you have never had a dilated eye exam before.

Your doctor may also recommend doing a test called an "optical coherence tomogram" (OCT). This test lets the doctor see the back of your eye.

If you get an OCT test, your eye doctor will take pictures of the inside of your eye with a special machine. The machine will not touch your eye. Your doctor may also dilate your pupils as part of an OCT test.

WHAT IS THE TREATMENT FOR AGE-RELATED MACULAR DEGENERATION?

There is no treatment for early AMD, so your eye doctor will probably just keep track of how your eyes are doing with regular eye exams. Eating healthy, getting regular exercise, and quitting smoking can also help.

If you are diagnosed with intermediate or late AMD, ask your eye doctor about treatment options and how the condition may affect your vision in the future.

If you have intermediate or late AMD, special dietary supplements (vitamins and minerals) may be able to stop it from getting worse.

For people with a type of late AMD called "wet" or "neovascular AMD," there are other treatments that may be able to stop further vision loss:

- Medicines called "anti-VEGF" drugs that the doctor injects in your eye
- Laser treatment, called "photodynamic therapy" (PDT)

HOW YOU CAN LIVE WITH VISION LOSS FROM AGE-RELATED MACULAR DEGENERATION

Not everyone with AMD develops late AMD or gets it in both eyes. But, if you do, living with vision loss from AMD can be challenging.

Having low vision means that even with glasses, contact lenses, medicine, or surgery, your vision loss makes it hard to do everyday tasks.

The good news is, there are things that can help—such as low vision devices and rehabilitation (training) programs.

Chapter 26 | Other Macular Disorders

Chapter Contents

Section 26.1 | **Macular Hole**

This section includes text excerpted from "Macular Hole," National Eye Institute (NEI), July 8, 2019.

WHAT IS A MACULAR HOLE?

A macular hole is a small break in the macula, located in the center of the eye's light-sensitive tissue called the "retina." The macula provides the sharp, central vision we need for reading, driving, and seeing fine detail.

A macular hole can cause blurred and distorted central vision. Macular holes are related to aging and usually occur in people over 60 years of age.

Is a Macular Hole the Same as Age-Related Macular Degeneration?

No. Macular holes and age-related macular degeneration (AMD) are two separate and distinct conditions, although the symptoms for each are similar. Both conditions are common in people 60 of age and over. An eye-care professional will know the difference.

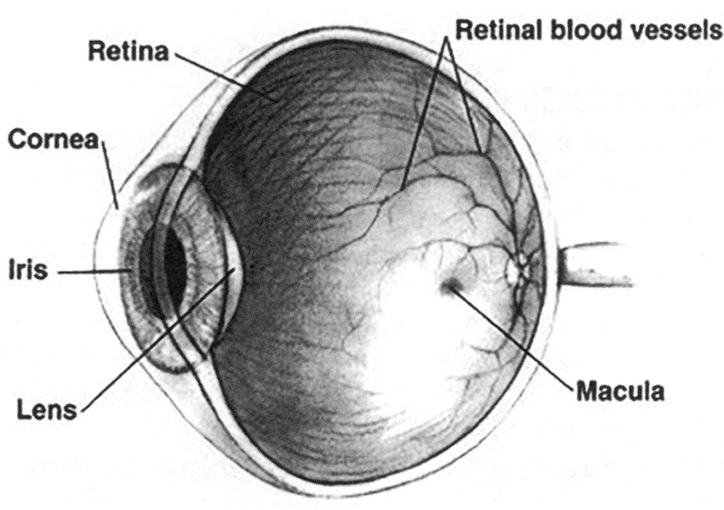

Figure 26.1. Macular Hole

ARE THERE DIFFERENT TYPES OF MACULAR HOLES?

Yes. There are three stages to a macular hole:

- **Foveal detachments (stage I).** Without treatment, about half of Stage I macular holes will progress.
- **Partial-thickness holes (stage II).** Without treatment, about 70 percent of Stage II macular holes will progress.
- **Full-thickness holes (stage III).**

The size of the hole and its location on the retina determine how much it will affect a person's vision. When a Stage III macular hole develops, most central and detailed vision can be lost. If left untreated, a macular hole can lead to a detached retina, a sight-threatening condition that should receive immediate medical attention.

WHAT ARE THE SYMPTOMS OF A MACULAR HOLE?

Macular holes often begin gradually. In the early stage of a macular hole, people may notice a slight distortion or blurriness in their straight-ahead vision. Straight lines or objects can begin to look bent or wavy. Reading and performing other routine tasks with the affected eye becomes difficult.

WHAT CAUSES A MACULAR HOLE

Most of the eye's interior is filled with vitreous, a gel-like substance that fills about 80 percent of the eye and helps it maintain a round shape. The vitreous contains millions of fine fibers that are attached to the surface of the retina. As we age, the vitreous slowly shrinks and pulls away from the retinal surface. Natural fluids fill the area where the vitreous has contracted and this is normal. In most cases, there are no adverse effects. Some patients may experience a small increase in floaters, which are little "cobwebs" or specks that seem to float about in your field of vision.

However, if the vitreous is firmly attached to the retina when it pulls away, it can tear the retina and create a macular hole. Also, once the vitreous has pulled away from the surface of the retina, some of the fibers can remain on the retinal surface and can contract. This increases tension on the retina and can lead to a macular hole. In either case, the fluid that has replaced the shrunken vitreous can then seep through the hole onto the macula, blurring and distorting central vision.

Macular holes can also occur in other eye disorders, such as high myopia (nearsightedness), injury to the eye, retinal detachment, and rarely, macular pucker.

Is My Other Eye at Risk?

If a macular hole exists in one eye, there is a 10 to 15 percent chance that a macular hole will develop in your other eye over your lifetime. Your doctor can discuss this with you.

WHAT IS THE TREATMENT FOR A MACULAR HOLE?

Although some macular holes can seal themselves and require no treatment, surgery is necessary in many cases to help improve vision. In this surgical procedure—called a "vitrectomy"—the vitreous gel is removed to prevent it from pulling on the retina and replaced with a bubble containing a mixture of air and gas. The bubble acts as an internal, temporary bandage that holds the edge of the macular hole in place as it heals. Surgery is performed under local anesthesia and often on an outpatient basis.

Following surgery, patients must remain in a face-down position, normally for a day or two but sometimes for as long as two-to-three weeks. This position allows the bubble to press against the macula and be gradually reabsorbed by the eye, sealing the hole. As the bubble is reabsorbed, the vitreous cavity refills with natural eye fluids.

Maintaining a face-down position is crucial to the success of the surgery. Because this position can be difficult for many people, it is important to discuss this with your doctor before surgery.

What Are the Risks of Macular Hole Surgery?

The most common risk following macular hole surgery is an increase in the rate of cataract development. In most patients, a cataract can progress rapidly, and often becomes severe enough to require removal. Other less common complications include infection and retinal detachment either during surgery or afterward, both of which can be immediately treated.

For a few months after surgery, patients are not permitted to travel by air. Changes in air pressure may cause the bubble in the eye to expand, increasing pressure inside the eye.

How Successful Is Macular Hole Surgery?

Vision improvement varies from patient to patient. People who have had a macular hole for less than six months have a better chance of recovering vision than those who have had one for a longer period. Discuss vision recovery with your doctor before your surgery. Vision recovery can continue for as long as three months after surgery.

What If I Cannot Remain in a Face-Down Position after the Macular Hole Surgery?

If you cannot remain in a face-down position for the required period after surgery, vision recovery may not be successful. People who are unable to remain in a face-down position for this length of time may not be good candidates for a vitrectomy. However, there are a number of devices that can make the "face-down" recovery period easier on you. There are also some approaches that can decrease the amount of "face-down" time. Discuss these with your doctor.

Section 26.2 | Macular Pucker

This section includes text excerpted from "Macular Pucker," National Eye Institute (NEI), July 8, 2019.

WHAT IS A MACULAR PUCKER?

A macular pucker is a scar tissue that has formed on the eye's macula, located in the center of the light-sensitive tissue called the "retina." The macula provides the sharp, central vision we need for reading, driving, and seeing fine detail. A macular pucker can cause blurred and distorted central vision.

Macular pucker is also known as "epiretinal membrane," "preretinal membrane," "cellophane maculopathy," "retina wrinkle," "surface wrinkling retinopathy," "premacular fibrosis," and "internal limiting membrane" (ILM) disease.

Is a Macular Pucker the Same as Age-Related Macular Degeneration?

No. A macular pucker and age-related macular degeneration (AMD) are two separate and distinct conditions, although the symptoms for each are similar. An eye-care professional will know the difference.

Is a Macular Pucker Similar to a Macular Hole?

Although both have similar symptoms—distorted and blurred vision—macular pucker and a macular hole are different conditions. They both result from tugging on the retina from a shrinking vitreous. When the vitreous separates from the retina, usually as part of the aging process, it can cause microscopic damage to the retina. As the retina heals itself, the resulting scar tissue can cause a macular pucker. Rarely, a macular pucker will develop into a macular hole. An eye-care professional can readily tell the difference between macular pucker and macular hole.

WHAT ARE THE SYMPTOMS OF THE MACULAR PUCKER?

Vision loss from a macular pucker can vary from no loss to severe loss, although severe vision loss is uncommon. People with a macular pucker may notice that their vision is blurry or mildly distorted, and straight lines can appear wavy. They may have difficulty in seeing fine detail and reading small print. There may be a gray area in the center of your vision, or perhaps even a blind spot.

WHAT ARE THE CAUSES OF A MACULAR PUCKER?

Most of the eye's interior is filled with vitreous, a gel-like substance that fills about 80 percent of the eye and helps it maintain a round shape. The vitreous contains millions of fine fibers that are attached to the surface of the retina. As we age, the vitreous slowly shrinks and pulls away from the retinal surface. This is called a "vitreous detachment," and is normal. In most cases, there are no adverse effects, except for a small increase in floaters, which are little "cobwebs" or specks that seem to float about in your field of vision.

However, sometimes when the vitreous pulls away from the retina, there is microscopic damage to the retina's surface (Note: This is not a macular hole). When this happens, the retina begins a healing process to the damaged area and forms scar tissue, or an epiretinal membrane, on the surface of the retina. This scar tissue is firmly attached to the retina surface. When the scar tissue contracts, it causes the retina to wrinkle, or pucker, usually without any effect on central vision. However, if the scar tissue has formed over the macula, our sharp, central vision becomes blurred and distorted.

WHAT IS THE TREATMENT FOR A MACULAR PUCKER?

A macular pucker usually requires no treatment. In many cases, the symptoms of vision distortion and blurriness are mild, and no treatment is necessary. People usually adjust to the mild visual distortion, since it does not affect activities of daily life, such as reading and driving. Neither eye drops, medications, nor nutritional supplements will improve vision distorted from macular pucker. Sometimes the scar tissue—which causes a macular pucker—separates from the retina, and the macular pucker clears up.

Rarely, vision deteriorates to the point where it affects daily routine activities. However, when this happens, surgery may be recommended. This procedure is called a "vitrectomy," in which the vitreous gel is removed to prevent it from pulling on the retina and replaced with a salt solution (because the vitreous is mostly water, you will notice no change between the salt solution and the normal vitreous). Also, the scar tissue which causes the wrinkling is removed. A vitrectomy is usually performed under local anesthesia.

After the operation, you will need to wear an eye patch for a few days or weeks to protect the eye. You will also need to use medicated eye drops to protect against infection.

How Successful Is Macular Pucker Surgery?

Surgery to repair a macular pucker is very delicate, and while vision improves in most cases, it does not usually return to normal. On average, about half of the vision lost from a macular pucker is restored; some people have significantly more vision restored, some less. In most cases, vision distortion is significantly reduced. Recovery of vision can take up to three months. Patients should talk with their eye-care professional about whether treatment is appropriate.

What Are the Risks of Macular Pucker Surgery?

The most common complication of a vitrectomy is an increase in the rate of cataract development. Cataract surgery may be needed within a few years after the vitrectomy. Other, less common complications are retinal detachment either during or after surgery, and infection after surgery. Also, the macular pucker may grow back, but this is rare.

Chapter 27 | Glaucoma

Chapter Contents

Section 27.1 | **Do Not Let Glaucoma Steal Your Sight!**

This section contains text excerpted from the following sources: Text in this section begins with excerpts from "Don't Let Glaucoma Steal Your Sight!" Centers for Disease Control and Prevention (CDC), December 6, 2018; Text beginning with the heading "What Is Glaucoma?" is excerpted from "Glaucoma," National Eye Institute (NEI), March 11, 2020.

Half of people with glaucoma do not know they have it. Get a healthy start this year by learning about glaucoma and taking steps to reduce your risk of vision loss!

KNOW THE FACTS ABOUT GLAUCOMA

- Glaucoma is a group of diseases that damage the eye's optic nerve and can result in vision loss and even blindness.
- About 3 million Americans have glaucoma. It is the second leading cause of blindness worldwide.
- Open-angle glaucoma, the most common form, results in increased eye pressure. There are often no early symptoms, which is why 50 percent of people with glaucoma do not know they have the disease.
- There is no cure (yet) for glaucoma, but if it is diagnosed early, you can preserve your vision and prevent vision loss. Taking action to preserve your vision health is the key.

WHAT IS GLAUCOMA?

Glaucoma is a group of eye diseases that can cause vision loss and blindness by damaging a nerve in the back of your eye called the "optic nerve."

The symptoms can start so slowly that you may not notice them. The only way to find out if you have glaucoma is to get a comprehensive dilated eye exam.

There is no cure for glaucoma, but early treatment can often stop the damage and protect your vision.

WHAT CAUSES GLAUCOMA

Scientists are not sure what causes the most common types of glaucoma, but many people with glaucoma have high eye pressure (intraocular pressure)—and treatments that lower eye pressure help to slow the disease.

There is no way to prevent glaucoma. That is why eye exams are so important—so you and your doctor can find it before it affects your vision.

WHAT ARE THE SYMPTOMS OF GLAUCOMA?

At first, glaucoma does not usually have any symptoms. That is why half of the people with glaucoma do not even know they have it.

Over time, you may slowly lose vision, usually starting with your side (peripheral) vision—especially the part of your vision that is closest to your nose. Because it happens so slowly, many people cannot tell that their vision is changing, especially at first.

But, as the disease gets worse, you may start to notice that you cannot see things off to the side anymore. Without treatment, glaucoma can eventually cause blindness.

ARE YOU AT RISK FOR GLAUCOMA?

Anyone can get glaucoma, but some people are at higher risk. You are at higher risk if you:

- Are over 60 years of age
- Are African American or Hispanic/Latinx and over 40 years of age
- Have a family history of glaucoma

Talk with your doctor about your risk for glaucoma, and ask how often you need to get checked.

When to Get Help Right Away

Angle-closure glaucoma can cause these sudden symptoms:

- Intense eye pain
- Upset stomach (nausea)
- Red-eye
- Blurry vision
- If you have these symptoms, go to your doctor or an emergency room now.

HOW DOES THE EYE DOCTOR CHECK FOR GLAUCOMA?

Eye doctors can check for glaucoma as part of a comprehensive dilated eye exam. The exam is simple and painless—your doctor will give you some eye drops to dilate (widen) your pupil and then check your eyes for glaucoma and other eye problems. The exam includes a visual field test to check your peripheral (side) vision.

WHAT IS THE TREATMENT FOR GLAUCOMA?

Doctors use a few different types of treatment for glaucoma, including medicines (usually eye drops), laser treatment, and surgery.

If you have glaucoma, it is important to start treatment right away. While it will not undo any damage to your vision, treatment can stop it from getting worse.

- **Medicines**. Prescription eye drops are the most common treatment. They lower the pressure in your eye and prevent damage to your optic nerve.
- **Laser treatment.** To lower the pressure in your eye, doctors can use lasers to help the fluid drain out of your eye. It is a simple procedure that your doctor can do in the office.
- **Surgery.** If medicines and laser treatments do not work, your doctor might suggest surgery. There are several different types of surgery that can help the fluid drain out of the eye.

Talk over your options with your doctor. While glaucoma is a serious disease, treatment works well. Remember these tips:

- If your doctor prescribes medicine, be sure to take it every day.
- Tell your doctor if your treatment causes side effects.
- See your doctor for regular checkups.
- If you are having trouble with everyday activities because of your vision loss, ask your doctor about low vision services or devices that could help.
- Encourage family members to get checked for glaucoma, since it can run in families.

Section 27.2 | **Glaucoma Types**

This section includes text excerpted from "Types of Glaucoma," National Eye Institute (NEI), June 26, 2019.

Glaucoma is a group of eye diseases that are usually characterized by damage to the optic nerve and gradual vision loss that starts with losing peripheral (side) vision. People who have high eye pressure are at higher risk for glaucoma.

Each type of glaucoma is different—but most have no early symptoms, so it is important to get tested regularly, especially if you are at higher risk.

PRIMARY GLAUCOMA

When experts do not know what causes a type of glaucoma, that type is called "primary glaucoma."

Open-Angle Glaucoma

Open-angle glaucoma is the most common type in the United States, where 9 in 10 people with glaucoma have the open-angle type. Many people do not have any symptoms until they start to lose their vision, and people may not notice vision loss right away.

Experts are not sure what causes open-angle glaucoma, but it may be caused by pressure building up in your eye. If the fluid in your eye cannot drain fast enough, it creates pressure that pushes on a nerve in the back of your eye (the optic nerve).

Over time, the pressure damages the optic nerve, which affects your vision. This can eventually lead to blindness—in fact, open-angle glaucoma causes almost 2 in 10 cases of blindness in African Americans. People with high blood pressure are also at a higher risk for this type.

Treatment options for open-angle glaucoma include medicines, laser treatment, and surgery.

Normal-Tension Glaucoma

Normal-tension glaucoma is a type of open-angle glaucoma that happens in people with normal eye pressure. About one in three people with open-angle glaucoma have the normal-tension type.

You may be at higher risk for normal-tension glaucoma if you:

- Are of Japanese ancestry
- Have a family history of normal-tension glaucoma
- Have had certain heart problems, such as an irregular heartbeat
- Have low blood pressure

Experts do not know what causes normal-tension glaucoma, but research shows that treatments that lower eye pressure can help slow the disease and stop vision loss. Treatment options for normal-tension glaucoma include medicines, laser treatment, and surgery.

Angle-Closure Glaucoma

Angle-closure glaucoma, also called "narrow-angle" or "acute glaucoma," is a medical emergency. Go to the doctor or emergency room immediately if you suddenly have:

- Intense pain in your eye
- Nausea
- Red eyes
- Blurred vision

In this type of glaucoma, the outer edge of the iris (the colored part of your eye) blocks fluid from draining out of the front of the eye. The fluid builds up quickly, causing a sudden increase in eye pressure. If it is not treated, angle-closure glaucoma can cause blindness in just a few days.

A doctor can use laser treatment and give you medicine to help the fluid drain. This can lower eye pressure and protect your vision. Your doctor might treat both eyes to prevent future problems, even if you only have angle-closure glaucoma in one eye.

Another type of angle-closure glaucoma, sometimes called "slow" or "chronic angle-closure glaucoma," happens more slowly and might not have any symptoms. Your doctor can treat this type with medicines, laser treatments, or surgery.

Congenital Glaucoma

Some babies are born with glaucoma—this is called "congenital glaucoma." About 1 out of 10,000 babies born in the United States have a defect (problem) in the eye that keeps fluid from draining normally.

In these cases, you can usually notice the symptoms right away. Children with congenital glaucoma:

- Have cloudy eyes
- Are sensitive to light
- Make extra tears
- May have eyes that are larger than normal

Surgery works very well to treat congenital glaucoma. If a doctor does surgery early enough, children with congenital glaucoma usually will not have any permanent vision loss.

Several other types of glaucoma can also develop in children. Any glaucoma that affects babies or children is called "pediatric glaucoma."

SECONDARY GLAUCOMA

Sometimes glaucoma is caused by another medical condition—this is called "secondary glaucoma."

Neovascular Glaucoma

Neovascular glaucoma happens when the eye makes extra blood vessels that cover the part of your eye where fluid would normally drain. It is usually caused by another medical condition, such as diabetes or high blood pressure.

If you have neovascular glaucoma, you may notice:

- Pain or redness in your eye
- Vision loss

This type of glaucoma can be hard to treat. Doctors need to treat the underlying cause (such as diabetes or high blood pressure) and use glaucoma treatments to lower the eye pressure that results from it. Treatment options include medicines, laser treatment, and surgery.

Pigmentary Glaucoma

Pigment dispersion syndrome happens when the pigment (color) from your iris (the colored part of your eye) flakes off. The loose pigment may block fluid from draining out of your eye, which can increase your eye pressure and cause pigmentary glaucoma.

Young, white men who are near-sighted are more likely to have pigment dispersion syndrome than others. If you have this condition, you may have blurry vision or see rainbow-colored rings around lights, especially when you exercise.

Doctors can treat pigmentary glaucoma by lowering your eye pressure, but there are very limited options available to prevent pigment from detaching from the iris. Treatment options include medicines, laser treatment, and surgery.

Exfoliation Glaucoma

Exfoliation glaucoma (sometimes called "pseudoexfoliation") is a type of open-angle glaucoma that happens in some people with exfoliation syndrome, a condition that causes extra material to detach from parts of the eye and block fluid from draining.

Research shows that genetics may play a role in exfoliation glaucoma. You are at higher risk if someone else in your family has exfoliation glaucoma.

This type of glaucoma can progress faster than primary open-angle glaucoma, and often causes higher eye pressure. This means that it is especially important for people who are at risk to get eye exams regularly. Treatment options include medicines, laser treatment, and surgery.

Uveitic Glaucoma

Uveitic glaucoma can happen in people who have uveitis, a condition that causes inflammation (irritation and swelling) in the eye. About 2 in 10 people with uveitis will develop uveitic glaucoma.

Experts are not sure how uveitis causes uveitic glaucoma, but they think that it may happen because uveitis can cause inflammation and scar tissue in the middle of the eye. This may damage or block the part of the eye where fluid drains out, causing high eye pressure and leading to uveitic glaucoma.

In some cases, the medicines that treat uveitis may also cause uveitic glaucoma, or make it worse. This is because corticosteroid medicines may cause increased eye pressure as a side effect.

Chapter 28 | Other Disorders of the Optic Nerve

Chapter Contents

Section 28.1 | **Neuromyelitis Optica**

This section includes text excerpted from "Neuromyelitis Optica Information Page," National Institute of Neurological Disorders and Stroke (NINDS), June 27, 2019.

Neuromyelitis optica (NMO) is an autoimmune disease of the central nervous system (CNS) that predominantly affects the optic nerves and spinal cord. It is sometimes also referred to as NMO spectrum disorder. In NMO, the body's immune system mistakenly attacks healthy cells and proteins in the body, most often those in the spinal cord and eyes. Individuals with NMO develop optic neuritis, which causes pain in the eye and vision loss. Individuals also develop transverse myelitis, which causes weakness or paralysis of arms and legs, and numbness, along with loss of bladder and bowel control. Magnetic resonance imaging (MRI) of the spine often shows an abnormality that extends over long segments of the spinal cord. Individuals may also develop episodes of severe nausea and vomiting, with hiccups from the involvement of a part of the brain that controls vomiting.

The disease is caused by abnormal autoantibodies that bind to a protein called "aquaporin-4." Binding of the aquaporin-4 antibody activates other components of the immune system, causing inflammation and damage to these cells. This also results in the brain and spinal cord the loss of myelin, the fatty substance that acts as insulation around nerve fibers and helps nerve signals move from cell to cell.

Neuromyelitis optica is different from multiple sclerosis (MS). Attacks are usually more severe in NMO than in MS, and NMO is treated differently than MS. Most individuals with NMO experience clusters of attacks days to months or years apart, followed by partial recovery during periods of remission. Women are more often affected by NMO than men. African Americans are at greater risk of the disease than are Caucasians. The onset of NMO varies from childhood to adulthood, with two peaks, one in childhood and the other in adults in their 40s.

TREATMENT OF NEUROMYELITIS OPTICA

There is no cure for NMO. In June 2019, the U.S. Food and Drug Administration (FDA) approved eculizumab injection to reduce the number of relapses in adults who are anti-aquaporin-4 (AQP4) antibody positive. NMO relapses and attacks are often treated with corticosteroid drugs and plasma exchange (also called "plasmapheresis," a process used to remove harmful antibodies from the bloodstream). Immunosuppressive drugs used to prevent attacks include mycophenolate mofetil, rituximab, and azathioprine. Pain, stiffness, muscle spasms, and bladder and bowel control problems can be managed with medications and therapies. Individuals with a major disability will require the combined efforts of physical and occupational therapists, along with social services professionals to address complex rehabilitation needs.

PROGNOSIS OF NEUROMYELITIS OPTICA

Most individuals with NMO have an unpredictable, relapsing course of disease with attacks occurring months or years apart. Disability is cumulative, the result of each attack damaging new areas of the central nervous system. Some individuals are severely affected by NMO and can lose vision in both eyes and the use of their arms and legs. Most individuals experience some degree of permanent limb weakness or vision loss from NMO. However, reducing the number of attacks with immunosuppressive medications may help prevent the accumulation of disability. Rarely, muscle weakness can be severe enough to cause breathing difficulties and may require the use of artificial ventilation.

Section 28.2 | **Coloboma of Optic Nerve**

This section includes text excerpted from "Coloboma of Optic Nerve," Genetic and Rare Diseases Information Center (GARD), National Center for Advancing Translational Sciences (NCATS), October 28, 2015. Reviewed March 2020.

Coloboma of the optic nerve is a congenital eye abnormality in which the optic nerve (which carries images of what the eye sees to the brain) is incompletely formed. The condition may occur in one or both eyes. The degree of visual impairment varies widely depending on the severity and structures involved. Serious detachments of the retina commonly occur in affected people, with a high risk for extensive retinal detachment. The coloboma may be associated with other features, such as a small eye (microphthalmia) with or without a cyst; small cornea (microcornea); or coloboma of other eye structures. Although the condition is present from birth, diagnosis may be delayed since the coloboma is inside the eye and not visible by simple inspection. Coloboma of the optic nerve may occur sporadically, maybe due to a genetic mutation and be inherited, or may occur as a feature of an underlying syndrome or other genetic condition.

CAUSES OF COLOBOMA OF OPTIC NERVE

Colobomas are due to incomplete development of the eye. During the second month of development in utero, a seam-like structure called the "optic fissure" closes up to form the structures of the eye. When it does not fuse normally, it results in a coloboma in the affected location of the eye.

A coloboma may occur sporadically, it may be inherited and due to mutations in various genes, or may occur as a feature of an underlying syndrome or other genetic condition. When an underlying syndrome or genetic condition is present, the cause is assumed to be the same as that of the underlying condition. For example, when an optic nerve coloboma occurs as part of renal coloboma syndrome, it is caused by mutations in the *PAX2* gene. Certain environmental factors affecting early development may also increase the risk of colobomas in general.

Many genes involved in early eye development may be responsible for colobomas in general. While some of these genes have been identified, most of them remain unknown. Most genetic mutations associated with colobomas have been identified only in very small numbers of affected people. Autosomal dominant inheritance has been reported. One gene that has been associated with coloboma of the optic nerve specifically is the *PAX6* gene.

The *PAX6* gene is part of a "family" of genes that are needed for forming tissues and organs during embryonic development, and for maintaining normal function of certain cells after birth. The genes in this family give the body instructions to make proteins that help control the activity of that particular genes. It is thought that the PAX6 protein turns on (activates) genes involved in forming the eyes before birth and regulating the actions of genes within many eye structures.

TREATMENT OF COLOBOMA OF OPTIC NERVE

There is no treatment, as of now, to correct an optic nerve coloboma, but low vision aids may be helpful for some people.

Section 28.3 | Septo-Optic Dysplasia

This section contains text excerpted from the following sources: Text in this section begins with excerpts from "Septo-Optic Dysplasia," Genetics Home Reference (GHR), National Institutes of Health (NIH), March 17, 2020; Text beginning with the heading "Treatment of Septo-Optic Dysplasia" is excerpted from "Septo-Optic Dysplasia Information Page," National Institute of Neurological Disorders and Stroke (NINDS), March 27, 2019.

Septo-optic dysplasia (SOD) is a disorder of early brain development. Although its signs and symptoms vary, this condition is traditionally defined by three characteristic features: underdevelopment (hypoplasia) of the optic nerves, abnormal formation of structures along the midline of the brain, and pituitary hypoplasia.

The first major feature, optic nerve hypoplasia, is the underdevelopment of the optic nerves, which carry visual information from the eyes to the brain. In affected individuals, the optic nerves are abnormally small and make fewer connections than usual between the eyes and the brain. As a result, people with optic nerve hypoplasia have impaired vision in one or both eyes. Optic nerve hypoplasia can also be associated with unusual side-to-side eye movements (nystagmus) and other eye abnormalities.

The second characteristic feature of septo-optic dysplasia is the abnormal development of structures separating the right and left halves of the brain. These structures include the corpus callosum, which is a band of tissue that connects the two halves of the brain, and the septum pellucidum, which separates the fluid-filled spaces called "ventricles" in the brain. In the early stages of brain development, these structures may form abnormally or fail to develop at all. Depending on which structures are affected, abnormal brain development can lead to intellectual disability and other neurological problems.

The third major feature of this disorder is pituitary hypoplasia. The pituitary is a gland at the base of the brain that produces several hormones. These hormones help control growth, reproduction, and other critical body functions. Underdevelopment of the pituitary can lead to a shortage (deficiency) of many essential hormones. Most commonly, pituitary hypoplasia causes growth hormone deficiency, which results in slow growth and unusually short stature. Severe cases cause panhypopituitarism, a condition in which the pituitary produces no hormones. Panhypopituitarism is associated with slow growth, low blood sugar (hypoglycemia), genital abnormalities, and problems with sexual development.

SIGNS AND SYMPTOMS OF SEPTO-OPTIC DYSPLASIA

The signs and symptoms of septo-optic dysplasia can vary significantly. Some researchers suggest that septo-optic dysplasia should actually be considered a group of related conditions rather than a single disorder. About one-third of people diagnosed with septo-optic dysplasia have all three major features; most affected individuals have two of the major features. In rare cases, septo-optic dysplasia is associated with additional signs and symptoms, including recurrent seizures (epilepsy), delayed development, and abnormal movements.

CAUSES OF SEPTO-OPTIC DYSPLASIA

In most cases of septo-optic dysplasia, the cause of the disorder is unknown. Researchers suspect that a combination of genetic and environmental factors may play a role in causing this disorder. Proposed environmental risk factors include viral infections, specific medications, and a disruption in blood flow to certain areas of the brain during critical periods of development.

At least three genes have been associated with septo-optic dysplasia, although mutations in these genes appear to be rare causes of this disorder. The three genes, *HESX1*, *OTX2*, and *SOX2*, all play important roles in embryonic development. In particular, they are essential for the formation of the eyes, the pituitary gland, and structures at the front of the brain (the forebrain) such as the optic nerves. Mutations in any of these genes disrupt the early development of these structures, which leads to the major features of septo-optic dysplasia.

TREATMENT OF SEPTO-OPTIC DYSPLASIA

Treatment for SOD is symptomatic. Hormone deficiencies may be treated with hormone replacement therapy. The optical problems associated with SOD are generally not treatable. Vision, physical, and occupational therapies may be required.

PROGNOSIS OF SEPTO-OPTIC DYSPLASIA

The prognosis for individuals with SOD varies according to the presence and severity of symptoms.

Section 28.4 | **Optic Atrophy 1 and Optic Neuritis**

This section contains text excerpted from the following sources: Text under the heading "Optic Atrophy 1" is excerpted from "Optic Atrophy 1," Genetic and Rare Diseases Information Center (GARD), National Center for Advancing Translational Sciences (NCATS), May 15, 2018; Text under the heading "Optic Neuritis" is excerpted from "Optic Neuritis," Genetic and Rare Diseases Information Center (GARD), National Center for Advancing Translational Sciences (NCATS), January 11, 2011. Reviewed March 2020.

OPTIC ATROPHY 1

Optic atrophy 1, also known as "optic atrophy type 1," (OPA1) is a disease that affects the optic nerve. The optic nerve carries signals from the eye to the brain about what is seen. People with optic atrophy type 1 have an optic nerve that has lost some tissue (atrophy). This atrophy causes the optic nerve not to work as well as it should, which affects the vision.

Signs and Symptoms of Optic Atrophy Type 1

Signs and symptoms of optic atrophy type 1 include vision loss, difficulty distinguishing colors, and an abnormally pale appearance (pallor) of the optic nerve. The vision loss typically begins at four to six years of age. The disease can occur in people of any ethnicity but seems to be more common in people of Danish descent.

Other symptoms of optic atrophy type 1 may include sensorineural hearing loss, difficulty coordinating movements (ataxia) and muscle disease (myopathy). When people have optic atrophy type 1 and signs and symptoms other than vision loss, it is known as "autosomal dominant optic atrophy plus syndrome" (ADOA Plus).

Causes of Optic Atrophy Type 1

Optic atrophy type 1 is caused by a genetic change (pathogenic variant or mutation) in the *OPA1* gene. The disease is inherited in an autosomal dominant manner.

Diagnosis and Treatment of Optic Atrophy Type 1

Optic atrophy type 1 may be suspected when a person has signs and symptoms of the disease on an exam done by an ophthalmologist. Genetic testing may be used to confirm the diagnosis. Treatment for optic atrophy type 1 may include vision and hearing aids when necessary.

What Is the Long-Term Outlook for People with Optic Atrophy 1?

In general, people with optic atrophy type 1 have worsening vision loss over time. However, some people only have mild vision loss, and for some people, the vision loss does not worsen with time. Vision loss can interfere with daily life, but it is not expected to shorten a person's lifespan.

The long-term outlook for people with optic atrophy type 1 may depend on the severity of vision loss and if there are any other symptoms, such as hearing loss or muscle weakness. About 20 percent of people with a genetic change (pathogenic variant or mutation) in the *OPA1* gene have symptoms other than vision loss.

In some cases, people with optic atrophy type 1 may experience anxiety and depression due to the symptoms of the disease. It is important to contact your doctor if you have concerns that you or a family member is suffering from anxiety or depression.

OPTIC NEURITIS

Optic neuritis is an inflammation of the optic nerve, the nerve that carries the visual signal from the eye to the brain. The condition may cause sudden, reduced vision in the affected eye(s).

Causes of Optic Neuritis

While the cause of optic neuritis is unknown, it has been associated with autoimmune diseases, infections, multiple sclerosis (MS), drug toxicity and deficiency of vitamin B_{12}.

Diagnosis of Optic Neuritis

The diagnosis of optic neuritis is usually based on clinical findings and ophthalmologic examination. A careful history, including information about recent illness, fever, or immunizations is helpful. An eye exam should be conducted with an assessment of visual acuity, pupil reactions, color vision, and peripheral vision. The optic nerve should be examined with ophthalmoscopy for inflammation and swelling. Additional tests may include magnetic resonance imaging (MRI) of the brain, spinal tap, and blood tests.

Treatment of Optic Neuritis

Vision often returns to normal within two to three weeks without treatment. In some cases, corticosteroids are given to speed recovery. If known, the underlying cause should be treated.

Chapter 29 | Disorders of the Retina

Chapter Contents

Section 29.1 | **Retinal Detachment**

This section includes text excerpted from "Retinal Detachment," National Eye Institute (NEI), June 26, 2019.

WHAT IS RETINAL DETACHMENT?

Retinal detachment is an eye problem that happens when your retina (a light-sensitive layer of tissue in the back of your eye) is pulled away from its normal position at the back of your eye.

WHAT ARE THE SYMPTOMS OF RETINAL DETACHMENT?

If only a small part of your retina has detached, you may not have any symptoms.

But, if more of your retina is detached, you may not be able to see as clearly as normal, and you may notice other sudden symptoms, including:

- A lot of new gray or black specks floating in your field of vision (floaters)
- Flashes of light in one eye or both eyes
- A dark shadow or "curtain" on the sides or in the middle of your field of vision

Retinal detachment can be a medical emergency. If you have symptoms of a detached retina, it is important to go to your eye doctor or the emergency room right away.

The symptoms of retinal detachment often come on quickly. If the retinal detachment is not treated right away, more of the retina can detach—which increases the risk of permanent vision loss or blindness.

ARE YOU AT RISK FOR RETINAL DETACHMENT?

Anyone can have a retinal detachment, but some people are at higher risk. You are at higher risk if:

- You or a family member has had a retinal detachment before

- You have had a serious eye injury
- You have had eye surgery, such as surgery to treat cataracts

Some other problems with your eyes may also put you at higher risk, including:

- Diabetic retinopathy (a condition in people with diabetes that affects blood vessels in the retina)
- Extreme nearsightedness (myopia), especially degenerative myopia
- Posterior vitreous detachment (when the gel-like fluid in the center of the eye pulls away from the retina)
- Certain other eye diseases, including retinoschisis or lattice degeneration

If you are concerned about your risk for retinal detachment, talk with your eye doctor.

WHAT CAUSES RETINAL DETACHMENT

There are many causes of retinal detachment, but the most common causes are aging or an eye injury.

There are three types of retinal detachment: rhegmatogenous, tractional, and exudative. Each type happens because of a different problem that causes your retina to move away from the back of your eye.

HOW YOU CAN PREVENT RETINAL DETACHMENT

There is no way to prevent retinal detachment—but you can lower your risk by wearing safety goggles or other protective eyewear when doing risky activities such as playing sports.

If you experience any symptoms of retinal detachment, go to your eye doctor or the emergency room right away. Early treatment can help prevent permanent vision loss.

It is also important to get comprehensive dilated eye exams regularly. A dilated eye exam can help your eye doctor find a small retinal tear or detachment early before it starts to affect your vision.

HOW DOES THE EYE DOCTOR CHECK FOR RETINAL DETACHMENT?

If you see any warning signs of a retinal detachment, your eye doctor can check your eyes with a dilated eye exam. The exam is simple and painless—your doctor will give you some eye drops to dilate (widen) your pupil and then look at your retina at the back of your eye.

If your eye doctor still needs more information after a dilated eye exam, you may get an ultrasound or an optical coherence tomography (OCT) scan of your eye. Both of these tests are painless and can help your eye doctor see the exact position of your retina.

WHAT IS THE TREATMENT FOR RETINAL DETACHMENT?

Depending on how much of your retina is detached and what type of retinal detachment you have, your eye doctor may recommend laser surgery, freezing treatment, or other types of surgery to fix any tears or breaks in your retina and reattach your retina to the back of your eye. Sometimes, your eye doctor will use more than one of these treatments at the same time.

- **Freeze treatment (cryopexy) or laser surgery**. If you have a small hole or tear in your retina, your doctor can use a freezing probe or a medical laser to seal any tears or breaks in your retina. You can usually get these treatments in the eye doctor's office.
- **Surgery**. If a larger part of your retina is detached from the back of your eye, you may need surgery to move your retina back into place. You will probably get these surgeries in a hospital.

Treatment for retinal detachment works well, especially if the detachment is found early. In some cases, you may need a second treatment or surgery if your retina detaches again—but treatment is ultimately successful for about 9 in 10 people.

Section 29.2 | **Retinitis Pigmentosa**

This section includes text excerpted from "Retinitis Pigmentosa," National Eye Institute (NEI), July 10, 2019.

WHAT IS RETINITIS PIGMENTOSA?

Retinitis pigmentosa (RP) is a group of rare, genetic disorders that involve a breakdown and loss of cells in the retina—which is the light-sensitive tissue that lines the back of the eye. Common symptoms include difficulty seeing at night and a loss of side (peripheral) vision.

How Common Is Retinitis Pigmentosa?

Retinitis pigmentosa is considered a rare disorder. Although current statistics are not available, it is generally estimated that the disorder affects roughly 1 in 4,000 people, both in the United States and worldwide.

WHAT CAUSES RETINITIS PIGMENTOSA

Retinitis pigmentosa is an inherited disorder that results from harmful changes in any one of more than 50 genes. These genes carry the instructions for making proteins that are needed in cells within the retina, called "photoreceptors." Some of the changes, or mutations, within genes are so severe that the gene cannot make the required protein, limiting the cell's function. Other mutations produce a protein that is toxic to the cell. Still, other mutations lead to an abnormal protein that does not function properly. In all three cases, the result is damage to the photoreceptors.

What Are Photoreceptors?

Photoreceptors are cells in the retina that begin the process of seeing. They absorb and convert light into electrical signals. These signals are sent to other cells in the retina and ultimately through the optic nerve to the brain where they are processed into the images we see. There are two general types of photoreceptors, called "rods and cones." Rods are in the outer regions of the retina, and allow us to see in dim and dark light. Cones reside mostly in the central portion of the retina, and allow us to perceive fine visual detail and color.

How Is Retinitis Pigmentosa Inherited?

To understand how RP is inherited, it is important to know a little more about genes and how they are passed from parent to child. Genes are bundled together on structures called "chromosomes." Each cell in your body contains 23 pairs of chromosomes. One copy of each chromosome is passed by a parent at conception through egg and sperm cells. The X and Y chromosomes, known as "sex chromosomes," determine whether a person is born female (XX) or male (XY). The 22 other paired chromosomes, called "autosomes," contain the vast majority of genes that determine nonsex traits. RP can be inherited in one of three ways:

AUTOSOMAL RECESSIVE INHERITANCE

In autosomal recessive inheritance, it takes two copies of the mutant gene to give rise to the disorder. An individual with a recessive gene mutation is known as a "carrier." When two carriers have a child, there is a:

- One in four chance the child will have the disorder
- One in two chance the child will be a carrier
- One in four chance the child will neither have the disorder nor be a carrier

AUTOSOMAL DOMINANT INHERITANCE

In this inheritance pattern, it takes just one copy of the gene with a disorder-causing mutation to bring about the disorder. When a parent has a dominant gene mutation, there is a one in two chance that any children will inherit this mutation and the disorder.

X-LINKED INHERITANCE

In this form of inheritance, mothers carry the mutated gene on one of their X chromosomes and pass it to their sons. Because females have two X chromosomes, the effect of a mutation on one X chromosome is offset by the normal gene on the other X chromosome. If a mother is a carrier of an X-linked disorder there is a:

- One in two chance of having a son with the disorder
- One in two chance of having a daughter who is a carrier

WHAT ARE THE SYMPTOMS OF RETINITIS PIGMENTOSA?

In the early stages of RP, rods are more severely affected than cones. As the rods die, people experience night blindness and a progressive loss of the visual field, the area of space that is visible at a given instant without moving the eyes. The loss of rods eventually leads to a breakdown and loss of cones. In the late stages of RP, as cones die, people tend to lose more of the visual field, developing tunnel vision. They may have difficulty performing essential tasks of daily living, such as reading, driving, walking without assistance, or recognizing faces and objects.

How Does Retinitis Pigmentosa Progress?

The symptoms of RP typically appear in childhood. Children often have difficulty getting around in the dark. It can also take abnormally long periods of time to adjust to changes in lighting. As their visual field becomes restricted, patients often trip over things and appear clumsy. People with RP often find bright lights uncomfortable, a condition known as, "photophobia." Because there are many gene mutations that cause the disorder, its progression can differ greatly from person to person. Some people retain central vision and a restricted visual field into their 50s, while others experience significant vision loss in early adulthood. Eventually, most individuals with RP will lose most of their sight.

HOW DOES THE DOCTOR CHECK FOR RETINITIS PIGMENTOSA?

Retinitis pigmentosa is diagnosed in part through an examination of the retina. An eye-care professional will use an ophthalmoscope, a tool that allows for a wider, clear view of the retina. This typically reveals abnormal, dark pigment deposits that streak the retina.

These pigment deposits are in part why the disorder was named "retinitis pigmentosa." Other tests for RP include:

- **Electroretinogram (ERG).** An ERG measures the electrical activity of photoreceptor cells. This test uses gold foil or a contact lens with electrodes attached. A flash of light is sent to the retina and the electrodes measure rod and cone cell responses. People with RP have a decreased electrical activity, reflecting the declining function of photoreceptors.
- **Visual field testing.** To determine the extent of vision loss, a clinician will give a visual field test. The person watches as a dot of light moves around the half-circle (180°) of space directly in front of the head and to either side. The patient pushes a button to indicate that she or he can see the light. This process results in a map of their visual field and their central vision.
- **Genetic testing.** In some cases, a clinician takes a deoxyribonucleic acid (DNA) sample from the person to give a genetic diagnosis. In this way, a person can learn about the progression of their particular form of the disorder.

WHAT IS THE TREATMENT FOR RETINITIS PIGMENTOSA?

A clinical trial sponsored by the National Eye Institute (NEI) found that a daily dose of 15,000 international units of vitamin A palmitate modestly slowed the progression of the disorder in adults. Because there are so many forms of RP, it is difficult to predict how any one patient will respond to this treatment. Talk to an eye-care professional to determine if taking vitamin A is right for you or your child.

An artificial vision device called the "Argus II" has also shown promise for restoring some vision to people with late-stage RP. The Argus II, developed by Second Sight with NEI support, is a prosthetic device that functions in place of lost photoreceptor cells. It consists of a light-sensitive electrode that is surgically implanted on the retina. A pair of glasses with a camera wirelessly transmits signals to the electrode that are then relayed to the brain. Although it does not restore normal vision, in clinical studies, the Argus II enabled people with RP to read large letters and navigate environments without the use of a cane or guide dog. In 2012, the U.S. Food and Drug Administration (FDA) granted a humanitarian device exemption for use of the Argus II to treat late-stage RP. This means the device has not proven effective, but the FDA has determined that its probable benefits outweigh its risks to health. The Argus II is eligible for Medicare payment.

LIVING WITH VISION LOSS

A number of services and devices are available to help people with vision loss carry out daily activities and maintain their independence. In addition to an eye-care professional, it is important to have help from a team of experts, which may include occupational therapists, orientation and mobility specialists, certified low vision therapists, and others.

Children with RP may benefit from low vision aids that maximize existing vision. For example, there are special lenses that magnify the central vision to expand the visual field and eliminate glare. Computer programs that read text are readily available. Closed-circuit televisions with a camera can adjust the text to suit one's vision. Portable lighting devices can adjust a dark or dim environment. Mobility training can teach people to use a cane or a guide dog, and eye-scanning techniques can help people to optimize remaining vision. Once a child is diagnosed, she or he will be referred to a low vision specialist, for a comprehensive evaluation. Parents may also want to meet with the child's school administrators and teachers to make sure that necessary accommodations are put in place.

For parents of children with RP, one challenge is to determine when a child might need to learn to use a cane or a guide dog. Having regular eye examinations to measure the progress of the disorder will help parents make informed decisions regarding low vision services and rehabilitation.

Section 29.3 | Retinoblastoma

This section includes text excerpted from "Retinoblastoma Treatment (PDQ®)–Patient Version," National Cancer Institute (NCI), December 20, 2019.

Retinoblastoma is a disease in which malignant (cancer) cells form in the tissues of the retina. The retina is made of nerve tissue that lines the inside wall of the back of the eye. It receives light and converts the light into signals that travel down the optic nerve to the brain. The brain decodes the signals so that you can see the image.

Retinoblastoma may be in one eye (unilateral) or in both eyes (bilateral). Cavitary retinoblastoma is a rare type of retinoblastoma in which cavities (hollow spaces) form within the tumor. Although retinoblastoma may occur at any age, it occurs most often in children younger than two years.

A child with a family history of retinoblastoma should have regular eye exams beginning early in life to check for retinoblastoma unless it is known that the child does not have the *RB1* gene change. Early diagnosis of retinoblastoma may mean the child will need less intense treatment. Talk with your child's doctor about the type of eye exam, how often eye exams are done, and at what age eye exams to check for retinoblastoma can stop.

FORMS OF RETINOBLASTOMA

A child is thought to have the heritable (inherited) form of retinoblastoma when there is a certain mutation (change) in the *RB1* gene. The mutation in the *RB1* gene may be passed from the parent to the child, or it may occur in the egg or sperm before conception or soon after conception.

Other factors that suggest the child may have the heritable form of retinoblastoma include the following:

- There is a family history of retinoblastoma.
- There is more than one tumor in the eye.
- There is a tumor in both eyes.

After heritable retinoblastoma has been diagnosed and treated, new tumors may continue to form for a few years. Regular eye exams to check for new tumors are usually done every 2 to 4 months for at least 28 months.

Most cases of retinoblastoma are the nonheritable form. Nonheritable retinoblastoma is not passed down from parents. This type of retinoblastoma is caused by mutations in the *RB1* gene that occur by chance after a child is born. Nonheritable retinoblastoma usually occurs in one eye.

A CHILD WITH HERITABLE RETINOBLASTOMA

A child with heritable retinoblastoma has an increased risk of a pineal tumor in the brain. When retinoblastoma and a brain tumor occur at the same time, it is called "trilateral retinoblastoma." The brain tumor is usually diagnosed between 20 and 36 months of age. Regular screening using MRI (magnetic resonance imaging) may be done for a child thought to have heritable retinoblastoma or for a child with retinoblastoma in one eye and a family history of the disease. CT (computerized tomography) scans are usually not used for routine screening in order to avoid exposing the child to ionizing radiation. Heritable retinoblastoma also increases the child's risk of other types of cancer, such as lung cancer, bladder cancer, or melanoma in later years. Regular follow-up exams are important.

Genetic testing can determine whether a child has the heritable or nonheritable form of retinoblastoma. It is not always clear from the family medical history whether a condition is inherited. Certain families may benefit from genetic counseling and genetic testing. Genetic counselors and other specially trained health professionals can help parents understand the following:

- Their family medical history
- Their options for *RB1* gene testing
- The risk of retinoblastoma for the child and the child's brothers or sisters
- The risks and benefits of learning genetic information

Genetic counselors can also help people cope with their genetic testing results, including how to discuss the results with family members.

Once it is known that the child has heritable retinoblastoma, other family members can be screened for the *RB1* mutation. For one specific mutation, the risk of retinoblastoma in a sibling may depend partly on whether the mutation is inherited from the mother or from the father.

SIGNS AND SYMPTOMS OF RETINOBLASTOMA

These and other signs and symptoms may be caused by retinoblastoma or by other conditions. Check with a doctor if your child has any of the following:

- Pupil of the eye that appears white instead of red when light shines into it. This may be seen in flash photographs of the child.
- Eyes that appear to be looking in different directions (crossed eyes)
- Pain or redness in the eye
- Infection around the eye
- Eyeball that is larger than normal
- Colored part of the eye and pupil look cloudy

TESTS AND PROCEDURES USED TO DIAGNOSE RETINOBLASTOMA

- **Physical exam and health history**. An exam of the body to check general signs of health, including checking for signs of disease, such as lumps or anything else that seems unusual. A history of the patient's health habits and past illnesses and treatments will also be taken. The doctor will ask if there is a family history of retinoblastoma.
- **Eye exam with dilated pupil**. An exam of the eye in which the pupil is dilated (opened wider) with medicated eye drops to allow the doctor to look through the lens and pupil to the retina. The inside of the eye, including the retina and the optic nerve, is examined with a light. In young children, this exam may be done under anesthesia. There are several types of eye exams that are done with the pupil dilated:

  - **Ophthalmoscopy**. An exam of the inside of the back of the eye to check the retina and optic nerve using a small magnifying lens and a light.
  - **Fluorescein angiography**. A procedure to look at blood vessels and the flow of blood inside the eye. An orange fluorescent dye called "fluorescein" is injected into a blood vessel in the arm and goes into the bloodstream. As the dye travels through blood vessels of the eye, a special camera takes pictures of the retina and choroid to find any blood vessels that are blocked or leaking.
- ***RB1* gene test**. A laboratory test in which a sample of blood or tissue is tested for a change in the *RB1* gene.
- **Ultrasound exam of the eye**. A procedure in which high-energy sound waves (ultrasound) are bounced off the internal tissues of the eye to make echoes. Eye drops are used to numb the eye and a small probe that sends and receives sound waves is placed gently on the surface of the eye. The echoes make a picture of the inside of the eye and the distance from the cornea to the retina is measured. The picture, called a "sonogram," shows on the screen of the ultrasound monitor. The picture can be printed to be looked at later.
- **Magnetic resonance imaging (MRI)**. A procedure that uses a magnet, radio waves, and a computer to make a series of detailed pictures of areas inside the body, such as the eye. This procedure is also called "nuclear magnetic resonance imaging" (NMRI).

Retinoblastoma can usually be diagnosed without a biopsy.

When retinoblastoma is in one eye, it sometimes forms in the other eye. Exams of the unaffected eye are done until it is known that the retinoblastoma is the nonheritable form.

PROGNOSIS AND TREATMENT OPTIONS

The prognosis and treatment options depend on the following:

- Whether the cancer is in one or both eyes

- The size and number of tumors
- Whether the tumor has spread to the area around the eye, to the brain, or to other parts of the body
- The age of the child
- How likely it is that vision can be saved in one or both eyes
- Whether second type of cancer has formed
- Whether the cancer is newly diagnosed or has recurred

Section 29.4 | Retinopathy of Prematurity

This section includes text excerpted from "Retinopathy of Prematurity," National Eye Institute (NEI), July 10, 2019.

WHAT IS RETINOPATHY OF PREMATURITY?

Retinopathy of prematurity (ROP) is a potentially blinding eye disorder that primarily affects premature infants weighing about 2¾ pounds (1250 grams) or less who are born before 31 weeks of gestation (a full-term pregnancy has a gestation of 38 to 42 weeks). The smaller a baby is at birth, the more likely that the baby is to develop ROP. This disorder—which usually develops in both eyes—is one of the most common causes of visual loss in childhood and can lead to lifelong vision impairment and blindness. ROP was first diagnosed in 1942.

How Many Infants Have Retinopathy of Prematurity?

Advances in neonatal care, smaller and more premature infants are being saved. These infants are at a much higher risk for ROP. Not all babies who are premature develop ROP. There are approximately 3.9 million infants born in the United States each year; of those, about 28,000 weigh 2¾ pounds or less. About 14,000 to 16,000 of these infants are affected by some degree of ROP. The disease improves and leaves no permanent damage in milder cases of ROP. About 90 percent of all infants with ROP are in the milder category and do not need treatment. However, infants with more severe disease can develop impaired vision or even blindness. About 1,100 to 1,500 infants annually develop ROP that is severe enough to require medical treatment. About 400 to 600 infants each year in the United States become legally blind from ROP.

ARE THERE DIFFERENT STAGES OF RETINOPATHY OF PREMATURITY?

Yes. ROP is classified in five stages, ranging from mild (stage I) to severe (stage V):

- **Stage I**—Mildly abnormal blood vessel growth. Many children who develop stage I improve with no treatment and eventually develop normal vision. The disease resolves on its own without further progression.
- **Stage II**—Moderately abnormal blood vessel growth. Many children who develop stage II improve with no treatment and eventually develop normal vision. The disease resolves on its own without further progression.
- **Stage III**—Severely abnormal blood vessel growth. The abnormal blood vessels grow toward the center of the eye instead of following their normal growth pattern along the surface of the retina. Some infants who develop stage III improve with no treatment and eventually develop normal vision. However, when infants have a certain degree of Stage III and "plus disease" develops, treatment is considered. "Plus disease" means that the blood vessels of the retina have become enlarged and twisted, indicating a worsening of the disease. Treatment at this point has a good chance of preventing retinal detachment.
- **Stage IV**—Partially detached retina. Traction from the scar produced by bleeding, abnormal vessels pulls the retina away from the wall of the eye.
- **Stage V**—Completely detached retina and the end-stage of the disease. If the eye is left alone at this stage, the baby can have severe visual impairment and even blindness.

Most babies who develop ROP have stages I or II. However, in a small number of babies, ROP worsens, sometimes very rapidly. Untreated ROP threatens to destroy vision.

CAN RETINOPATHY OF PREMATURITY CAUSE OTHER COMPLICATIONS?

Yes. Infants with ROP are considered to be at higher risk for developing certain eye problems later in life, such as retinal detachment, myopia (nearsightedness), strabismus (crossed eyes), amblyopia (lazy eye), and glaucoma. In many cases, these eye problems can be treated or controlled.

WHAT CAUSES RETINOPATHY OF PREMATURITY

Retinopathy of prematurity occurs when abnormal blood vessels grow and spread throughout the retina, the tissue that lines the back of the eye. These abnormal blood vessels are fragile and can leak, scarring the retina and pulling it out of position. This causes a retinal detachment. Retinal detachment is the main cause of visual impairment and blindness in ROP.

Several complex factors may be responsible for the development of ROP. The eye starts to develop at about 16 weeks of pregnancy when the blood vessels of the retina begin to form at the optic nerve in the back of the eye. The blood vessels grow gradually toward the edges of the developing retina, supplying oxygen and nutrients. During the last 12 weeks of pregnancy, the eye develops rapidly. When a baby is born full-term, the retinal blood vessel growth is mostly complete (retina usually finishes growing a few weeks to a month after birth). But, if a baby is born prematurely before these blood vessels have reached the edges of the retina, normal vessel growth may stop. The edges of the retina—the periphery—may not get enough oxygen and nutrients.

Scientists believe that the periphery of the retina then sends out signals to other areas of the retina for nourishment. As a result, new abnormal vessels begin to grow. These new blood vessels are fragile and weak and can bleed, leading to retinal scarring. When these scars shrink, they pull on the retina, causing it to detach from the back of the eye.

ARE THERE OTHER RISK FACTORS FOR RETINOPATHY OF PREMATURITY?

In addition to birth weight and how early a baby is born, other factors contributing to the risk of ROP include anemia, blood transfusions, respiratory distress, breathing difficulties, and the overall health of the infant.

An ROP epidemic occurred in the 1940s and early 1950s when hospital nurseries began using excessively high levels of oxygen in incubators to save the lives of premature infants. During this time, ROP was the leading cause of blindness in children in the United States. In 1954, scientists funded by the National Institutes of Health (NIH) determined that the relatively high levels of oxygen routinely given to premature infants at that time were an important risk factor, and that reducing the level of oxygen given to premature babies reduced the incidence of ROP. With newer technology and methods to monitor the oxygen levels of infants, oxygen use as a risk factor has diminished in importance.

Although it had been suggested as a factor in the development of ROP, researchers supported by the National Eye Institute (NEI) determined that lighting levels in hospital nurseries has no effect on the development of ROP.

WHAT IS THE TREATMENT FOR RETINOPATHY OF PREMATURITY?

The most effective proven treatments for ROP are laser therapy or cryotherapy. Laser therapy "burns away" the periphery of the retina, which has no normal blood vessels. With cryotherapy, physicians use an instrument that generates freezing temperatures to briefly touch spots on the surface of the eye that overlie the periphery of the retina. Both laser treatment and cryotherapy destroy the peripheral areas of the retina, slowing or reversing the abnormal growth of blood vessels. Unfortunately, the treatments also destroy some side vision. This is done to save the most important part of our sight—the sharp, central vision we need for "straight ahead" activities, such as reading, sewing, and driving.

Both laser treatments and cryotherapy are performed only on infants with advanced ROP, particularly stage III with "plus disease." Both treatments are considered invasive surgeries on the eye, and doctors do not know the long-term side effects of each.

In the later stages of ROP, other treatment options include:

- **Scleral buckle**. This involves placing a silicone band around the eye and tightening it. This keeps the vitreous gel from pulling on the scar tissue and allows the retina to flatten back down onto the wall of the eye. Infants who have had a sclera buckle need to have the band removed months or years later since the eye continues to grow; otherwise, they will become nearsighted. Sclera buckles are usually performed on infants with stage IV or V.
- **Vitrectomy**. Vitrectomy involves removing the vitreous and replacing it with a saline solution. After the vitreous has been removed, the scar tissue on the retina can be peeled back or cutaway, allowing the retina to relax and lay back down against the eyewall. Vitrectomy is performed only at stage V.

What Happens If Treatment Does Not Work

While ROP treatment decreases the chances for vision loss, it does not always prevent it. Not all babies respond to ROP treatment, and the disease may get worse. If treatment for ROP does not work, a retinal detachment may develop. Often, only part of the retina detaches (stage IV). When this happens, no further treatments may be needed, since a partial detachment may remain the same or go away without treatment. However, in some instances, physicians may recommend treatment to try to prevent further advancement of the retinal detachment (stage V). If the center of the retina or the entire retina detaches, central vision is threatened, and surgery may be recommended to reattach the retina.

Section 29.5 | **Juvenile Retinoschisis**

This section includes text excerpted from "Juvenile Retinoschisis," Genetic and Rare Diseases Information Center (GARD), National Center for Advancing Translational Sciences (NCATS), February 27, 2016. Reviewed March 2020.

Juvenile retinoschisis is an eye condition characterized by an impaired vision that begins in childhood and occurs almost exclusively in males. The condition affects the retina, which is a specialized light-sensitive tissue that lines the back of the eye. This affects the sharpness of vision. Central vision is more commonly affected. Vision often deteriorates early in life, but then usually becomes stable until late adulthood. The second decline in vision typically occurs in a man's fifties or sixties. Sometimes severe complications occur, including separation of the retinal layers (retinal detachment) or leakage of blood vessels in the retina (vitreous hemorrhage). These can lead to blindness. Juvenile retinoschisis is caused by mutations in the *RS1* gene. It is inherited in an X-linked recessive pattern. Low-vision aids can be helpful. Surgery may be needed for some complications.

CAUSES OF JUVENILE RETINOSCHISIS

Mutations in the *RS1* gene cause most cases of juvenile retinoschisis. The *RS1* gene provides instructions for producing a protein called "retinoschisin," which is found in the retina. Studies suggest that retinoschisin plays a role in the development and maintenance of the retina, perhaps playing a role in cell adhesion (the attachment of cells together).

RS1 gene mutations lead to a reduced amount or complete absence of retinoschisin, which can cause tiny splits (schisis) or tears to form in the retina. This damage often forms a "spoke-wheel" pattern in the macula, which can be seen during an eye examination. In about half of individuals, these abnormalities are seen in the area of the macula, affecting visual acuity. In the other half, the sides of the retina are affected, resulting in impaired peripheral vision.

Some individuals with juvenile retinoschisis do not have a mutation in the *RS1* gene. In these individuals, the cause of the disorder is unknown.

INHERITANCE OF JUVENILE RETINOSCHISIS

Juvenile retinoschisis is inherited in an x-linked recessive pattern. The gene associated with this condition is located on the X chromosome, one of the two sex chromosomes. In males (who have only one X chromosome), one altered copy of the gene in each cell is sufficient to cause the condition. In females (who have two X chromosomes), a mutation must be present in both copies of the gene to cause the disorder. Males are affected by X-linked recessive disorders much more frequently than females. A striking characteristic of X-linked inheritance is that fathers cannot pass X-linked traits to their sons.

In X-linked recessive inheritance, a female with one mutated copy of the gene (mutation) in each cell is called a "carrier." She can pass on the mutation, but usually does not experience signs and symptoms of the condition. Carrier women have a 50 percent chance of passing the mutation to their children, males who inherit the mutation will be affected; females who inherit the mutation will be carriers and will nearly always have normal vision. Carrier testing for at-risk female relatives and prenatal testing for pregnancies at increased risk are possible if the disease-causing mutation in the family is known.

TREATMENT OF JUVENILE RETINOSCHISIS

There is no specific treatment for juvenile retinoschisis. Low vision services are designed to benefit those whose ability to function is compromised by impaired vision. Public-school systems are mandated by federal law to provide an appropriate education for children who have vision impairment. Surgery may be required to address the infrequent complications of vitreous hemorrhage and retinal detachment. Affected individuals should avoid high-contact sports and other activities that can cause head trauma to reduce the risk of retinal detachment and vitreous hemorrhage.

Section 29.6 | Choroideremia

This section includes text excerpted from "Choroideremia," Genetics Home Reference (GHR), National Institutes of Health (NIH), March 17, 2020.

WHAT IS CHOROIDEREMIA?

Choroideremia is a condition characterized by progressive vision loss that mainly affects males. The first symptom of this condition is usually an impairment of night vision (night blindness), which can occur in early childhood. A progressive narrowing of the field of vision (tunnel vision) follows, as well as a decrease in the ability to see details (visual acuity). These vision problems are due to an ongoing loss of cells (atrophy) in the specialized light-sensitive tissue that lines the back of the eye (retina) and a nearby network of blood vessels (the choroid). The vision impairment in choroideremia worsens over time, but the progression varies among affected individuals. However, all individuals with this condition will develop blindness, most commonly in late adulthood.

FREQUENCY OF CHOROIDEREMIA

The prevalence of choroideremia is estimated to be 1 in 50,000 to 100,000 people. However, it is likely that this condition is underdiagnosed because of its similarities to other eye disorders. Choroideremia is thought to account for approximately, four percent of all blindness.

CAUSES OF CHOROIDEREMIA

Mutations in the *CHM* gene cause choroideremia. The *CHM* gene provides instructions for producing the Rab escort protein-1 (REP-1). As an escort protein, REP-1 attaches to molecules called "Rab proteins" within the cell and directs them to the membranes of various cell compartments (organelles). Rab proteins are involved in the movement of proteins and organelles within cells (intracellular trafficking). Mutations in the *CHM* gene lead to an absence of REP-1 protein or the production of a REP-1 protein that cannot carry out its protein escort function. This lack of functional REP-1 prevents Rab proteins from reaching and attaching (binding) to the organelle membranes. Without the aid of Rab proteins in intracellular trafficking, cells die prematurely.

The REP-1 protein is active (expressed) throughout the body, as is a similar protein, REP-2. Research suggests that when REP-1 is absent or nonfunctional, REP-2 can perform the protein escort duties of REP-1 in many of the body's tissues. Very little REP-2 protein is present in the retina, however, so it cannot compensate for the loss of REP-1 in this tissue. Loss of REP-1 function and subsequent misplacement of Rab proteins within the cells of the retina causes the progressive vision loss characteristic of choroideremia.

Chapter 30 | **Disorders of the Vitreous**

Chapter Contents

Section 30.1 | Floaters

This section includes text excerpted from "Floaters," National Eye Institute (NEI), July 5, 2019.

WHAT ARE FLOATERS?

Floaters are little "cobwebs" or specks that float about in your field of vision. They are small, dark, shadowy shapes that can look like spots, thread-like strands, or squiggly lines. They move as your eyes move and seem to dart away when you try to look at them directly. They do not follow your eye movements precisely and usually drift when your eyes stop moving.

Most people have floaters and learn to ignore them; they are usually not noticed until they become numerous or more prominent. Floaters can become apparent when looking at something bright, such as white paper or a blue sky.

Floaters and Retinal Detachment

Sometimes a section of the vitreous pulls the fine fibers away from the retina all at once, rather than gradually, causing many new floaters to appear suddenly. This is called a "vitreous detachment," which in most cases is not sight-threatening and requires no treatment.

However, a sudden increase in floaters, possibly accompanied by light flashes or peripheral (side) vision loss, could indicate a retinal detachment. A retinal detachment occurs when any part of the retina, the eye's light-sensitive tissue, is lifted or pulled from its normal position at the back wall of the eye.

A retinal detachment is a serious condition and should always be considered an emergency. If left untreated, it can lead to permanent visual impairment within two or three days or even blindness in the eye.

Those who experience a sudden increase in floaters, flashes of light in peripheral vision, or a loss of peripheral vision should have an eye-care professional examine their eyes as soon as possible.

WHAT CAUSES FLOATERS

Floaters occur when the vitreous, a gel-like substance that fills about 80 percent of the eye and helps it maintain a round shape, slowly shrinks.

As the vitreous shrinks, it becomes somewhat stringy, and the strands can cast tiny shadows on the retina. These are floaters.

In most cases, floaters are part of the natural aging process and simply an annoyance. They can be distracting at first, but eventually tend to "settle" at the bottom of the eye, becoming less bothersome. They usually settle below the line of sight and do not go away completely.

However, there are other, more serious causes of floaters, including infection, inflammation (uveitis), hemorrhaging, retinal tears, and injury to the eye.

ARE YOU AT RISK FOR FLOATERS?

Floaters are more likely to develop as we age and are more common in people who are very nearsighted, have diabetes, or who have had a cataract operation.

WHAT IS THE TREATMENT FOR FLOATERS?

For people who have floaters that are simply annoying, no treatment is recommended.

On rare occasions, floaters can be so dense and numerous that they significantly affect vision. In these cases, a vitrectomy, a surgical procedure that removes floaters from the vitreous, may be needed.

A vitrectomy removes the vitreous gel, along with its floating debris, from the eye. The vitreous is replaced with a salt solution. Because the vitreous is mostly water, you will not notice any change between the salt solution and the original vitreous.

This operation carries significant risks to sight because of possible complications, which include retinal detachment, retinal tears, and cataract. Most eye surgeons are reluctant to recommend this surgery unless the floaters seriously interfere with vision.

Section 30.2 | **Vitreous Detachment**

This section includes text excerpted from "Vitreous Detachment," National Eye Institute (NEI), July 11, 2019.

WHAT IS VITREOUS DETACHMENT?

Most of the eye's interior is filled with vitreous, a gel-like substance that helps the eye maintain a round shape. There are millions of fine fibers intertwined within the vitreous that are attached to the surface of the retina, the eye's light-sensitive tissue. As we age, the vitreous slowly shrinks, and these fine fibers pull on the retinal surface. Usually, the fibers break, allowing the vitreous to separate and shrink from the retina. This is a vitreous detachment.

In most cases, a vitreous detachment, also known as a "posterior vitreous detachment," is not sight-threatening and requires no treatment.

ARE YOU AT RISK FOR VITREOUS DETACHMENT?

A vitreous detachment is a common condition that usually affects people over 50 years of age, and is very common after 80 years of age. People who are nearsighted are also at increased risk. Those who have a vitreous detachment in one eye are likely to have one in the other, although it may not happen until years later.

WHAT ARE THE SYMPTOMS OF VITREOUS DETACHMENT?

As the vitreous shrinks, it becomes somewhat stringy, and the strands can cast tiny shadows on the retina that you may notice as floaters, which appear as little "cobwebs" or specks that seem to float about in your field of vision. If you try to look at these shadows they appear to quickly dart out of the way.

One symptom of a vitreous detachment is a small but sudden increase in the number of new floaters. This increase in floaters may be accompanied by flashes of light (lightning streaks) in your peripheral, or side vision. In most cases, either you will not notice a vitreous detachment, or you will find it merely annoying because of the increase in floaters.

HOW DOES VITREOUS DETACHMENT AFFECT VISION?

Although a vitreous detachment does not threaten sight, once in a while some of the vitreous fibers pull so hard on the retina that they create a macular hole to or lead to a retinal detachment. Both of these conditions are sight-threatening and should be treated immediately.

If left untreated, a macular hole or detached retina can lead to permanent vision loss in the affected eye. Those who experience a sudden increase in floaters or an increase in flashes of light in peripheral vision should have an eye-care professional examine their eyes as soon as possible.

HOW DOES THE EYE DOCTOR CHECK FOR VITREOUS DETACHMENT?

The only way to diagnose the cause of the problem is by a comprehensive dilated eye examination. If the vitreous detachment has led to a macular hole or detached retina, early treatment can help prevent loss of vision.

Chapter 31 | **Disorders of the Uvea**

Chapter Contents

Section 31.1 | **Uveal Coloboma**

This section includes text excerpted from "Coloboma," National Eye Institute (NEI), August 14, 2019.

WHAT IS A COLOBOMA?

Coloboma comes from a Greek word which means "curtailed." It is used to describe conditions where normal tissue in or around the eye is missing from birth.

To understand coloboma, it is useful to be familiar with the normal structure and appearance of the eye, and the terms related to the different parts of the eye.

WHAT ARE THE DIFFERENT TYPES OF COLOBOMA?

There are different kinds of coloboma, depending on which part of the eye is missing. Coloboma can affect the:

- Eyelid
- Lens
- Macula

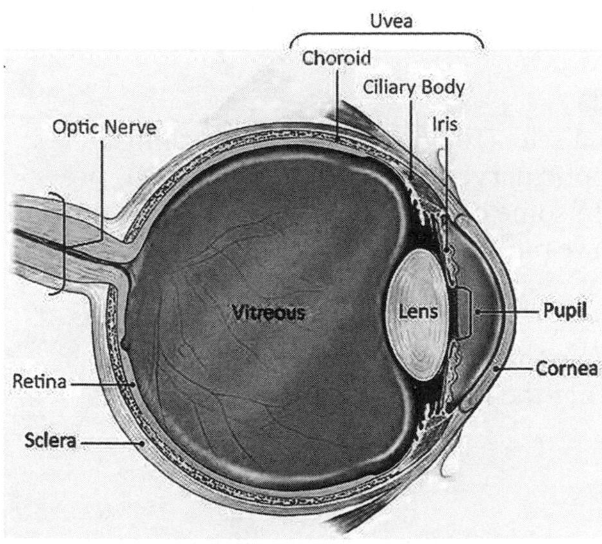

Figure 31.1. Diagram of the Eye

- Optic nerve
- Uvea

Eyelid Coloboma

In eyelid coloboma, a piece of either the upper or lower eyelid is absent. Eyelid coloboma may be part of a genetic syndrome or happen as a result of a disruption of eyelid development in a baby. A syndrome is a specific grouping of birth defects or symptoms present in one person.

Lens Coloboma

In this type of coloboma, a piece of the lens is absent. The lens, which helps focus light on the retina, will typically appear with a notch.

Macular Coloboma

This happens when the center of the retina, called the "macula," does not develop normally. The macula is responsible for daylight, fine and color vision. Macular coloboma may be caused when normal eye development is interrupted or following an inflammation of the retina during the development of the baby.

Optic Nerve Coloboma

Optic nerve coloboma refers to one of two distinct things:

- An abnormal optic nerve that is deeply "excavated" or hollowed out. In some cases, it can also be referred to as an "optic nerve pit." The optic nerve is the bundle of nerve fibers that relays the light signals from the eye to the brain.
- A uveal coloboma that is large enough to involve the optic nerve, either the inferior portion or, the entire optic disc.

Uveal Coloboma

This coloboma can present as an iris coloboma (the iris is the colored part of the eye), with the traditional "keyhole" or "cat-eye" appearance to the iris, and/or as a chorioretinal coloboma where the retina in the lower inside corner of the eye is missing.

HOW COMMON IS UVEAL COLOBOMA?

Uveal coloboma is a rare condition that is not always well documented. Depending on the study and where the study was conducted, a majority of estimates range from 0.4 to 5 cases per 10,000 births. Some cases may go unnoticed because uveal coloboma does not always affect vision or the outside appearance of the eye.

Uveal coloboma is a significant cause of blindness. Studies estimate that 5 to 10 percent of blind European children have uveal coloboma or uveal coloboma-related malformations.

WHAT CAUSES UVEAL COLOBOMA

It is believed that uveal coloboma is primarily genetic in origin. "Genetic" means that the coloboma was caused by a gene that was not working properly when the eye was forming. Sometimes coloboma is part of a specific genetic syndrome, for which the genetics are known. For instance, coloboma is one feature of CHARGE syndrome, which is associated with a change in, or complete deletion of a gene called "*CHD7*" in most cases.

Researchers have found genes associated with eye malformation in the microphthalmia, anophthalmia, coloboma (MAC) spectrum in up to 20 percent of cases. To date, however, we still do not know which genes explain most cases of coloboma.

Some researchers have proposed that certain environmental factors may contribute to developing coloboma, either in humans or in animals. These findings have been published over time in the research literature, but there has been no systematic analysis of possible links. For instance, it is known that babies exposed to alcohol during pregnancy can develop coloboma—but they also have other anomalies. There are no known strong links between environmental exposures and isolated coloboma.

It is always possible that coloboma happens strictly by chance. In summary, there is little data to presently say why coloboma happened to a person in a family where no one else is affected.

How Does Uveal Coloboma Happen?

To understand how uveal coloboma happens, we first have to understand how the eye forms in the developing baby. The eyes start as stalks coming out of the brain. The tip of each stalk will become the eye itself, while the rest of the stalk will become the optic nerve linking the eye to the brain. There is a seam at the bottom of each stalk, where blood vessels originally run. This seam is known as the "optic fissure," or the "choroidal fissure," or the "embryonic fissure." Starting in the fifth week of gestation (pregnancy), this seam must close. The closure starts roughly in the middle of the developing eye and runs in both directions. This process is finished by the seventh week of gestation. If for some reason, the closure does not happen, a uveal coloboma is formed.

Depending on where the closure did not happen, the baby can have an iris coloboma (front of the fissure), a chorioretinal coloboma (back of the fissure), or any combination of these. Uveal coloboma can affect one eye (unilateral) or both eyes (bilateral). The condition can be the same in both eyes (symmetric) or different in both eyes (asymmetric). A uveal coloboma may go from front to back (continuous) or have "skip lesions." The fact that the seam runs at the bottom of the stalk is the reason why uveal coloboma is always located in the lower inside corner of the eye.

How Is Uveal Coloboma Inherited?

Isolated coloboma can follow all possible patterns of single gene inheritance, namely autosomal dominant, autosomal recessive and X-linked. In one family, however, coloboma will follow only one pattern. For instance, in case of an autosomal dominant pattern, a person with coloboma would have a one in two chance of passing on the coloboma to each of her or his offspring. In families with a single case of coloboma, it is not possible to say what pattern of inheritance is involved; therefore, it is not possible to give an exact recurrence risk number. The recurrence risk of coloboma computed from averaging data across many families (empiric risk) is about 10 percent. This is an imperfect number, as it mixes information from families where this risk may be close to zero percent with information from families where the actual risk maybe 25 percent or even 50 percent.

The topic of inheritance of coloboma is complicated by several factors:

- Sometimes a person who is at risk for developing coloboma may not develop the condition, or it may be so minor that it goes unnoticed. This may appear in family history as an inconsistent, noninterpretable pattern of inheritance.
- Knowing the pattern of inheritance of coloboma in a family does not give information on how the vision of an at-risk person will be affected. The location (front versus back of the eye), side (left eye, right eye, or both) and size of the coloboma cannot be predicted.
- There may be more than one gene involved in being at risk for coloboma, and environmental factors might play a role.

For coloboma due to a known syndrome, such as CHARGE syndrome, inheritance is based on what is known about the genetic basis of that particular syndrome. However, it is rarely, if ever, possible to say whether coloboma will be a feature of the syndrome in a person inheriting the genetic background responsible for this syndrome.

WHAT ARE THE SYMPTOMS OF UVEAL COLOBOMA?

There may or may not be any symptoms related to coloboma; it all depends on the amount and location of the missing tissue. People with a coloboma affecting the macula and the optic nerve will likely have reduced vision. In general, it is difficult to exactly predict what level of vision a baby will have only by looking at how much of the retina is missing. A more precise estimate of the level of vision can be obtained over time, as the child grows and can perform more vision tests.

People with a coloboma affecting any part of the retina will have what is called a "field defect." A field defect means that a person is a missing vision in a specific location. Because coloboma is located in the lower part of the retina, vision in the upper part of the field of vision will be missing. This may or may not be noticeable to the affected person and may or may not affect performing daily activities.

A person with a coloboma affecting the front of the eye only will not have any decreased vision from it. Some people, however, have reported being more sensitive to light.

ARE THERE OTHER DISEASES OR CONDITIONS ASSOCIATED WITH COLOBOMA?

In the Eye

Coloboma is sometimes found in association with other eye features. These may include:

- Difference in eye color between the two eyes (heterochromia)
- Small eye (microphthalmia)
- Increased thickness of the cornea. The cornea is the clear front part of the eye.
- Clouding of the lens (cataract)
- Elevated pressure in the eye (glaucoma)
- Retinal malformation (retinal dysplasia)
- Nearsightedness (myopia) or farsightedness (hyperopia)
- Involuntary eye movements (nystagmus)
- Protrusion of the back of the eyeball (posterior staphyloma)

In Other Parts of the Body

Coloboma may be an isolated feature or may be found with other features. Sometimes these other features may be few and minor, such as skin tags near the ear. Sometimes they may be more numerous and severe, such as a heart or a kidney defect. A few of these associations may be genetic syndromes. These include (but are not limited to):

- CHARGE syndrome

- Cat-Eye syndrome (CES)
- Kabuki syndrome (KS)
- 13q deletion syndrome
- Wolf-Hirschhorn syndrome (WHS)

WHAT IS THE TREATMENT FOR UVEAL COLOBOMA?

Patients with uveal coloboma should have yearly follow-up exams by an eye-care professional. However, there is no medication or surgery that can cure or reverse coloboma and make the eye whole again. Treatment consists of helping patients adjust to vision problems and make the most of the vision they have by:

- Correcting any refractive error with glasses or contact lenses
- Maximizing the vision of the most affected eye in asymmetric cases. This may involve patching or using drops to temporarily blur vision in the stronger eye for a limited period of time.
- Ensuring that amblyopia (lazy eye) does not develop in childhood in case of asymmetry. Sometimes amblyopia treatment (patching, glasses and/or drops) can improve vision in eyes even with severe colobomas.
- Treating any other eye condition that may be present with coloboma, such as cataracts
- Treating any complications that might arise from a retinal coloboma later in life, such as the growth of new blood vessels at the back of the eye (neovascularization) and/or retinal detachment. These complications are rare, in the order of 1 to 2 percent based on our experience.
- Using low vision devices, as needed
- Making use of rehabilitation services, such as early intervention programs
- Offering genetic counseling to the patient and family members

If the eye with the coloboma is very small (microphthalmia), other follow-ups may be needed. Conformers and expanders may be used to help support the face and encourage the eye socket to grow. Children may also be fitted for a prosthetic (artificial) eye to improve appearance. As the face develops, new conformers will need to be made.

For people who wish to alter the appearance of a coloboma affecting the front of the eye, two options are available:

- Colored contact lenses that make the black part of the eye (pupil) round.
- Surgery to make the pupil rounder. This procedure pulls and sutures together the lower edges of the iris.

IS GENETIC TESTING AVAILABLE FOR UVEAL COLOBOMA?

Testing may be available in cases where the coloboma is part of a specific genetic syndrome. This testing would look for the gene(s) causing that syndrome. Genetic testing is done on a blood sample and may involve looking at the patient's chromosomes or looking at one or more specific genes on some of the chromosomes.

To date, there is no high yield clinical test for uveal coloboma since at least 80 percent of cases remain unexplained. Genes that have been associated with uveal coloboma may be part of broader panel tests for conditions, such as anophthalmia, microphthalmia, anterior segment dysgenesis and/or developmental eye diseases. However, results from such testing will be negative in the majority of cases.

Section 31.2 | **Uveal Melanoma**

This section includes text excerpted from "Intraocular (Uveal) Melanoma Treatment (PDQ®)—Patient Version," National Cancer Institute (NCI), October 2, 2019.

WHAT IS UVEAL MELANOMA?

Intraocular melanoma begins in the middle of three layers of the wall of the eye. The outer layer includes the white sclera (the white of the eye) and the clear cornea at the front of the eye. The inner layer has a lining of nerve tissue, called the "retina," which senses light and sends images along the optic nerve to the brain.

The middle layer, where intraocular melanoma forms, is called the "uvea" or "uveal tract," and has three main parts:

Iris

The iris is the colored area at the front of the eye (the eye color). It can be seen through the clear cornea. The pupil is in the center of the iris and it changes size to let more or less light into the eye. Intraocular melanoma of the iris is usually a small tumor that grows slowly and rarely spreads to other parts of the body.

Ciliary body

The ciliary body is a ring of tissue with muscle fibers that change the size of the pupil and the shape of the lens. It is found behind the iris. Changes in the shape of the lens help the eye focus. The ciliary body also makes the clear fluid that fills the space between the cornea and the iris. Intraocular melanoma of the ciliary body is often larger and more likely to spread to other parts of the body than intraocular melanoma of the iris.

Choroid

The choroid is a layer of blood vessels that bring oxygen and nutrients to the eye. Most intraocular melanomas begin in the choroid. Intraocular melanoma of the choroid is often larger and more likely to spread to other parts of the body than intraocular melanoma of the iris.

Intraocular melanoma is rare cancer that forms from cells that make melanin in the iris, ciliary body, and choroid. It is the most common eye cancer in adults.

RISK FACTORS OF UVEAL MELANOMA

Anything that increases your risk of getting a disease is called a "risk factor." Having a risk factor does not mean that you will get cancer; not having risk factors does not mean that you will not get cancer. Talk with your doctor if you think you may be at risk.

Risk factors for intraocular melanoma include the following:

- Having a fair complexion, which includes the following:
  - Fair skin that freckles and burns easily, does not tan, or tans poorly
  - Blue or green or other light-colored eyes
- Older age
- Being white

SIGNS OF UVEAL MELANOMA

Intraocular melanoma may not cause early signs or symptoms. It is sometimes found during a regular eye exam when the doctor dilates the pupil and looks into the eye. Signs and symptoms may be caused by intraocular melanoma or by other conditions. Check with your doctor if you have any of the following:

- Blurred vision or other change in vision
- Floaters (spots that drift in your field of vision) or flashes of light
- A dark spot on the iris
- A change in the size or shape of the pupil
- A change in the position of the eyeball in the eye socket

TESTS USED TO DIAGNOSE UVEAL MELANOMA

The following tests and procedures may be used:

- **Physical exam and history**. An exam of the body to check general signs of health, including checking for signs of disease, such as lumps or anything else that seems unusual. A history of the patient's health habits and past illnesses and treatments will also be taken.
- **An eye exam with dilated pupil.** An exam of the eye in which the pupil is dilated (enlarged) with medicated eye drops to allow the doctor to look through the lens and pupil to the retina. The inside of the eye, including the retina and the optic nerve, is checked. Pictures may be taken over time to keep track of changes in the size of the tumor. There are several types of eye exams:

- **Ophthalmoscopy.** An exam of the inside of the back of the eye to check the retina and optic nerve using a small magnifying lens and a light.
- **Slit-lamp biomicroscopy.** An exam of the inside of the eye to check the retina, optic nerve, and other parts of the eye using a strong beam of light and a microscope.
- **Gonioscopy.** An exam of the front part of the eye between the cornea and iris. A special instrument is used to see if the area where fluid drains out of the eye is blocked.

- **Ultrasound exam of the eye.** A procedure in which high-energy sound waves (ultrasound) are bounced off the internal tissues of the eye to make echoes. Eye drops are used to numb the eye and a small probe that sends and receives sound waves is placed gently on the surface of the eye. The echoes make a picture of the inside of the eye and the distance from the cornea to the retina is measured. The picture, called a "sonogram," shows on the screen of the ultrasound monitor.
- **High-resolution ultrasound biomicroscopy (UBM).** A procedure in which high-energy sound waves (ultrasound) are bounced off the internal tissues of the eye to make echoes. Eye drops are used to numb the eye and a small probe that sends and receives sound waves is placed gently on the surface of the eye. The echoes make a more detailed picture of the inside of the eye than a regular ultrasound. The tumor is checked for its size, shape, and thickness, and for signs that the tumor has spread to nearby tissue.
- **Transillumination of the globe and iris**. An exam of the iris, cornea, lens, and ciliary body with a light placed on either the upper or lower lid.
- **Fluorescein angiography (FA)**. A procedure to look at blood vessels and the flow of blood inside the eye. An orange fluorescent dye (fluorescein) is injected into a

blood vessel in the arm and goes into the bloodstream. As the dye travels through the blood vessels of the eye, a special camera takes pictures of the retina and choroid to find any areas that are blocked or leaking.

- **Indocyanine green angiography (IGA).** A procedure to look at blood vessels in the choroid layer of the eye. A green dye (indocyanine green) is injected into a blood vessel in the arm and goes into the bloodstream. As the dye travels through the blood vessels of the eye, a special camera takes pictures of the retina and choroid to find any areas that are blocked or leaking.
- **Ocular coherence tomography (OCT).** An imaging test that uses light waves to take cross-section pictures of the retina, and sometimes the choroid, to see if there is swelling or fluid beneath the retina.

FACTORS AFFECTING PROGNOSIS AND TREATMENT OPTIONS

The prognosis and treatment options depend on the following:

- How the melanoma cells look under a microscope
- The size and thickness of the tumor
- The part of the eye the tumor is in (iris, ciliary body, or choroid)
- Whether the tumor has spread within the eye or to other places in the body
- Whether there are certain changes in the genes linked to intraocular melanoma
- The patient's age and general health
- Whether the tumor has recurred (come back) after treatment

Section 31.3 | **Uveitis**

This section includes text excerpted from "Uveitis," National Eye Institute (NEI), July 11, 2019.

WHAT IS UVEITIS?

Uveitis is a general term describing a group of inflammatory diseases that produces swelling and destroys eye tissues. These diseases can slightly reduce vision or lead to severe vision loss.

The term "uveitis" is used because the diseases often affect a part of the eye called the "uvea." Nevertheless, uveitis is not limited to the uvea. These diseases also affect the lens, retina, optic nerve, and vitreous, producing reduced vision or blindness.

Uveitis may be caused by problems or diseases occurring in the eye or it can be part of an inflammatory disease affecting other parts of the body. It can happen at all ages and primarily affects people between 20 to 60 years old. Uveitis can last for a short (acute) or a long (chronic) time. The severest forms of uveitis reoccur many times.

Eye-care professionals may describe the disease more specifically as:

- Anterior uveitis
- Intermediate uveitis
- Posterior uveitis
- Panuveitis uveitis

Eye-care professionals may also describe the disease as infectious or noninfectious uveitis.

WHAT IS UVEA AND WHAT PARTS OF THE EYE ARE MOST AFFECTED BY UVEITIS?

The uvea is the middle layer of the eye which contains much of the eye's blood vessels. This is one way that inflammatory cells can enter the eye. Located between the sclera, the eye's white outer coat, and the inner layer of the eye, called the "retina," the uvea consists of the iris, ciliary body, and choroid:

- **Iris**. The colored circle at the front of the eye. It defines eye color, secretes nutrients to keep the lens healthy, and controls the amount of light that enters the eye by adjusting the size of the pupil.
- **Ciliary body**. It is located between the iris and the choroid. It helps the eye focus by controlling the shape of the lens and it provides nutrients to keep the lens healthy.
- **Choroid**. A thin, spongy network of blood vessels, which primarily provides nutrients to the retina.

Uveitis disrupts vision by primarily causing problems with the lens, retina, optic nerve, and vitreous:

- **Lens**. Transparent tissue that allows light into the eye.
- **Retina**. The layer of cells on the back, inside part of the eye that converts light into electrical signals sent to the brain.
- **Optic nerve**. A bundle of nerve fibers that transmits electrical signals from the retina to the brain.
- **Vitreous**. The fluid-filled space inside the eye.

WHAT CAUSES UVEITIS

Uveitis is caused by inflammatory responses inside the eye.

Inflammation is the body's natural response to tissue damage, germs, or toxins. It produces swelling, redness, heat, and destroys tissues as certain white blood cells (WBCs) rush to the affected part of the body to contain or eliminate the insult.

Uveitis may be caused by:

- An attack from the body's own immune system (autoimmunity)
- Infections or tumors occurring within the eye or in other parts of the body
- Bruises to the eye
- Toxins that may penetrate the eye

The disease will cause symptoms, such as decreased vision, pain, light sensitivity, and increased floaters. In many cases the cause is unknown.

What Diseases Are Associated with Uveitis?

Uveitis can be associated with many diseases including:

- Acquired immunodeficiency syndrome (AIDS)
- Ankylosing spondylitis (AS)
- Behcet syndrome (BS)
- Cytomegalovirus (CMV) retinitis
- Herpes zoster infection
- Histoplasmosis
- Kawasaki disease (KS)
- Multiple sclerosis (MS)
- Psoriasis
- Reactive arthritis
- Rheumatoid arthritis (RA)
- Sarcoidosis
- Syphilis
- Toxoplasmosis
- Tuberculosis (TB)
- Ulcerative colitis (UC)
- Vogt Koyanagi Harada's disease (VKH)

WHAT ARE THE TYPES OF UVEITIS?

Uveitis is usually classified by where it occurs in the eye.

What Is Anterior Uveitis?

Anterior uveitis occurs in the front of the eye. It is the most common form of uveitis, predominantly occurring in young and middle-aged people. Many cases occur in healthy people and may only affect one eye but some are associated with rheumatologic, skin, gastrointestinal, lung, and infectious diseases.

What Is Intermediate Uveitis?

Intermediate uveitis is commonly seen in young adults. The center of the inflammation often appears in the vitreous. It has been linked to several disorders including, sarcoidosis and multiple sclerosis.

What Is Posterior Uveitis?

Posterior uveitis is the least common form of uveitis. It primarily occurs in the back of the eye, often involving both the retina and the choroid. It is often called "choroiditis" or "chorioretinitis." There are many infectious and noninfectious causes of posterior uveitis.

What Is Panuveitis?

Panuveitis is a term used when all three major parts of the eye are affected by inflammation. Behcet's disease is one of the most well-known forms of panuveitis and it greatly damages the retina.

Intermediate, posterior, and panuveitis are the most severe and highly recurrent forms of uveitis. They often cause blindness if left untreated.

WHAT ARE THE SYMPTOMS OF UVEITIS?

Uveitis can affect one or both eyes. Symptoms may develop rapidly and can include:

- Blurred vision
- Dark, floating spots in the vision (floaters)
- Eye pain
- Redness of the eye
- Sensitivity to light (photophobia)

Anyone suffering eye pain, severe light sensitivity, and any change in vision should immediately be examined by an ophthalmologist.

The signs and symptoms of uveitis depend on the type of inflammation.

Acute anterior uveitis (AAU) may occur in one or both eyes and in adults is characterized by eye pain, blurred vision, sensitivity to light, a small pupil, and redness.

Intermediate uveitis causes blurred vision and floaters. Usually, it is not associated with pain.

Posterior uveitis can produce vision loss. This type of uveitis can only be detected during an eye examination.

HOW DOES THE EYE DOCTOR CHECK FOR UVEITIS?

The diagnosis of uveitis includes a thorough examination and the recording of the patient's complete medical history. Laboratory tests may be done to rule out an infection or an autoimmune disorder.

A central nervous system (CNS) evaluation will often be performed on patients with a subgroup of intermediate uveitis, called "pars planitis," to determine whether they have multiple sclerosis which is oftcn associated with pars planitis.

The eye exams used include:

- **An eye chart or visual acuity (VA) test**. This test measures whether a patient's vision has decreased.
- **A funduscopic exam**. The pupil is widened (dilated) with eye drops and then a light is shown through with an instrument called an "ophthalmoscope" to noninvasively inspect the back, inside part of the eye.
- **Ocular pressure**. An instrument, such a tonometer or a tonopen, measures the pressure inside the eye. Drops that numb the eye may be used for this test.
- **Slit-lamp exam**. A slit lamp noninvasively inspects much of the eye. It can inspect the front and back parts of the eye and some lamps may be equipped with a tonometer to measure eye pressure. A dye called "fluorescein," which makes blood vessels easier to see may be added to the eye during the examination. The dye only temporarily stains the eye.

WHAT IS THE TREATMENT FOR UVEITIS?

Uveitis treatments primarily try to eliminate inflammation, alleviate pain, prevent further tissue damage, and restore any loss of vision. Treatments depend on the type of uveitis a patient displays. Some, such as using corticosteroid eye drops and injections around the eye or inside the eye, may exclusively target the eye whereas other treatments, such as immunosuppressive agents taken by mouth, may be used when the disease is occurring in both eyes, particularly in the back of both eyes.

An eye-care professional will usually prescribe steroidal anti-inflammatory medication that can be taken as eye drops, swallowed as a pill, injected around or into the eye, infused into the blood intravenously, or released into the eye via a capsule that is surgically implanted inside the eye. Long-term steroid use may produce side effects, such as stomach ulcers, osteoporosis (bone thinning), diabetes, cataracts, glaucoma, cardiovascular disease (CVD), weight gain, fluid retention, and Cushing syndrome. Usually, other agents are started if it appears that patients need moderate or high doses of oral steroids for more than three months.

Other immunosuppressive agents that are commonly used include medications, such as methotrexate, mycophenolate, azathioprine, and cyclosporine. These treatments require regular blood tests to monitor for possible side effects. In some cases, biologic response modifiers (BRM), or biologics, such as adalimumab, infliximab, daclizumab, abatacept, and rituximab are used. These drugs target specific elements of the immune system. Some of these drugs may increase the risk of having cancer.

Anterior Uveitis Treatments

Anterior uveitis may be treated by:

- Taking eye drops that dilate the pupil to prevent muscle spasms in the iris and ciliary body
- Taking eye drops containing steroids, such as prednisone, to reduce inflammation

Intermediate, Posterior, and Panuveitis Treatments

Intermediate, posterior, and panuveitis are often treated with injections around the eye, medications given by mouth, or, in some instances, time-release capsules that are surgically implanted inside the eye. Other immunosuppressive agents may be given. A doctor must make sure a patient is not fighting an infection before proceeding with these therapies.

A National Eye Institute (NEI)-funded study, called the "Multicenter Uveitis Treatment Trial" (MUST), compared the safety and effectiveness of conventional treatment for these forms of uveitis, which suppresses a patient's entire immune system, with a new local treatment that exclusively suppressed inflammation in the affected eye. Conventionally-treated patients were initially given high doses of prednisone, a corticosteroid medication, for one to four weeks which were then reduced gradually to low doses whereas locally-treated patients had a capsule that slowly released fluocinolone, another corticosteroid medication, surgically inserted in their affected eyes. Both treatments improved vision to a similar degree, with patients gaining almost one line on an eye chart. The conventional treatment produced few side effects. In contrast, the implant produced more eye problems, such as abnormally high eye pressure, glaucoma, and cataracts. Although both treatments decreased inflammation in the eye, the implant did so faster and to a greater degree. Nevertheless, visual improvements were similar to those of patients given conventional treatment.

Part 5 | Eye Injuries and Disorders of the Surrounding Structures

Chapter 32 | **Eye Injuries**

Chapter Contents

Section 32.1 | Black Eye

"Black Eye," © 2017 Omnigraphics. Reviewed March 2020.

WHAT IS A BLACK EYE?

A black eye (periorbital hematoma) is an impact injury that causes broken blood vessels in the tissue around the eye. This results in a bruise and swelling caused by the accumulation of blood and fluids beneath the skin. The skin around the eye is very loose, allowing this area to swell quickly as fluids build up. Despite the common name "black eye," there is usually no injury to the eye itself.

CAUSES OF BLACK EYE

Black eyes are usually caused by an object forcefully hitting the eye or nose. Depending on the location of the blow, one or two black eyes may develop. A strike to the nose typically results in two black eyes. Black eyes can also be caused by surgeries performed on the face, nose, jaw, and some types of dental work.

SYMPTOMS OF BLACK EYE

The term "black eye" is a good indication of the most visible symptoms of this type of injury. Because the area around the eye can bruise easily and turns a dark color quickly, a black eye is easily recognizable. However, dark bruising around the eye is not the only symptom of a black eye. Symptoms of a typical black eye can include:

- Bruising around the eye or nose that appears red, purple, yellow, green, or black
- Swelling around the eye that sometimes causes the eye to close completely
- Pain around the eye or nose
- Blurry vision

A more serious injury to the eye, face, or head can result in additional symptoms, such as:

- Loss of vision
- Seeing double or double vision

- Persistent, severe headache
- Blood collecting on the surface of the eyeball
- Blood or fluid flowing from the eye, ear, or nose
- Inability to move the eye or to look in different directions without turning the head
- Signs of injury to the head or face, including cuts or bruises elsewhere on the face
- Broken teeth
- Broken bones in the face
- Nausea or vomiting
- Dizziness
- Inability to walk
- Unexplained or sudden behavioral changes
- Loss of consciousness or fainting

DIAGNOSIS OF BLACK EYE

One of the most important factors in diagnosing a black eye is to determine whether the injury is limited to the soft tissue around the eye, or if a more critical head injury has occurred. A doctor or other healthcare provider will typically perform a physical examination to make this determination. Vision is checked by moving an object in front of the patient's face and asking them to follow the movement with their eyes. A light shined in the eye will test for proper dilation of the pupil. Special devices may be used to see inside the eye, in order to examine the retina or cornea for any injuries. An examination of the face and head will help determine if there have been any injuries to the skull or facial bones. Further testing may be performed by x-ray or other types of medical imaging.

The occurrence of two black eyes, especially after a forceful blow to the back of the head, may indicate a severe skull fracture. This is a very serious injury that can be life-threatening. Immediate medical attention should be sought if two black eyes appear at the same time.

TREATMENT OF BLACK EYE

Most black eyes heal on their own within a few days. A black eye can be treated at home with ice packs used for 20 minutes at a time, once every hour. If no improvement is seen after a few days, or if pain, swelling, or bruising persists, medical treatment should be sought. If any of the more serious symptoms described above occur, medical treatment should be sought immediately.

PREVENTION OF BLACK EYE

Black eyes are most commonly caused by sports injuries or accidents. The best method of protection is to always make use of proper safety equipment, such as helmets, goggles, or other protective equipment.

COMPLICATIONS OF BLACK EYE

Although most black eyes are surface injuries that heal on their own, there are several serious complications that can develop from this type of injury.

- **Hyphema**—bleeding inside the eye, between the back of the cornea and the front of the iris. This is a medical emergency that can lead to vision loss if left untreated.
- **Subconjunctival hemorrhage**—the white of the eye appears bright red due to bleeding in the eye.
- **Skull fracture**—broken bones in the skull.
- **Damage to the eyeball**—cuts or scratches on the surface of the eye, or object embedded in the eyeball.
- **Persistent swelling, severe pain, changes in vision**—these symptoms can indicate a more serious problem and medical attention should be sought.
- **Infection**—signs of infection include fever, warmth around the eye, persistent redness, and/or drainage.
- **Retinal detachment**—changes in vision, dizziness, nausea, migraine headaches, seeing flashing lights in the field of vision.
- **Traumatic uveitis and iritis**—pain during exposure to bright light, spots appearing to float in the field of vision, blurred vision, irregularly shaped pupil, redness in the iris.

- **Glaucoma**—a forceful blow to the eye can cause undetected bleeding inside the eye that produces increased pressure on the optic nerve.
- **Orbital floor fracture**—a forceful blow to the eye can push the eyeball back into the eye socket, resulting in pinching of the optic nerve and the muscles that help the eye move. This is a medical emergency that can result in loss of vision if left untreated.

References

1. Cunha, John P. "Black Eye," MedicineNet.com. June 1, 2015.
2. Hellem, Amy. "Is a Black Eye Serious?" AllAboutVision.com. January 2017.
3. Moss, Dr. Hart. "A Black Eye—How Long Does It Take to Heal?" EyeHealthWeb. n.d.
4. Porter, Daniel. "Black Eye Diagnosis," American Academy of Ophthalmology (AAO). March 1, 2017.

Section 32.2 | **Orbital Blowout Fracture**

An orbital blowout fracture is a fracture on the orbital floor (the bones at the bottom of the orbit, or eye socket) of the eyes. The eye socket is the skull cavity that holds the eye and protects the eyeball. This protective structure results in the eyeball being left undamaged in the event of many traumas. However, the force from the blow itself can spread throughout the orbit and result in a blowout, or breakage, of the orbital floor.

HOW TO IDENTIFY A BLOWOUT

When a severe blow occurs to the eye, the doctor will recommend a computed tomography (CT) scan of the eye and brain, which will show any areas of damage. A fracture in the orbital floor can be seen clearly with the help of a CT scan. The scan also allows the doctor to see sinus cavities—which is important because, during most orbital blowout fractures, associated blood and fluid seep into the maxillary sinus cavity.

CAUSES OF BLOWOUT FRACTURES

Any large object with a lot of force coming in contact with the eye socket can cause a blowout fracture. This kind of fracture commonly occurs from motor-vehicle accidents; a sports injury that occurs while playing baseball, softball, racquetball, or tennis; and when a fist or elbow makes contact with the eye.

SYMPTOMS OF AN ORBITAL BLOWOUT FRACTURE

Following are some of the symptoms that may indicate an orbital blowout fracture:

- Pain while looking up and down
- Tenderness around the eye
- Sunken eye
- Severe swelling of the eyelid and face
- Redness of the sclera (the white part of the eye)
- Nosebleed

There may be instances in which the orbital floor breaks but is not completely fractured. If this occurs, then it is possible that one of the eye muscles can become trapped between the bones, causing vertical double vision or restricted eye movement when looking up and down. Additionally, the nerve that innervates the cheeks and upper lip can become damaged, causing numbness.

Patients are often visibly shaken due to extreme swelling, bruising, and the trauma they experienced.

TYPES OF ORBITAL BLOWOUT FRACTURE

An orbital blowout fracture can occur in one or more of the orbital walls:

Inferior blowout fracture—this most common type of orbital blowout fracture affects the floor of the orbit (maxillary sinus roof). In children, the fracture recoils to its original position and traps contents of the orbit, a condition called "trapdoor fracture."

Medial blowout fracture—the second most common type in orbital blowout fracture occurs when the trauma is to the "orbital lamina," one of the main elements of a medial orbital wall.

Superior blowout fracture—this uncommon type of orbital blowout fracture is usually seen in patients with pneumatization of the orbital roof. This type of fracture may involve only the sinus or the anterior cranial fossa (the largest of the three cranial fossa situated over the nasal and orbital cavities), or the entire orbital roof.

Lateral blowout fracture—this type of orbital blowout fracture occurs rarely, since the bone in this region is very thick and surrounded by muscles. If there is a fracture, it is either associated with the orbital rim or other serious craniofacial injuries (injuries of the face or skull).

TREATMENT AND PROGNOSIS

If the blowout is minor, it usually heals with time and does not pose any permanent threats. The list that follows includes some immediate treatments and remedies to consider while enduring a simple blowout:

- Treat the affected area with an ice pack to reduce swelling.
- Use a nasal decongestant to drain the blood and fluid that may get accumulated in the sinuses.
- Avoid blowing the nose so that the pressure does not push the sinus content into the orbit.
- Use oral steroids and antibiotics in some rare cases to decrease swelling or scarring and prevent infections.

In cases in which the risk of a chronic impairment outweighs the risk of surgery, surgical treatment might be considered. Also, those with persistent symptoms are usually advised to undergo surgery. The period during which the surgery must be done may vary but, usually, it should happen within two weeks of the injury. Possible indications that the injury might require surgery are:

- Significant enophthalmos—a posterior displacement of the eyeball within the orbit
- Significant diplopia—double vision (i.e., a perception of two images of a single object, which can be displaced horizontally, vertically, or diagonally)

- Muscle entrapment (especially in children affected by a trapdoor fracture)
- Large area fractures

Most orbital blowout fractures heal without causing any long-term concerns. However, after four weeks of injury, an eye examination is recommended to rule out any complications such as:

- Orbital cellulitis (inflammation of the eye tissue)
- Angle-recession glaucoma (glaucoma that develops following an eye trauma)
- Retinal tear or detachment

Most cases of an orbital blowout fracture have a good prognosis, since long-term issues are low.

An orbital blowout fracture can be a serious injury that is easily dismissed as a black eye or swollen eye. It is important to consult with a physician in order to identify the extent of the injury so that it does not pose a serious threat.

References

1. "Blowout Fracture," American Association for Pediatric Ophthalmology and Strabismus (AAPOS), March 2017.
2. "Orbital Blowout Fracture," Kabbani, Ayla Al and Gaillard, Frank, Radiopaedia.org, July 11, 2018.
3. "Orbital Blowout Fracture Symptoms and Treatments," Bedinghaus, Troy. L. Verywell Health, January 19, 2020.

Section 32.3 | **Foreign Object or Chemical in the Eye**

A foreign object in the eye can be any particle such as dirt, dust, or metal that enters the eye. This often happens while engaging in activities such as drilling, cutting, or grinding, or when a particle is carried by the wind. Similarly, chemicals can come into contact with the eye while cleaning, gardening, or during any type of work that involves chemicals. Most objects settle under the eyelid or on the surface of the eye.

SYMPTOMS OF A FOREIGN OBJECT OR CHEMICAL IN THE EYE

If there is a foreign object or chemical in the eye, immediate symptoms will be noticed. A person may experience:

- A feeling of pressure and discomfort
- A sensation that something is in the eye
- Eye pain
- Severe tearing
- Pain while looking at light
- Red or bloodshot eyes
- Excessive blinking

Situations in which a foreign object penetrates the eye are rare. Usually, this happens as a result of a high-speed impact, such as an explosion. Foreign objects that penetrate the eye are called "intraocular objects." Symptoms of an intraocular object include discharge of blood or fluid from the eye.

FOREIGN OBJECTS OR CHEMICALS THAT CAN ENTER THE EYE

When a foreign object or chemical enters the eye, it usually affects the cornea or the conjunctiva. Some common types of foreign objects or chemicals that enter the eye are:

- Foreign objects
    - Eyelashes
    - Sawdust
    - Dirt
    - Sand
    - Cosmetics
    - Contact lenses
    - Metal particles
    - Glass shards
- Chemical Substances
    - Vinegar
    - Nail-polish remover

- Cleaning products
- Pepper spray

EMERGENCY CARE FOR A FOREIGN OBJECT OR CHEMICAL IN THE EYE

If the eye is affected by a foreign object or chemical, it is necessary to take prompt action to help prevent infection and/or potential vision loss. This is particularly important in cases of an intraocular injury.

Do's and Don'ts

- Do not try to remove the object yourself, as this could cause serious damage. Get medical help immediately.
- Minimize eye movement.
- Wrap the eye with a clean cloth or bandage.
- Do not touch, rub, or press the eye.
- Avoid using any implements such as tweezers or cotton swabs.
- Flush the eyes with water or a sterile saline solution (available in any drugstore) for at least 15 to 30 minutes, checking it every five minutes to see if the foreign object or chemical has cleared out.
- For intraocular objects, cover the eye with a small cup taped in place to keep pressure off the eye.
- Try finding the container in which the chemical came in since the instruction might tell you what to do in case the product gets into your eye.

TREATMENT FOR A FOREIGN OBJECT OR CHEMICAL IN THE EYE

The doctor will examine the vision and arrange for an x-ray or CT scan to determine whether the object has entered the eyeball prior to removing the object. Scratches in the eye will heal by themselves but, in some cases, a doctor may recommend an eye patch.

In case in which there is a chemical in the eye, the doctor will flush the eye out and prescribe pain-relief medications. The doctor might recommend visiting an ophthalmologist, if required.

As your eye is healing, try not to rub or scratch it, even if it is itchy. If the pain worsens, seek advice about which pain-relief medicine to use. Avoid wearing contact lenses; use glasses instead. Wear dark glasses (sunglasses) for the next few days.

PREVENTIVE MEASURES THAT CAN BE TAKEN

If you work in an environment that is prone to airborne objects, such as wood chips, dust, metal fragments, or chemicals, that may come into contact with your eyes, it is necessary to wear a face visor or goggles to protect your eyes. Similarly, certain chores at home, such as gardening or cleaning with chemicals, require the use of eye protection.

Keep things such as needles, pins, coins, marbles, or the tops of ballpoint pens out of a child's reach. Also, teach children not to insert objects into their eyes.

Most injuries can be minor and should heal by themselves. However, if the object is not removed properly it may cause an infection or scarring. Also, if the surface of the eye is scratched, it may not heal properly and may develop a corneal ulcer (keratitis). Hence, if a foreign object or chemical gets into the eye, seek immediate medical attention in order to avoid any serious injuries or possible blindness.

References

1. "Foreign Object in the Eye," Healthline Media, September 13, 2012.
2. "Objects or Chemicals in the Eye," Healthdirect, November 2019.

Section 32.4 | Traumatic Brain Injury and Vision Loss

Traumatic brain injury (TBI) occurs when the brain is harmed by an external force, such as a violent blow to the head or an object penetrating the skull. More than 1.4 million Americans receive treatment for TBI every year, while millions more suffer mild brain injuries—such as a concussion—and do not seek medical treatment. TBI can disrupt normal brain functioning and produce sensory, cognitive, or physical impairments that may be temporary or permanent. Many people with a TBI, or even a mild head injury, experience problems with their eyes and vision.

Situations that cause TBI can also cause trauma to the eyes or vision system, resulting in sight-threatening conditions such as retinal detachment, vitreous hemorrhage, or optic nerve damage. In addition to injuring the eyes directly, however, TBI can also cause vision problems by damaging parts of the brain involved in processing visual input from the eyes, such as the occipital lobe. Vision involves not only seeing with the eyes, but also interpreting, making sense of, and developing appropriate responses to visual images. Vision accounts for around 85 percent of the sensory input that is processed by the brain, and it affects perception, cognition, learning, motor skills, and other systems in the body. As a result, vision problems related to TBI can have a significant impact on people's everyday activities and overall quality of life (QOL).

COMMON TYPES OF VISION PROBLEMS

An accident that injures the brain can also cause physical injury to the eyes and the vision system. Some of the potentially serious injuries that create vision problems include the following:

- **Retinal detachment.** The retina is a thin layer of photoreactive cells at the back of the eye that turns light images into nerve impulses and sends them to the brain for processing. A violent blow to the head can cause the retina to tear loose from the back of the eye. Without prompt medical treatment, retinal detachment can result in permanent blindness.
- **Optic nerve damage.** When TBI causes swelling of the brain, the increased pressure within the skull can cut off blood circulation to the optic nerve. Damage to the optic nerve can disrupt the flow of visual input from the eyes to the brain, sometimes resulting in permanent vision loss.

- **Vitreous hemorrhage.** The vitreous is a clear, jelly-like substance that fills the rear portion of the eye and allows light to pass through to the retina. A brain injury can break blood vessels in the eye and allow blood to enter the vitreous. Although such hemorrhages can disrupt vision temporarily, most cases clear up over time without causing permanent damage.

SYMPTOMS OF VISION PROBLEMS

Many other vision problems associated with TBI occur due to damage to parts of the brain involved in processing visual signals from the eyes. The symptoms vary depending on the extent of the injury, the parts of the brain that are affected, and the patient's individual recovery process. Some of the symptoms of vision problems that commonly result from TBIs include the following:

- Blurry vision
- Double vision
- Sensitivity to light
- Headaches when performing visual tasks
- Motion sickness, nausea, or vomiting when performing visual tasks
- Difficulty reading
- Difficulty with visual attention, concentration, comprehension, or memory
- Visual balance disorders
- Decreased peripheral vision or reduction of the visual field
- Inability to maintain visual contact or focus
- Difficulty with eye movements, including the ability to: change focus from near to distant objects; track moving objects; shift gaze quickly from one object to another; and achieve the eye teaming or alignment required for binocular vision and depth perception

IMPACT OF VISION PROBLEMS

The vision symptoms experienced by people with TBI can affect many aspects of their daily lives, including the ability to work, go to school, drive a car, participate in recreational activities, and perform self-care tasks. Some of the difficulties caused by dysfunction in the brain's ability to process visual images include the following:

- **Difficulty with reading or close work.** Many people with TBI or concussion experience blurry near vision, which can make it hard to read or look at a computer screen. They may find it difficult to focus on near objects, or text may appear to move or jump around.
- **Struggles with pain or discomfort.** Swelling inside the skull often causes headaches, eye pain, and nausea or motion sickness when performing visual tasks.
- **Issues with movement or balance.** Many people with TBI have trouble tracking moving objects with their eyes or judging the relative location of objects in space. They may feel as if the floor is tilted, or they may become dizzy when they turn around or lean to the side.
- **Difficulty processing and understanding visual information.** Injury to the occipital lobe can make it difficult for the brain to make sense of images seen by the eyes. People with TBI may find it difficult to scan for visual information, focus visual attention on objects, or recall visual information.
- **Anxiety or irritability in certain environments.** Visual problems associated with TBI may cause people to feel uncomfortable or distressed when confronted with certain visual input, such as bright lights, complex patterns, or rapid motion.
- **Struggles with loss of vision or visual field.** People with decreased vision, double vision, or visual field loss face a risk of physical harm from bumping into objects, being struck by objects, or tripping over objects.

TREATMENT OF VISION PROBLEMS

It is important to seek medical attention for any type of head injury that results in vision problems. Treatment for TBI-related vision problems depends on the type of problem and the underlying cause. An optometrist or ophthalmologist can provide treatment for eye issues that can be corrected with surgery, patching, corrective eyeglasses, magnifying eyeglasses, or special lenses, such as prism lenses. Eye doctors who specialize in visual problems related to TBI, such as neuro-ophthalmologists, may be needed for more complex problems involving the brain's visual processing center. Occupational therapists, vision-rehabilitation therapists, and low vision specialists can also provide exercises, training, and adaptive devices aimed at decreasing or eliminating TBI-related vision problems.

MANAGEMENT OF VISION PROBLEMS

People with TBI can also use a number of strategies to adapt or manage the associated vision problems. Some suggestions include the following:

- Take frequent breaks to give the eyes and brain a rest while reading, using a computer, watching television, or doing other vision-dependent activities.
- Use magnifying lenses or increase the print size and contrast on computer screens to make things easier to see.
- Avoid bright, fluorescent, and flashing lights or other visual input that might prove irritating to the eyes or brain.
- Wear tinted sunglasses to reduce glare and use glare-reducing filters on computer screens.
- Reduce visual input and overload by decluttering your home and work environment.
- Use adaptive devices such as talking appliances, audiobooks, screen-reading software and apps, and mobility canes to help with reduced vision or vision loss.

References

1. "About Vision Problems Associated with Brain Injuries," Optometrists Network, 2017.
2. Metcalf, Eric. "Head Injuries Can Lead to Serious Vision Problems," Everyday Health, January 20, 2009.
3. Politzer, Thomas. "Introduction to Vision and Brain Injury," Neuro-Optometric Rehabilitation Association (NORA), n.d.
4. Powell, Janet M., Alan Weintraub, Laura Dreer, and Tom Novack. "Vision Problems and Traumatic Brain Injury," Model Systems Knowledge Translation Center, 2014.

Chapter 33 | Eye Injury Prevention

According to the American Academy of Ophthalmology (AAO), an estimated 90 percent of eye injuries are preventable with the use of proper safety eyewear. Even a minor injury to the cornea—such as that from a small particle of dust or debris—can be painful and become a life-long issue, so take the extra precaution and always protect the eyes. If the eye is injured, seek emergency medical help immediately.

DANGERS AT HOME

When we think of eye protection, we tend to think of people wearing hard hats and lab coats. We often forget that even at home, we might find ourselves dealing with similar threats to our eyes. Dangerous chemicals that could burn or splash the eyes are not restricted to chemical laboratories. They are also in our garages and under our kitchen sinks. Debris and other air-borne irritants are present at home, too, whether one is doing a home construction project or working in the yard. The debris from a lawnmower or "weed wacker," for example, can be moving at high speeds and provide no time to react. Some sports also put the eyes at risk of injury from foreign objects moving at high speeds.

EFFECTIVE EYEWEAR

The best way to prevent injury to the eye is to always wear the appropriate eye protection. The U.S. Bureau of Labor Statistics

This chapter includes text excerpted from "Eye Injury Prevention," Federal Occupational Health (FOH), U.S. Department of Health and Human Services (HHS), May 20, 2012. Reviewed March 2020.

(BLS) reports that approximately three out of every five workers injured were either not wearing eye protection at the time of the accident or wearing the wrong kind of eye protection for the job. To be effective, eyewear must fit properly and be effectively designed to protect the eyes based on the activity being performed. The Occupational Safety Health Administration (OSHA) has standards that require employers to provide their workers with the appropriate eye protection.

WHEN TO WEAR PROTECTIVE EYEWEAR

According to the standards proposed by OSHA, you (or anyone who is watching you work) should always wear properly fitted eye protective gear, such as safety glasses with side protection/shields, when:

- Doing work that may produce particles, slivers, or dust from materials, such as wood, metal, plastic, cement, and drywall
- Hammering, sanding, grinding, or doing masonry work
- Working with power tools
- Working with chemicals, including common household chemicals, such as ammonia, oven cleaners, and bleach
- Using a lawnmower, riding mower, or other motorized gardening devices, such as string trimmers (also called "weed wacker" or "weed whip")
- Working with wet or powdered cement
- Welding (which requires extra protection such as a welding mask or helmet from sparks and ultraviolet (UV) radiation)
- "Jumping" the battery of a motor vehicle
- Being a bystander to any of the above

SPORTS

It is also recommended that you protect your eyes from injury when participating in certain sports, including:

- Indoor racket sports

- Paintball
- Baseball
- Basketball
- Hockey
- Cycling
- Riding or being a passenger on a motorcycle

SUN

The eyes also need to be protected from prolonged sun exposure, so have sunglasses with UV protection at hand. If you are putting on sunscreen, you should also be wearing sunglasses with UV protection. Vision is a gift. Make the extra effort to protect it.

Chapter 34 | **Workplace Eye Safety**

Chapter Contents

Section 34.1 | **Workplace Eye Injuries and Diseases**

This section contains text excerpted from the following sources: Text under the heading "Work-Related Eye Injuries in the United States" is excerpted from "NIOSHTIC-2 Publications Search—Work-Related Eye Injuries in the U.S.," Centers for Disease Control and Prevention (CDC), April 12, 2019; Text beginning with the heading "How Do Eye Injuries Happen to Workers?" is excerpted from "Eye Safety," Centers for Disease Control and Prevention (CDC), July 29, 2013. Reviewed March 2020.

WORK-RELATED EYE INJURIES IN THE UNITED STATES

Each day, nearly 2,000 U.S. workers have an eye injury that requires medical treatment. Characterizing these injuries aids the development of eye safety programs and the design of eye protection. Two national injury surveillance systems collect data on workplace eye injuries. The U.S. Bureau of Labor Statistics (BLS) Survey of Injuries and Illnesses captures data reported by private industry employers on medically-treated eye injuries involving a day or more away from work (DAFW). The National Institute for Occupational Safety and Health's (NIOSH) occupational supplement to the National Electronic Injury and Illness System (NEISS-Work) captures data on eye injuries treated in the U.S. hospital emergency departments. NEISS-Work data are based on worker reporting of work-relatedness at the time of treatment. Occupational eye injury rates have been declining. In 2007, there were 33,000 DAFW eye injuries (3% of all DAFW cases) at a rate of 3.5 injuries per 10,000 full-time workers (FTE) and 212,000 ED-treated occupational eye injuries (6% of all ED-treated cases) at a rate of 15 injuries per 10,000 FTE. Younger workers, males, and construction industry workers had the highest rates. Most injury events involved eye contact with an object such as scrap or debris or involved exposure to substances, such as chemicals. Although eye injury rates have decreased, the eye injury etiology remains largely the same. Increased use of eye protection may significantly influence the injury rate and patterns.

HOW DO EYE INJURIES HAPPEN TO WORKERS?

Striking or Scraping

The majority of eye injuries result from small particles or objects striking or scraping the eye such as dust, cement chips, metal slivers, and wood chips. These materials are often ejected by tools, windblown, or fall from above a worker. Large objects may also strike the eye or face, or a worker may run into an object causing blunt-force trauma to the eyeball or eye socket.

Penetration

Objects such as nails, staples, or slivers of wood or metal can go through the eyeball and result in a permanent loss of vision.

Chemical and Thermal Burns

Industrial chemicals or cleaning products are common causes of chemical burns to one or both eyes. Thermal burns to the eye also occur, often among welders. These burns routinely damage workers' eyes and surrounding tissue.

HOW DO WORKERS ACQUIRE EYE DISEASES?

Eye diseases are often transmitted through the mucous membranes of the eye as a result of direct exposure to things, such as blood splashes, and droplets from coughing or sneezing or from touching the eyes with a contaminated finger or object. Eye diseases can result in minor reddening or soreness of the eye or in a life-threatening disease, such as human immunodeficiency virus (HIV), hepatitis B virus, or avian influenza.

WHAT CAN WORKERS DO TO PREVENT EYE INJURY AND DISEASE?

Wear personal protective eyewear such as goggles, face shields, safety glasses, or full-face respirators.

The eye protection chosen for specific work situations depends upon the nature and extent of the hazard, the circumstances of exposure, other protective equipment used, and personal vision needs. Eye protection should be fit to an individual or adjustable to provide appropriate coverage. It should be comfortable and allow for sufficient peripheral vision.

WHAT CAN EMPLOYERS DO TO PREVENT WORK-RELATED EYE INJURY AND DISEASE?

Employers can ensure engineering controls are used to reduce eye injuries and to protect against ocular infection exposures. Employers can also conduct a hazard assessment to determine the appropriate type of protective eyewear appropriate for a given task.

Section 34.2 | Preventing Eye Injuries in the Workplace

This section contains text excerpted from the following sources: Text in this section begins with excerpts from "Eye Safety at Work Is Everyone's Business," National Eye Institute (NEI), March 12, 2006. Reviewed March 2020; Text beginning with the heading "Recommended Eye Protection" is excerpted from "Eye Safety," Centers for Disease Control and Prevention (CDC), July 29, 2013. Reviewed March 2020.

Each day, about 2,000 U.S. workers receive medical treatment because of eye injuries sustained at work. Workplace injury is a leading cause of eye trauma, vision loss, disability, and blindness, and can interfere with your ability to perform your job and carry out normal activities. Employers and workers need to be aware of the risks to sight, especially if they work in high-risk occupations. High-risk occupations include construction, manufacturing, mining, carpentry, auto repair, electrical work, plumbing, welding, and maintenance. The combination of removing or minimizing eye safety hazards and wearing proper eye safety protection can prevent many eye injuries. Personal protective eyewear, such as safety glasses with side shields, goggles, face shields, and/or welding helmets can protect you from common hazards including flying fragments, large chips, hot sparks, optical radiation, splashes from molten metals, objects, particles, and glare. The risk of eye injury and the need for preventive measures depend on your job and the conditions in your workplace. Employers can take several precautions to make the work environment as safe as possible and help reduce the risk of visual impairment and blindness caused by injury. They can

- Conduct an eye-hazard assessment
- Remove or reduce all eye hazards where possible

- Provide appropriate safety eye protection for the types of hazards at the worksite
- Require all employees in hazardous situations to wear the appropriate eye protection
- Keep eye protection in good condition and assist workers with attaining the proper fit
- Keep bystanders out of work areas and/or behind protective barriers
- Use caution flags to identify potential hazards such as hanging or protruding objects
- Provide emergency sterile eyewash solutions/stations near hazardous areas
- Provide post-first-aid instructions and information on how to get emergency aid

Eye safety should receive continuing attention in workplace educational programs. Procedures for handling eye injuries should also be established and reinforced.

Workers should have a comprehensive dilated eye examination on a regular basis (typically every two years) to help ensure good eye health. Maintaining healthy vision is important to avoid injuries on the job.

RECOMMENDED EYE PROTECTION

Before selecting appropriate eye protection for emergency workers at a site, assess the conditions and hazards and follow these recommendations:

- At a minimum, wear safety glasses with side protection.
- Wear goggles when more protection is needed.
- Consider using hybrid eye safety products with the comfort of glasses, the enclosure of goggles, and better breathability.
- Add a face shield over glasses or goggles for even greater protection.
- Use a full-facepiece respirator for the best overall protection.

- When cutting or welding, use a welding helmet, goggles, or welding respirator with the appropriate lens shade.
- Make sure that cutter's and welder's helpers, other workers, and bystanders are protected from the light and sparks coming from torch cutting or welding.

Section 34.3 | **Eye Protection for Infection Control**

This section includes text excerpted from "Eye Safety: Eye Protection for Infection Control," Centers for Disease Control and Prevention (CDC), July 29, 2013. Reviewed March 2020.

The Centers for Disease Control and Prevention (CDC) recommends eye protection for a variety of potential exposure settings where workers may be at risk of acquiring infectious diseases via ocular exposure. Workers should understand that regular prescription eyeglasses and contact lenses are not considered eye protection.

Infectious diseases can be transmitted through various mechanisms, among which are infections that can be introduced through the mucous membranes of the eye (conjunctiva). These include viruses and bacteria that can cause conjunctivitis (e.g., adenovirus, herpes simplex virus, *Staphylococcus aureus*) and viruses that can cause systemic infections, including bloodborne viruses (e.g., hepatitis B and C viruses, human immunodeficiency virus (HIV)), herpes viruses, and rhinoviruses. Infectious agents are introduced to the eye either directly (e.g., blood splashes, respiratory droplets generated during coughing or suctioning) or from touching the eyes with contaminated fingers or other objects.

Eye protection provides a barrier to infectious materials entering the eye and is often used in conjunction with other personal protective equipment (PPE) such as gloves, gowns, masks, or respirators.

INFECTION CONTROL QUESTIONS AND ANSWERS

What Types of Eye Protection Should Be Worn?

The eye protection chosen for specific work situations depends upon the circumstances of exposure, other PPE used, and personal vision needs. There is a wide variety in the types of protective eyewear, and appropriate selection should be based on a number of factors, the most important of which is the nature and extent of the hazard. Eye protection must be comfortable and allow for sufficient peripheral vision and must be adjustable to ensure a secure fit. It may be necessary to provide several different types, styles, and sizes. The selection of protective eyewear appropriate for a given task should be made from an evaluation of each activity, including regulatory requirements when applicable. These hazard assessments require a clear understanding of the work tasks, including knowledge of the potential routes of exposure and the opportunities for exposure in the task assessed (nature and extent of worker contact). Exposure incident reports should be reviewed to identify those incidents (whether or not infection occurred) that could have been prevented by the proper use of protective eyewear.

What Are Common Types of Eye Protection?

GOGGLES

Appropriately fitted, indirectly-vented goggles* with a manufacturer's antifog coating provide the most reliable practical eye protection from splashes, sprays, and respiratory droplets. Newer styles of goggles may provide better indirect airflow properties to reduce fogging, as well as better peripheral vision and more size options for fitting goggles to different workers. Many styles of goggles fit adequately over prescription glasses with minimal gaps. However, to be efficacious, goggles must fit snugly, particularly from the corners of the eye across the brow. While highly effective as eye protection, goggles do not provide splash or spray protection to other parts of the face.

**Directly-vented goggles may allow penetration by splashes or sprays; therefore, indirectly-vented or nonvented goggles are preferred for infection control.*

FACE SHIELDS

Face shields are commonly used as an infection control alternative to goggles.** As opposed to goggles, a face shield can also provide protection to other facial areas. To provide better face and eye protection from splashes and sprays, a face shield should have crown and chin protection and wrap around the face to the point of the ear, which reduces the likelihood that a splash could go around the edge of the shield and reach the eyes. Disposable face shields for medical personnel made of lightweight films that are attached to a surgical mask or fit loosely around the face should not be relied upon as optimal protection.

***In a chemical exposure or industrial setting, face shields should be used in addition to goggles, not as a substitute for goggles (ANSI Z87.1-2003 Practice for occupational and educational eye and face protection).*

SAFETY GLASSES

Safety glasses provide impact protection but do not provide the same level of splash or droplet protection as goggles and generally should not be used for infection control purposes.

FULL-FACE RESPIRATORS

Full-facepiece elastomeric respirators and powered air-purifying respirators (PAPRs) are designed and used for respiratory protection, but because of their design incidentally provide highly effective eye protection as well. Selection of this type of PPE should be based on an assessment of the respiratory hazard in an infection control situation, but will also provide, optimal eye protection.

Why Eye Protection Is Available for Prescription Lenses Users?

Many safety goggles or Plano (nonprescription) safety glasses fit comfortably over street eyewear and can provide satisfactory protection without impairing the fit of the prescription eyewear. Prescription safety glasses with side protection are available but do not protect against splashes or droplets as well as goggles. Special prescription inserts are available for goggles. When full-facepiece elastomeric negative pressure (i.e., nonpowered) respirators or tight-fitting powered air-purifying respirators (PAPRs) are indicated for respiratory protection, these devices require appropriate prescription inserts to avoid compromising the seal around the face; PAPRs designed with loose-fitting facepieces or with hoods that completely cover the head and neck may be more accommodating to prescription lens wearers.

Contact lenses, by themselves, offer no infection control protection. However, contact lenses may be worn with any of the recommended eye protection devices, including full-face respirators. Contact lens users should rigorously adhere to handwashing guidelines when inserting, adjusting, or removing contact lenses.

What Combination of Eye Protection and Other PPE Should Be Used?

Eye protection should be selected in the context of other PPE use requirements. Safety goggles may not fit properly when used with certain half-face respirators, and similarly, face shields may not fit properly over some respirators. Once PPE requirements have been established for a specific infection control situation, the selected PPE should be pretested to assure suitable fit and protection when used as an ensemble. Elastomeric, full-facepiece respirators and powered air-purifying respirators (PAPRs) have the advantage of incidentally providing optimal eye protection. In situations where all combinations of PPE may not be readily available to workers, judicious selection of complementary PPE is important to allow for appropriate protection.

How Should Potentially Contaminated Eye Protection Be Removed?

Eye protection should be removed by handling only the portion of this equipment that secures the device to the head (i.e., plastic temples, elasticized band, ties), as this is considered relatively "clean." The front and sides of the device (i.e., goggles, face shield) should not be touched, as these are the surfaces most likely to become contaminated by sprays, splashes, or droplets during patient care. Nondisposable eye protection should be placed in a designated receptacle for subsequent cleaning and disinfection. The sequence of PPE removal should follow a defined regimen that should be developed by infection control staff and take into consideration the need to remove other PPE.

Is It Safe for Others to Reuse My Eye Protection?

The eyewear described above is generally not disposable and must be disinfected before reuse. Where possible, each individual worker should be assigned her/his own eye protection to ensure appropriate fit and to minimize the potential of exposing the next wearer. A labeled container for used (potentially contaminated) eye protection should be available in the HCW change-out/locker room. Eye protection deposited here can be collected, disinfected, washed, and then reused.

How Should Eye Protection Be Disinfected?

Healthcare setting-specific procedures for cleaning and disinfecting used patient care equipment should be followed for reprocessing reusable eye protection devices. Manufacturers may be consulted for their guidance and experience in disinfecting their respective products. Contaminated eye protection devices should be reprocessed in an area where other soiled equipment is handled. Eye protection should be physically cleaned and disinfected with the designated hospital disinfectant, rinsed, and allowed to air dry. Gloves should be worn when cleaning and disinfecting these devices.

Chapter 35 | **Protecting Eyes from Sports Injuries**

Eye injuries are a leading cause of blindness in children in the United States—and most of these injuries happen while kids are playing sports. The good news is that wearing the right protective eyewear can prevent 9 in 10 sports-related eye injuries.

WHAT IS PROTECTIVE EYEWEAR?

Protective eyewear is an eyewear made of ultra-strong polycarbonate, a type of plastic that is very impact-resistant and also protects eyes from ultraviolet (UV) rays. Types of protective eyewear for sports include safety goggles, face guards, and special eyewear designed for specific sports. Regular eyeglasses, sunglasses, and contacts do not protect kids from eye injuries—but most protective eyewear can be made to match kids' glasses or contact prescriptions. Kids can also wear safety goggles over their regular glasses or contacts.

WHEN DO KIDS NEED TO USE PROTECTIVE EYEWEAR?

Kids need to use protective eyewear whenever they are practicing or playing a sport that raises their risk of eye injury. Some sports have a higher risk of eye injuries than others.

This chapter contains text excerpted from the following sources: Text in this chapter begins with excerpts from "Sports and Eye Safety: Tips for Parents and Teachers," National Eye Institute (NEI), July 1, 2019; Text under the heading "Simple Steps to Prevent Eye Injuries in Sports" is excerpted from "Simple Steps to Prevent Eye Injuries in Sports," Office of Disease Prevention and Health Promotion (ODPHP), U.S. Department of Health and Human Services (HHS), February 3, 2020.

Sports with a high risk of eye injury include:

- Baseball and softball
- Basketball
- Fencing
- Hockey
- Mountain biking
- Paintball
- Racquetball and squash

Sports with a moderate risk of eye injury include:

- Badminton
- Golf
- Soccer
- Tackle football
- Tennis

And sports with a low risk of eye injury include:

- Diving
- Gymnastics
- Road biking
- Skiing
- Swimming
- Track and field

Youth sports leagues do not always require players to use protective eyewear. That is why it is important for parents, teachers, and coaches to know the risks and make sure that all young athletes use protective eyewear when they are at risk for eye injuries.

WHAT KIND OF PROTECTIVE EYEWEAR DO KIDS NEED?

There are different types of protective eyewear that are best for different sports.

Kids need safety goggles with polycarbonate lenses when playing sports, such as:

- Baseball and softball (when fielding)
- Basketball

- Mountain biking
- Racquetball and squash

Kids need helmets with attached polycarbonate face guards or face masks when playing sports, such as:

- Baseball and softball (when batting)
- Hockey
- Tackle football

Kids need swim safety goggles with polycarbonate lenses when playing sports that happen in the water, such as:

- Surfing
- Water polo
- Water skiing or tubing

Kids may need other types of eye and face protection for sports such as fencing, lacrosse, and paintball, and when playing certain positions, such as goalie. If you are not sure what type of protective eyewear your child needs, ask your child's eye doctor or coach.

SIMPLE STEPS TO PREVENT EYE INJURIES IN SPORTS

Most athletes think of knee and shoulder problems when we talk about sports-related injuries. With fall sports in full swing, it is important to remember that eye injuries in sports are not only common, but they are potentially very serious.

According to the American Academy of Ophthalmology (AAO), sports account for approximately 100,000 eye injuries each year. Roughly 42,000 of those injuries require evaluation in emergency departments. In fact, a patient with a sports-related eye injury presents to a United States emergency room every 13 minutes. It is estimated that sports-related eye injuries cost between $175 million and $200 million per year.

Generally baseball, basketball and racquet sports cause the highest numbers of eye injuries. One of every three of these eye injuries in sports occurs in children. In kids between the ages of 5 and 14, baseball is the leading cause. Basketball is a common culprit in athletes aged 15 and older. And boxing and martial arts present a high risk for serious eye injuries.

These eye injuries can be mild ones, but serious injuries, such as orbital fractures, corneal abrasions, and detached retina can occur. Approximately 13,500 people become legally blind from sports-related eye injuries every year.

Fortunately, the AAO estimates that 90 percent of eye injuries are preventable. Athletes should remember these simple tips to avoid serious eye damage in sports:

- Wear appropriate eye protection, especially in basketball, racket sports, field hockey, and soccer. In baseball, ice hockey and men's lacrosse, an athlete should wear a helmet with a polycarbonate shield. Polycarbonate lenses are believed to be ten times more resistant to impact than other materials. All protective eyewear should comply with the American Society of Testing Materials (ASTM) standards.
- Wear additional protective eyewear, if you wear contact lenses or glasses. Contacts offer no protection against impacts to the eye. Glasses and sunglasses do not provide adequate protection and could shatter upon impact, increasing the danger to the eye.
- Wear eye protection for all sports if you are functionally one-eyed, meaning one eye has normal vision and the other is less than 20/40 vision.
- Inspect protective eyewear regularly and replace it when it appears worn or damaged.

Last, if an eye injury does occur, every athlete should consider going to an emergency department or consulting an ophthalmologist. Even a seemingly minor injury can actually be potentially serious and lead to loss of vision.

Remember, 90 percent of sports-related eye injuries can be prevented. Let us start taking steps to eliminate these injuries.

Chapter 36 | Eyelid Disorders

Chapter Contents

Section 36.1 | **Blepharitis**

This section includes text excerpted from "Blepharitis," National Eye Institute (NEI), July 2, 2019.

WHAT IS BLEPHARITIS?

Blepharitis is a common condition that causes inflammation of the eyelids. The condition can be difficult to manage because it tends to recur.

WHAT OTHER CONDITIONS ARE ASSOCIATED WITH BLEPHARITIS?

Complications from blepharitis include:

- **Stye.** A red tender bump on the eyelid that is caused by an acute infection of the oil glands of the eyelid.
- **Chalazion.** This condition can follow the development of a stye. It is a usually a painless firm lump caused by inflammation of the oil glands of the eyelid. A chalazion can be painful and red if there is also an infection.
- **Problems with the tear film.** Abnormal or decreased oil secretions that are part of the tear film can result in excess tearing or dry eye. Because tears are necessary to keep the cornea healthy, tear film problems can make people more at risk for corneal infections.

WHAT CAUSES BLEPHARITIS

Blepharitis occurs in two forms:

- **Anterior blepharitis** affects the outside front of the eyelid, where the eyelashes are attached. The two most common causes of anterior blepharitis are bacteria (*Staphylococcus*) and scalp dandruff.
- **Posterior blepharitis** affects the inner eyelid (the moist part that makes contact with the eye) and is caused by problems with the oil (meibomian) glands in this part of the eyelid. Two skin disorders can cause this form of blepharitis: acne rosacea, which leads to red and inflamed skin, and scalp dandruff (seborrheic dermatitis).

WHAT ARE THE SYMPTOMS OF BLEPHARITIS?

Symptoms of either form of blepharitis include a foreign body or burning sensation, excessive tearing, itching, sensitivity to light (photophobia), red and swollen eyelids, redness of the eye, blurred vision, frothy tears, dry eye, or crusting of the eyelashes on awakening.

WHAT IS THE TREATMENT FOR BLEPHARITIS?

Treatment for both forms of blepharitis involves keeping the lids clean and free of crusts. Warm compresses should be applied to the lid to loosen the crusts, followed by a light scrubbing of the eyelid with a cotton swab and a mixture of water and baby shampoo. Because blepharitis rarely goes away completely, most patients must maintain an eyelid hygiene routine for life. If the blepharitis is severe, an eye-care professional may also prescribe antibiotics or steroid eyedrops.

When scalp dandruff is present, a dandruff shampoo for the hair is recommended as well. In addition to the warm compresses, patients with posterior blepharitis will need to massage their eyelids to clean the oil accumulated in the glands. Patients who also have acne rosacea should have that condition treated at the same time.

Section 36.2 | **Benign Essential Blepharospasm**

This section contains text excerpted from the following sources: Text in this section begins with excerpts from "Benign Essential Blepharospasm," Genetics Home Reference (GHR), National Institutes of Health (NIH), March 17, 2020; Text beginning with the heading "Treatment for Benign essential blepharospasm" is excerpted from "Benign Essential Blepharospasm Information Page," National Institute of Neurological Disorders and Stroke (NINDS), March 27, 2019.

Benign essential blepharospasm (BEB) is a condition characterized by abnormal blinking or spasms of the eyelids. This condition is a type of dystonia, which is a group of movement disorders involving uncontrolled tensing of the muscles (muscle contractions), rhythmic shaking (tremors), and other involuntary movements. BEB is different from the common, temporary eyelid twitching that can be caused by fatigue, stress, or caffeine.

The signs and symptoms of BEB usually appear in mid to late adulthood and gradually worsen. The first symptoms of the condition include an increased frequency of blinking, dry eyes, and eye irritation that is aggravated by wind, air pollution, sunlight, and other irritants. These symptoms may begin in one eye, but they ultimately affect both eyes. As the condition progresses, spasms of the muscles surrounding the eyes cause involuntary winking or squinting. Affected individuals have increased difficulty keeping their eyes open, which can lead to severe vision impairment.

In more than half of all people with BEB, the symptoms of dystonia spread beyond the eyes to affect other facial muscles and muscles in other areas of the body. When people with BEB also experience involuntary muscle spasms affecting the tongue and jaw (oromandibular dystonia), the combination of signs and symptoms is known as "Meige syndrome."

FREQUENCY OF BENIGN ESSENTIAL BLEPHAROSPASM

Benign essential blepharospasm affects an estimated 20,000 to 50,000 people in the United States. For unknown reasons, it occurs in women more than twice as often as it occurs in men.

CAUSES OF BENIGN ESSENTIAL BLEPHAROSPASM

The causes of BEB are unknown, although the disorder likely results from a combination of genetic and environmental factors. Certain genetic changes probably increase the likelihood of developing this condition, and environmental factors may trigger the signs and symptoms in people who are at risk.

Studies suggest that this condition may be related to other forms of adult-onset dystonia, including uncontrolled twisting of the neck muscles (spasmodic torticollis) and spasms of the hand and finger muscles (writer's cramp). Researchers suspect that benign essential blepharospasm and similar forms of dystonia are associated with malfunction of the basal ganglia, which are structures deep within the brain that help start and control movement.

Although genetic factors are almost certainly involved in BEB, no genes have been clearly associated with the condition. Several studies have looked at the relationship between common variations (polymorphisms) in the *DRD5* and *TOR1A* genes and the risk of developing BEB. These studies have had conflicting results, with some showing an association and others finding no connection. Researchers are working to determine which genetic factors are related to this disorder.

TREATMENT OF BENIGN ESSENTIAL BLEPHAROSPASM

In most cases of BEB the treatment of choice is botulinum toxin injections which relax the muscles and stop the spasms. Other treatment options include medications (drug therapy) or surgery—either local surgery of the eye muscles or deep brain stimulation surgery.

PROGNOSIS OF BENIGN ESSENTIAL BLEPHAROSPASM

With botulinum toxin treatment, most individuals with BEB have substantial relief of symptoms. Although some may experience side effects, such as drooping eyelids, blurred or double vision, and eye dryness, these side effects are usually only temporary. The condition may worsen or expand to surrounding muscles; remain the same for many years; and, in rare cases, improve spontaneously.

Section 36.3 | Blepharospasm

This section includes text excerpted from "Blepharospasm," National Eye Institute (NEI), June 26, 2019.

WHAT IS BLEPHAROSPASM?

Blepharospasm is an abnormal, involuntary blinking or spasm of the eyelids.

WHAT CAUSES BLEPHAROSPASM

Blepharospasm is associated with an abnormal function of the basal ganglion from an unknown cause. The basal ganglion is the part of the brain responsible for controlling the muscles. In rare cases, heredity may play a role in the development of blepharospasm.

WHAT ARE THE SYMPTOMS OF BLEPHAROSPASM?

Most people develop blepharospasm without any warning symptoms. It may begin with a gradual increase in blinking or eye irritation. Some people may also experience fatigue, emotional tension, or sensitivity to bright light. As the condition progresses, the symptoms become more frequent, and facial spasms may develop. Blepharospasm may decrease or cease while a person is sleeping or concentrating on a specific task.

WHAT IS THE TREATMENT FOR BLEPHAROSPASM?

To date, there is no successful cure for blepharospasm, although several treatment options can reduce its severity.

In the United States and Canada, the injection of Oculinum (botulinum toxin, or Botox) into the muscles of the eyelids is an approved treatment for blepharospasm. Botulinum toxin, produced by the bacterium *Clostridium botulinum*, paralyzes the muscles of the eyelids.

Medications taken by mouth for blepharospasm are available but usually produce unpredictable results. Any symptom relief is usually short term and tends to be helpful in only 15 percent of the cases.

Myectomy, a surgical procedure to remove some of the muscles and nerves of the eyelids, is also a possible treatment option. This surgery has improved symptoms in 75 to 85 percent of people with blepharospasm.

Alternative treatments may include biofeedback, acupuncture, hypnosis, chiropractic, and nutritional therapy. The benefits of these alternative therapies have not been proven.

Section 36.4 | Blepharophimosis, Ptosis, and Epicanthus Inversus Syndrome

This section contains text excerpted from the following sources: Text in this section begins with excerpts from "Blepharophimosis, Ptosis, and Epicanthus Inversus Syndrome," Genetics Home Reference (GHR), National Institutes of Health (NIH), March 17, 2020; Text under the heading "Treatment of Blepharophimosis, Ptosis, and Epicanthus Inversus Syndrome" is excerpted from "Blepharophimosis-Epicanthus Inversus-Ptosis Syndrome," Genetic and Rare Diseases Information Center (GARD), National Center for Advancing Translational Sciences (NCATS), June 6, 2011. Reviewed March 2020.

Blepharophimosis, ptosis, and epicanthus inversus syndrome (BPES) is a condition that mainly affects development of the eyelids. People with this condition have a narrowing of the eye opening (blepharophimosis), droopy eyelids (ptosis), and an upward fold of the skin of the lower eyelid near the inner corner of the eye (epicanthus inversus). In addition, there is an increased distance between the inner corners of the eyes (telecanthus). Because of these eyelid abnormalities, the eyelids cannot open fully, and vision may be limited.

Other structures in the eyes and face may be mildly affected by BPES. Affected individuals are at an increased risk of developing vision problems, such as nearsightedness (myopia) or farsightedness (hyperopia) beginning in childhood. They may also have eyes that do not point in the same direction (strabismus) or "lazy eye" (amblyopia) affecting one or both eyes. People with blepharophimosis, ptosis, and epicanthus inversus syndrome may also have distinctive facial features including a broad nasal bridge, low-set ears, or a shortened distance between the nose and upper lip (a short philtrum).

There are two types of BPES, which are distinguished by their signs and symptoms. Both types I and II include the eyelid malformations and other facial features. Type I is also associated with an early loss of ovarian function (primary ovarian insufficiency (POI)) in women, which causes their menstrual periods to become less frequent and eventually stop before age 40. POI can lead to difficulty conceiving a child (subfertility) or a complete inability to conceive (infertility).

CAUSES OF BLEPHAROPHIMOSIS, PTOSIS, AND EPICANTHUS INVERSUS SYNDROME

Mutations in the *FOXL2* gene cause BPES types I and II. The *FOXL2* gene provides instructions for making a protein that is active in the eyelids and ovaries. The FOXL2 protein is likely involved in the development of muscles in the eyelids. Before birth and in adulthood, the protein regulates the growth and development of certain ovarian cells and the breakdown of specific molecules.

It is difficult to predict the type of BPES that will result from the many *FOXL2* gene mutations. However, mutations that result in a partial loss of FOXL2 protein function generally cause BPES type II. These mutations probably impair regulation of normal development of muscles in the eyelids, resulting in malformed eyelids that cannot open fully. Mutations that lead to a complete loss of FOXL2 protein function often cause BPES type I. These mutations impair the regulation of eyelid development as well as various activities in the ovaries, resulting in eyelid malformation and abnormally accelerated maturation of certain ovarian cells and the premature death of egg cells.

TREATMENT OF BLEPHAROPHIMOSIS, PTOSIS, AND EPICANTHUS INVERSUS SYNDROME

Management of blepharophimosis syndrome type 1 requires the input of several specialists including a clinical geneticist, pediatric ophthalmologist, eye plastic (oculoplastic) surgeon, endocrinologist, reproductive endocrinologist, and gynecologist.

Eyelid surgery should be discussed with an oculoplastic surgeon to decide on the method and timing that is best suited for the patient. Traditionally, surgical correction of the blepharophimosis, epicanthus inversus, and telecanthus (canthoplasty) is performed at ages three to five years, followed about a year later by ptosis correction (usually requiring a brow suspension procedure). If the epicanthal folds are small, a "Y-V canthoplasty" is traditionally used; if the epicanthal folds are severe, a "double Z-plasty" is used. Unpublished reports have indicated that advanced understanding of the lower eyelid position has allowed for more targeted surgery that results in a more natural appearance.

Chapter 37 | **Disorders of the Tear Duct**

Chapter Contents

Section 37.1 | Blocked Tear Duct (Dacryostenosis)

"Blocked Tear Duct (Dacryostenosis)," © 2020 Omnigraphics. March 2020.

Most tears come from the lacrimal glands, which are located above the eyes. The tears flow down the surface of the eyes to lubricate them, and then drain into tiny holes (puncta) in the corner of the upper and lower eyelids. These tears then travel through small canals in the lids (canaliculi) to a sac located where the lids attach to the side of the nose (lacrimal sac). They then travel down a duct (the nasolacrimal duct) before emptying into the nose, where they evaporate or are reabsorbed.

A blocked tear duct is when this ocular drainage system is either partially or fully clogged. Because of this blockage, the tears cannot drain normally, and this inability to drain causes watery, irritated, and chronically infected eyes.

CAUSES OF A BLOCKED TEAR DUCT

A person can be born with a blocked tear duct (congenital blocked tear duct) when the duct is not completely developed at birth. This can improve within the first year of life with no treatment necessary. In adults, this blockage may be due to an injury, infection, or tumor.

Other causes of a blocked tear duct include:

- Irregular development of the skull and face (craniofacial abnormalities), such as those affected by Down syndrome or other disorders
- Age-related conditions, such as narrowing of the punctal openings
- Nose trauma, such as a broken nose resulting in scar tissue blocking the tear duct
- Nasal polyps, which are growths on the lining of the nasal passage, or sinuses. Nasal polyps usually affect people with nasal allergies.

SYMPTOMS OF A BLOCKED TEAR DUCT

The main symptom of a blocked tear duct is excessive tearing (epiphora) that causes tears to overflow onto the face and cheeks.

In infants, this becomes noticeable during the first two or three weeks after their birth. Other symptoms include:

- Inflammation or swelling of the eye, tenderness and redness of the inside corner or around the eyes and nose
- Recurring eye infections
- Discharge of mucus from the eye
- Crusty eyelashes
- Blurry vision
- Blood-tinged tears
- Fever

DIAGNOSIS OF A BLOCKED TEAR DUCT

Ophthalmologists (eye doctors) diagnose a blocked tear duct through various tests. A complete eye examination is done, and the individual's medical history is discussed so that the doctor can learn about any possible causes.

Tests are performed to check how the ocular drainage system is working by flushing a special fluid into the opening of the affected tear duct. If the fluid is not tasted in the throat, then the person is diagnosed with a blocked tear duct. Other tests include an x-ray or a computed tomography (CT) scan of the tear duct, called the "dacryocystogram," although this test is rarely needed.

TREATMENT FOR A BLOCKED TEAR DUCT

In some cases, more than one treatment is required to completely open the blocked tear duct. A blocked tear duct in a newborn will mostly improve on its own during the first few months when their ocular drainage system matures and opens. Sometimes, the ophthalmologist may recommend using a special massage technique that opens the membrane covering the lower opening of the baby's nose.

When the blocked tear duct is the result of a facial injury, the drainage system usually will start working again a few months after the injury. The ophthalmologist may recommend waiting for a few months after the injury before considering surgery, since most blockages do not require treatment.

For infants and toddlers whose ducts are not opening up, or for adults whose ducts are partially blocked, a technique that uses dilation, probing, and irrigation may be used. For this technique, an instrument is used to dilate the punctal openings and a narrow probe is then guided through the openings into the tear drainage system through the nasal opening, and then removed. The drainage system is then flushed with a saline solution to clear out any residual blockage.

With a procedure called "stenting," or "intubation," tiny tubes are inserted through one or both puncta. These tubes go all the way through the drainage system and out through the nose, which helps to open up the blockages. The tubes are left in for three to four months and then removed.

A surgical procedure called the "dacryocystorhinostomy" is used in rare scenarios. By this method, a new route is created for the tears to drain out normally through the nose, by developing a new connection between the lacrimal sac and the nose.

If a tumor causes a blocked tear duct, then surgery may be done to remove it, or medications may be prescribed to shrink it.

Although in many cases a blocked tear duct cannot be prevented, proper treatment of nasal and eye infections or inflammations may reduce the risks of acquiring one. Using protective eyewear can help prevent a blockage that is caused by an injury.

References

1. "Blocked Tear Duct," Boyd, Kierstan. American Academy of Ophthalmology (AAO), March 1, 2015.
2. "Blocked Tear Duct," MedlinePlus, National Institutes of Health (NIH), August 5, 2018.

Section 37.2 | **Dacryocystitis**

Dacryocystitis is a condition that affects the lacrimal sac, a small chamber located near the inner corner of the eye that collects excess tears from the eye's surface and drains them into the nose through the nasolacrimal duct. When this drainage system is obstructed, bacteria may become trapped and cause an infection. Dacryocystitis is characterized by pain, swelling, irritation, redness, and infection of the lacrimal sac.

TYPES AND CAUSES OF DACRYOCYSTITIS

There are two main types of dacryocystitis: acute and chronic. Acute dacryocystitis appears suddenly due to the blockage of a tear duct. Some of the possible causes include sinus problems, physical injury, health conditions such as tuberculosis (TB), or a cyst or tumor. The blockage causes tears and mucus to accumulate in the lacrimal sac, which creates a breeding ground for bacteria. Chronic dacryocystitis is a persistent, long-lasting condition characterized primarily by excessive watering of the eyes. It may result from an acute case that is not managed properly or from a congenital (present from birth) narrowing or obstruction of the nasolacrimal duct.

SYMPTOMS OF DACRYOCYSTITIS

The symptoms of chronic dacryocystitis are often limited to excessive tear production in one eye. They may also include one or more of the following common symptoms of acute dacryocystitis:

- Pain, redness, and swelling in the inner corner of the eye
- Crusting around the eyelids and eyelashes
- A painful lump or abscess between the eye and nose
- Oozing of pus from the corner of the eye
- Discharge of pus upon applying pressure to the lacrimal sac

- Swelling that makes it difficult to open the eye
- Fever

DIAGNOSIS OF DACRYOCYSTITIS

To diagnose dacryocystitis, an ophthalmologist will evaluate the patient's symptoms and examine the eye to determine whether the drainage system is obstructed. The examination is likely to include looking at the eye and eyelid with a microscope, flushing fluid through the nasolacrimal duct, and taking a sample of fluid discharge from the lacrimal sac to check for bacteria.

TREATMENT OF DACRYOCYSTITIS

For acute dacryocystitis caused by a bacterial infection, an eye doctor will typically prescribe an oral antibiotic or a topical antibiotic in the form of ointment or eyedrops. Other recommended forms of treatment include applying a warm compress to the lacrimal sac several times a day and gently massaging the nasolacrimal duct to clear out pus and debris. If the symptoms are severe and include feelings of illness along with a fever, the patient should seek emergency treatment at a hospital. Intravenous antibiotics may be needed to prevent the development of potentially fatal complications, such as orbital cellulitis.

For chronic dacryocystitis—or acute dacryocystitis that is caused by a blockage—the eye doctor may recommend a surgical procedure called "dacryocystorhinostomy" (DCR). DCR is intended to bypass the obstruction in the nasolacrimal duct and restore the flow of tears from the lacrimal sac into the nose. The procedure uses a minimally invasive technique called "endonasal approach," which involves inserting an endoscope through the nose into the nasal cavity. The surgeon uses a laser attached to the endoscope to create a hole between the lacrimal sac and the nose and then inserts a tube to facilitate the drainage of tears.

In another type of surgical treatment, known as "balloon dacryoplasty," the surgeon inserts a tiny balloon into the nasolacrimal duct and inflates it to widen a congenital narrowing or blockage.

It does not have as high a success rate as DCR, however, and is not recommended for treating acute dacryocystitis.

References

1. Garrity, James. "Dacryocystitis," MSD Manuals, 2017.
2. Kerkar, Pramod. "Dacryocystitis: Types, Causes, Symptoms, Treatment, Surgery," EPainAssist, September 24, 2015.
3. Roth, Ashley. "Everything You Need to Know about Dacryocystitis," EyeHealthWeb, September 2016.

Chapter 38 | Computer Vision Syndrome

Chapter Contents

Section 38.1 | **Blue-Light Hazard**

This section includes text excerpted from "SSL Technology Fact Sheet: Optical Safety of LEDs," U.S. Department of Energy (DOE), June 2013. Reviewed March 2020.

The safety of light-emitting diode (LED) lighting with regard to human health has occasionally been the subject of scrutiny. One such concern is photoretinitis—photochemical damage to the retina—which can result from too much exposure to violet and blue light. This is known as "blue-light hazard." The risk of blue-light hazard is sometimes associated with LEDs, even though LEDs that emit white light do not contain significantly bluer than any other source at the same color temperature. According to current international standards, no light source that emits white light and is used in general lighting applications is considered hazardous to the retina for healthy adults. That said, the optical safety of specialty lamps or colored sources must be considered on a case-by-case basis, and light sources used around susceptible populations, such as infants or adults with certain types of eye disease, require additional evaluation.

THE EFFECTS OF OPTICAL RADIATION

Light is a physical (and psychological) stimulus that has many effects on the human body. Besides enabling vision, light entrains our circadian rhythms—body processes, such as our sleep/wake cycle, appetite, body temperature fluctuations, and more. Visible light is just one portion of the electromagnetic spectrum. It is sandwiched between ultraviolet (UV) and infrared (IR) radiation, which have shorter and longer wavelengths, respectively. Collectively, this radiant energy is referred to as optical radiation, with wavelengths ranging from 200 to 3,000 nm. The complete electromagnetic spectrum also includes radio waves, x-rays, gamma rays, and microwaves, among other types of radiant energy.

Optical radiation falls on the skin and eyes, where the energy is transformed via photochemical processes or thermal reactions. While this sensory interaction is an essential part of human perception, too much radiant energy can damage tissue. Shorter wavelengths (UV) can cause sunburn, or may even have effects at a cellular/deoxyribonucleic acid (DNA) level. Longer wavelengths (IR) are perceived as heat; again, too much can lead to discomfort or injury. Among the six defined optical radiation hazards, the only one that is practically applicable to LEDs is blue-light hazard; by design, LEDs used for lighting do not emit UV or IR radiation.

Regardless of the source type, the blue component cannot be removed from white light that is appropriate for interior environments. Besides being necessary for proper visual appearance and color rendering, blue light is essential for nonvisual photoreception, such as regulating our circadian rhythms.

The amount of blue light in typical architectural lighting products is not hazardous. Even when the light intensity gets uncomfortably high, the risk is mitigated by natural defense mechanisms, including aversion response (blinking, head movement, and pupil constriction) and continuous eye movement (saccades), which protect the retina from overexposure. Without these, the sun could damage our eyes.

The radiation to which our eyes and skin are exposed can cause both acute and long-term effects.

IS ALL BLUE LIGHT THE SAME?

Light at any given wavelength is the same regardless of what it was emitted from (or reflected off); that is, there is no physical difference in the stimulus, or the resulting visual and nonvisual effects whether the light is from an LED lamp, incandescent lamp, CFL, or any other source. At the same time, visible light is a continuous spectrum of wavelengths. "Blue light" is a simplified term generally referring to the range of radiant energy between violet and cyan, having wavelengths of approximately 400 to 500 nm.

Most sources emit light over a range of wavelengths—including blue—rather than any one specifically. Additionally, our visual system is based on photoreceptors with broad response ranges that integrate spectral information. Hazardous radiation is similarly defined using functions that account for the variable effects across different wavelengths. For example, the blue-light hazard weighting function extends from approximately 380 to 540 nm, with a peak at 435 to 440 nm. Accordingly, it is important to consider the effects of energy over a range of wavelengths, rather than any local peak.

What we consider "white light" can be made up of many different combinations of wavelengths, and have many different tints. It is also possible that two light sources that look identical to a human observer are comprised of different spectral content—this is known as "metamerism." Importantly, there is a basic balance of long- and short-wavelength energy that must occur for a source to appear a certain shade of white, referred to as color temperature, although the specific spectral content may be somewhat different.

DO LIGHT-EMITTING DIODES EMIT MORE BLUE LIGHT?

Often, investigations into the effect of short-wavelength radiation—be it on humans or artwork—suggest that LEDs are dangerous because they emit more blue light than other sources like incandescent bulbs or CFLs. While it is true that most LED products that emit white light include a blue LED pump, the proportion of blue light in the spectrum is not significantly higher for LEDs than it is for any other light source at the same correlated color temperature (CCT). This is exemplified by comparing the blue-light hazard efficacy (KB,v)—the blue-light hazard potential per lumen—of sources with similar CCTs. Other calculations could be performed using a different measure of blue content, and as long as the weighting.

HOW MUCH LIGHT IS A CONCERN?

Given that CCT is highly predictive of blue light content, it is possible to use photobiological safety standards to determine a threshold for hazard based on CCT.

Importantly, a product must exceed the threshold for both the luminance and illuminance conditions to be considered hazardous. The hazard from the sun, is mitigated by humans' natural aversion response, so injury is unlikely.

WHAT SITUATIONS ARE CONCERNS?

The white-light architectural lighting products do not pose a risk for blue-light hazard, based on the 500-lux evaluation criterion prescribed by photobiological safety standards. Several situations require further attention, including:

- Nonwhite light sources (e.g., blue LEDs)
- Applications where infants could be in close proximity to bright light sources, since they have not yet developed aversion responses
- Applications where those suffering from lupus or eye disease may be exposed to high light levels
- Applications where intentional exposure to bright light is expected, or viewing conditions may be outside the norm

While these scenarios may require additional investigation, they are not necessarily hazardous.

CONCLUSIONS

Light-emitting diode products are no more hazardous than other lighting technologies that have the same CCT. Furthermore, white-light products used in general lighting service applications are not considered a risk for blue-light hazard according to current international standards. Sensitive individuals may have additional concerns, and colored light sources should be evaluated on a case-by-case basis.

Section 38.2 | **How To Prevent Computer Eyestrain**

This section includes text excerpted from "Computer Workstations eTool," Occupational Safety and Health Administration (OSHA), March 15, 2008. Reviewed March 2020.

MONITORS

Viewing Distance

POTENTIAL HAZARDS

Monitors placed too close or too far away may cause you to assume awkward body positions that may lead to eyestrain.

- Viewing distances that are too long can cause you to lean forward and strain to see small text. This can fatigue the eyes and place stress on the torso because the backrest is no longer providing support.
- Viewing distances that are too short may cause your eyes to work harder to focus (convergence problems) and may require you to sit in awkward postures. For instance, you may tilt your head backward or push your chair away from the screen, causing you to type with outstretched arms.

POSSIBLE SOLUTIONS

- Sit at a comfortable distance from the monitor where you can easily read all text with your head and torso in an upright posture and your back supported by your chair. Generally, the preferred viewing distance is between 20 and 40 inches (50 and 100 cm) from the eye to the front surface of the computer screen. **NOTE:** Text size may need to be increased for smaller monitors.
  - Make more room for the back of the monitor by pulling the desk away from the wall or divider.
  - Provide a flat-panel display, which is not as deep as a conventional monitor and requires less desk space.
  - Place monitor in the corner of a work area. Corners often provide more desk depth than a straight run of desk top.
  - Move back and install an adjustable keyboard tray to create a deeper working surface.

Viewing Angle-Height and Side-to-Side

POTENTIAL HAZARDS

Working with your head and neck turned to the side for a prolonged period loads neck muscles unevenly and increases fatigue and pain.

POSSIBLE SOLUTIONS

- Position your computer monitor directly in front of you, so your head, neck and torso face forward when viewing the screen. Monitors should not be farther than 35 degrees to the left or right.
- If you work primarily from printed material, place the monitor slightly to the side and keep the printed material directly in front. Keep printed materials and monitors as close as possible to each other.

POTENTIAL HAZARDS

A display screen that is too high or low will cause you to work with your head, neck, shoulders, and even your back in awkward postures. When the monitor is too high, for example, you have to work with your head and neck tilted back. Working in these awkward postures for a prolonged period fatigues the muscles that support the head.

POSSIBLE SOLUTIONS

- The top of the monitor should be at or slightly below eye level. The center of the computer monitor should normally be located 15 to 20 degrees below horizontal eye level.
- The entire visual area of the display screen should be located so the downward viewing angle is never greater than 60 degrees when you are in any of the four reference postures. In the reclining posture the straight forward line of sight will not be parallel with the floor, which may increase the downward viewing angle. Using very large monitors also may increase the angle.

- Remove some or all of the equipment (computer case, surge protector, etc.) on which the monitor may be placed. Generally, placing the monitor on top of the computer case will raise it too high for all but the tallest users.
- Elevate your line of sight by raising your chair. Be sure that you have adequate space for your thighs under the desk and that your feet are supported.

POTENTIAL HAZARDS

Bifocal users typically view the monitor through the bottom portion of their lenses. This causes them to tilt the head backward to see a monitor that may otherwise be appropriately placed. As with a monitor that is too high, this can fatigue muscles that support the head.

POSSIBLE SOLUTIONS

- Lower the monitor (below recommendations for nonbifocal users) so you can maintain appropriate neck postures. You may need to tilt the monitor screen up toward you.
- Raise the chair height until you can view the monitor without tilting your head back. You may have to raise the keyboard and use a foot rest.
- Use a pair of single-vision lenses with a focal length designed for computer work. This will eliminate the need to look through the bottom portion of the lens.

Viewing Time

POTENTIAL HAZARDS

Viewing the monitor for long periods of time may cause eye fatigue and dryness. Users often blink less while viewing the monitor.

POSSIBLE SOLUTIONS

- Rest your eyes periodically by focusing on objects that are farther away (for example, a clock on a wall 20 feet away).

- Stop, look away, and blink at regular intervals to moisten the eyes.
- Alternate duties with other noncomputer tasks such as filing, phone work, or customer interaction to provide periods of rest for the eyes.

Viewing Clarity

POTENTIAL HAZARDS

Monitors that are tilted significantly either toward or away from the operator may distort objects on the screen, making them difficult to read. Also, when the monitor is tilted back, overhead lights may create glare on the screen. This can result in eyestrain and sitting in awkward postures to avoid eye glare.

POSSIBLE SOLUTIONS

- Tilt the monitor so it is perpendicular to your line of sight, usually by tilting the screen no more than 10 to 20 degrees. This is most easily done if the monitor has a riser/swivel stand. A temporary solution involves tilting the monitor back slightly by placing a book under the front edge. **NOTE:** Tilting the monitor back may create glare on the screen from ceiling lighting and a glare screen may be needed.
- Monitor support surfaces should allow the user to modify viewing distances and tilt and rotation angles.

POTENTIAL HAZARDS

Factors that reduce image quality make viewing more difficult and may lead to eye strain. These factors include:

- Electromagnetic fields caused by other electrical equipment located near computer workstations, which can result in display quality distortions.
- Dust accumulation, which is accelerated by magnetic fields associated with computer monitors and can reduce contrast and degrade viewing conditions.

POSSIBLE SOLUTIONS

- Computer workstations should be isolated from other equipment that may have electrostatic potentials in excess of +/- 500 volts.
- Computer monitors should be periodically cleaned and dusted.

WORKSTATION ENVIRONMENT

Lighting

POTENTIAL HAZARD

Bright lights shining on the display screen "wash out" images, making it difficult to clearly see your work. Straining to view objects on the screen can lead to eye fatigue.

POSSIBLE SOLUTIONS

- Place rows of lights parallel to your line of sight.
- Provide light diffusers so that desk tasks (writing, reading papers) can be performed while limiting direct brightness on the computer screen.
- Remove the middle bulbs of 4-bulb fluorescent light fixtures to reduce the brightness of the light to levels more compatible with computer tasks if diffusers or alternative light sources are not available. **NOTE:** A standard florescent light fixture on a nine-foot ceiling with four, 40-watt bulbs will produce approximately 50 foot-candles of light at the desktop level.
- Provide supplemental task/desk lighting to adequately illuminate writing and reading tasks while limiting brightness around monitors.
- Generally, for paper tasks and offices with CRT displays, office lighting should range between 20 and 50 foot-candles. If LCD monitors are in use, higher levels of light are usually needed for the same viewing tasks (up to 73 foot-candles).

POTENTIAL HAZARD

Bright light sources behind the display screen can create contrast problems, making it difficult to clearly see your work.

POSSIBLE SOLUTIONS

- Use blinds or drapes on windows to eliminate bright light. Blinds and furniture placement should be adjusted to allow light into the room, but not directly into your field of view. **NOTE:** Vertical blinds work best for East/West facing windows and horizontal blinds for North/South facing windows.
- Use indirect or shielded lighting where possible and avoid intense or uneven lighting in your field of vision. Ensure that lamps have glare shields or shades to direct light away from your line of sight.
- Reorient the workstation so bright lights from open windows are at right angles with the computer screen.

POTENTIAL HAZARD

High contrast between light and dark areas of the computer screen, horizontal work surface, and surrounding areas can cause eye fatigue and headaches.

POSSIBLE SOLUTION

- For computer work, use well-distributed diffuse light. The advantage of diffuse lighting is that:
  - There are fewer hot spots (or glare surfaces) in the visual field.
  - The contrasts created by the shape of objects tend to be softer.
- Use light, matte colors and finishes on walls and ceilings to better reflect indirect lighting and reduce dark shadows and contrast.

Glare

POTENTIAL HAZARD

Direct light sources (for example, windows, overhead lights) that cause reflected light to show up on the monitor make images more difficult to see, resulting in eye strain and fatigue.

POSSIBLE SOLUTIONS

- Place the face of the display screen at right angles to windows and light sources. Position task lighting (for example, a desk lamp) so the light does not reflect on the screen.
- Clean the monitor frequently. A layer of dust can contribute to glare.
- Use blinds or drapes on windows to help reduce glare. **NOTE:** Vertical blinds work best for East/West facing windows and horizontal blinds for North/South facing windows.
- Use glare filters that attach directly to the surface of the monitor to reduce glare. Glare filters, when used, should not significantly decrease screen visibility. Install louvers, or "egg crates," in overhead lights to re-direct lighting.
- Use barriers or light diffusers on fixtures to reduce glare from overhead lighting.

POTENTIAL HAZARD

- **NOTE:** Generally, a large number of low powered lamps rather than a small number of high powered lamps will result in less glare.

Reflected light from polished surfaces, such as a keyboards, may cause annoyance, discomfort, or loss in visual performance and visibility.

POSSIBLE SOLUTIONS

To limit reflection from walls and work surfaces around the screen, paint them with a medium colored, nonreflective paint. Arrange workstations and lighting to avoid reflected glare on the display screen or surrounding surfaces.

Tilt down the monitor slightly to prevent it from reflecting overhead light.

Set the computer monitor for dark characters on a light background; they are less affected by reflections than are light characters on a dark background.

Ventilation

Potential Hazards

- Users may experience discomfort from poorly designed or malfunctioning ventilation systems, for example, air conditioners or heaters that directly "dump" air on users.
- Dry air can dry the eyes (especially if the user wears contact lenses).
- Poor air circulation can result in stuffy or stagnant conditions.
- Temperatures above or below standard comfort levels can affect comfort and productivity.

Possible Solutions

- Do not place desks, chairs, and other office furniture directly under air conditioning vents unless the vents are designed to redirect the air flow away from these areas.
- Use diffusers or blocks to redirect and mix air flows from ventilation systems.
    - Keep air flow rates within three and six inches per second (7.5 and 15 centimeters per second). These air flow rates are barely noticeable or not noticeable at all.
- Keep relative humidity of the air between 30 and 60 percent.
- The recommended ambient indoor temperatures range between 68°F and 74°F (20°C and 23.5°C) during heating season and between 73°F and 78°F (23°C and 26°C) during the cooling season.

POTENTIAL HAZARD

Exposure to chemicals, volatile organic compounds (VOCs), ozone, and particles from computers and their peripherals (for example, laser printers) may cause discomfort or health problems.

POSSIBLE SOLUTIONS

- Enquire about the potential for a computer or its components to emit pollutants. Those that do should be placed in well-ventilated areas.

- Maintain proper ventilation to ensure that there is an adequate supply of fresh air.
- Allow new equipment to "air out" in a well-ventilated area prior to installing.

Part 6 | Congenital and Other Disorders That Affect Vision

Chapter 39 | **Hereditary Disorders Affecting Vision**

Chapter Contents

Section 39.1 | **Achromatopsia**

This section includes text excerpted from "Achromatopsia," Genetics Home Reference (GHR), National Institutes of Health (NIH), March 17, 2020.

Achromatopsia is a condition characterized by partial or total absence of color vision. People with complete achromatopsia cannot perceive any colors; they see only black, white, and shades of gray. Incomplete achromatopsia is a milder form of the condition that allows some color discrimination.

Achromatopsia also involves other problems with vision, including increased sensitivity to light and glare (photophobia), involuntary back-and-forth eye movements (nystagmus), and significantly reduced sharpness of vision (low visual acuity). Affected individuals can also have farsightedness (hyperopia) or, less commonly, nearsightedness (myopia). These vision problems develop in the first few months of life.

Achromatopsia is different from the more common forms of color vision deficiency (also called "color blindness"), in which people can perceive color but have difficulty distinguishing between certain colors, such as red and green.

FREQUENCY OF ACHROMATOPSIA

Achromatopsia affects an estimated 1 in 30,000 people worldwide. Complete achromatopsia is more common than incomplete achromatopsia.

Complete achromatopsia occurs frequently among Pingelapese islanders, who live on one of the Eastern Caroline Islands of Micronesia. Between 4 and 10 percent of people in this population have a total absence of color vision.

CAUSES OF ACHROMATOPSIA

Achromatopsia results from changes in one of several genes: *CNGA3*, *CNGB3*, *GNAT2*, *PDE6C*, or *PDE6H*. A particular *CNGB3* gene mutation underlies the condition in Pingelapese islanders.

Achromatopsia is a disorder of the retina, which is the light-sensitive tissue at the back of the eye. The retina contains two types of light receptor cells, called "rods and cones." These cells transmit visual signals from the eye to the brain through a process called "phototransduction." Rods provide vision in low light (night vision). Cones provide vision in bright light (daylight vision), including color vision.

Mutations in any of the genes listed above prevent cones from reacting appropriately to light, which interferes with phototransduction. In people with complete achromatopsia, cones are nonfunctional, and vision depends entirely on the activity of rods. The loss of cone function leads to a total lack of color vision and causes other vision problems. People with incomplete achromatopsia retain some cone function. These individuals have limited color vision, and their other vision problems tend to be less severe.

Some people with achromatopsia do not have identified mutations in any of the known genes. In these individuals, the cause of the disorder is unknown. Other genetic factors that have not been identified likely contribute to this condition.

Section 39.2 | **Alström Syndrome**

This section includes text excerpted from "Alström Syndrome," Genetic and Rare Diseases Information Center (GARD), National Center for Advancing Translational Sciences (NCATS), June 22, 2016. Reviewed March 2020.

Alström syndrome is a rare genetic disorder that affects many body systems. Symptoms develop gradually, beginning in infancy, and can be variable. In childhood, the disorder is generally characterized by vision and hearing abnormalities, childhood obesity, and heart disease (cardiomyopathy). Over time, diabetes mellitus, liver problems, and slowly progressive kidney dysfunction which can lead to kidney failure may develop. Alström syndrome is caused by mutations in the *ALMS1* gene. It is inherited in an autosomal recessive manner. While there is no specific treatment for Alström syndrome, symptoms can be managed by a team of specialists with the goal of improving the quality of life (QOL) and increasing the lifespan.

SYMPTOMS OF ALSTRÖM SYNDROME

The signs and symptoms of Alström syndrome vary among affected individuals. The age that symptoms begin also varies. Symptoms may first appear anywhere from infancy to early adulthood.

Signs and symptoms may include:

- Vision abnormalities, specifically cone-rod dystrophy and cataracts
- Progressive sensorineural hearing loss in both ears and chronic infection or inflammation of the middle ear
- Heart disease that enlarges and weakens the heart muscle (dilated cardiomyopathy)
- Excessive eating (hyperphagia) and rapid weight gain leading to obesity
- Insulin resistance leading to high levels of insulin in the blood (hyperinsulinemia) and type 2 diabetes mellitus
- Elevated levels of fats (lipids) in the blood (hyperlipidemia)
- Fatty liver that may progress to significant liver disease
- Short stature
- Skin findings including abnormally increased coloration and "velvety" thickening of the skin in certain areas of the body (acanthosis nigricans)
- Lower hormone levels produced by the male testes or the female ovaries (hypogonadism)

Alström syndrome can also cause serious or life-threatening medical problems involving the liver, kidneys, bladder, and lungs.

INHERITANCE OF ALSTRÖM SYNDROME

Alström syndrome is inherited in an autosomal recessive manner. This means, to be affected, a person must have a mutation in both copies of the *ALMS1* gene in each cell.

Affected people inherit one mutated copy of the gene from each parent, who is referred to as a carrier. Carriers of an autosomal recessive condition typically do not have any signs or symptoms (they are unaffected). When two carriers of an autosomal recessive condition have children, each child has a:

- 25 percent (1 in 4) chance to be affected
- 50 percent (1 in 2) chance to be an unaffected carrier like each parent
- 25 percent (1 in 4) chance to be unaffected and not be a carrier

DIAGNOSIS OF ALSTRÖM SYNDROME

Genetic testing of the *ALMS1* gene is available for Alström syndrome. Although genetic testing is not necessary to make a diagnosis of Alström syndrome, it can be helpful to confirm a diagnosis. If a mutation is not identified in both copies of the *ALMS1* gene of an individual suspected to have Alström syndrome, it does not rule out the diagnosis.

Alström syndrome is diagnosed based on clinical findings (signs and symptoms), medical history, and family history. Making a diagnosis can be complicated by the variation in the age of symptom onset from one individual to another. Genetic testing is not necessary to make the diagnosis of Alström syndrome, although it can be useful to confirm a diagnosis.

TREATMENT OF ALSTRÖM SYNDROME

While there is no specific treatment for Alström syndrome, symptoms can be managed by a team of specialists with the goal of improving the quality of life (QOL) and increasing the lifespan.

PROGNOSIS OF ALSTRÖM SYNDROME

The prognosis for Alström syndrome varies depending on the progression of symptoms, specifically heart and kidney disease. The lifespan and overall QOL for individuals with Alström syndrome can be improved by early diagnosis, treatment, surveillance, and proper management of symptoms.

Section 39.3 | **Axenfeld-Rieger Syndrome**

This section includes text excerpted from "Axenfeld-Rieger Syndrome," Genetic and Rare Diseases Information Center (GARD), National Center for Advancing Translational Sciences (NCATS), June 22, 2016. Reviewed March 2020.

WHAT IS AXENFELD-RIEGER SYNDROME?

Axenfeld-Rieger syndrome is a group of disorders that mainly affects the development of the eye. Common eye symptoms include cornea defects and iris defects. People with this syndrome may have an off-center pupil (corectopia) or extra holes in the eyes that can look like multiple pupils (polycoria). About 50 percent of people with this syndrome develop glaucoma, a condition that increases pressure inside of the eye, and may cause vision loss or blindness.

Even though Axenfeld-Rieger syndrome is primarily an eye disorder, this syndrome can affect other parts of the body. Most people with this syndrome have distinctive facial features and many have issues with their teeth, including unusually small teeth (microdontia) or fewer than normal teeth (oligodontia). Some people have extra folds of skin around their belly button, heart defects, or other more rare birth defects.

There are three types of Axenfeld-Rieger syndrome and each has a different genetic cause. Axenfeld-Rieger syndrome type 1 is caused by mutations in the *PITX2* gene. Axenfeld-Rieger syndrome type 3 is caused by mutations in the *FOXC1* gene. The gene that causes Axenfeld-Rieger syndrome type 2 is not known, but it is located on chromosome 13. Axenfeld-Rieger syndrome has an autosomal dominant pattern of inheritance. Treatment depends on the symptoms.

WHAT ARE THE SIGNS AND SYMPTOMS OF AXENFELD-RIEGER SYNDROME?

Axenfeld-Rieger syndrome is an eye disorder. People with this disorder typically have cornea defects, which is the clear cover on the front of the eye. They may have a cloudy cornea or posterior embryotoxin, which is when you can see an opaque ring around the outer edge of the cornea. People with this disorder can also have issues with their iris, which is the colored part of the eye. They typically have iris stands, which is a connective tissue that connects the iris with the lens. There may be issues with the pupils as well, which is the black opening in the eye. One of the pupils may be in the wrong location (corectopia), the pupils may be abnormally large or small, or there may be extra pupils (polycoria).

About 50 percent of people with this syndrome develop glaucoma, which is a condition that increases pressure inside of the eye. This may cause vision loss or blindness. People with this syndrome can also have strabismus (cross-eye), cataracts (cloudy lens), macular degeneration (an eye disorder that causes vision loss), or coloboma (a hole in a structure in the eye).

Even though Axenfeld-Rieger syndrome is primarily an eye disorder, people with this syndrome can also have symptoms that affect other parts of the body. These symptoms mostly involve the teeth and facial bones. Symptoms affecting the teeth include cone-shaped teeth (peg-like incisors), missing teeth (oligodontia), small teeth (microdontia), and abnormal spacing of the teeth. Symptoms affecting the facial bones may include an underdeveloped jaw, a protruding lower lip, and widely spaced eyes. Other symptoms include extra folds of skin around the belly button, heart defects, or other more rare birth defects.

HOW IS AXENFELD-RIEGER SYNDROME INHERITED?

Axenfeld-Rieger syndrome is inherited in an autosomal dominant manner.

There are two copies of every gene in our body. In autosomal dominant conditions, if there is a mutation in just one copy of that gene, then that person will develop the condition. This mutation can be inherited from a parent, or it can happen by chance for the first time in that one person, which is called a "*de novo* mutation."

Each child of an individual with Axenfeld-Rieger syndrome has a 50 percent chance of inheriting the mutation. Children who inherit the mutation will have Axenfeld-Rieger syndrome, although their symptoms could be more or less severe than their parent's.

Section 39.4 | **Bardet-Biedl Syndrome**

This section includes text excerpted from "Bardet-Biedl Syndrome," Genetic and Rare Diseases Information Center (GARD), National Center for Advancing Translational Sciences (NCATS), August 27, 2018.

Bardet-Biedl syndrome (BBS) is an inherited condition that affects many parts of the body. People with this syndrome have progressive visual impairment due to cone-rod dystrophy, extra fingers or toes (polydactyly), truncal obesity, decreased function of the male gonads (hypergonadism), kidney abnormalities, and learning difficulties. Mutations in many genes are known to cause BBS and inheritance is usually autosomal recessive. Treatment depends on the symptoms present in each person.

SYMPTOMS OF BARDET-BIEDL SYNDROME

Bardet-Biedl syndrome affects many parts of the body. Signs and symptoms can vary among affected individuals, even within the same family. The major features include:

- Progressive vision loss due to deterioration of the retina. This usually begins in mid-childhood with problems with night vision, followed by the development of blind spots in peripheral vision. Blind spots become bigger with time and eventually merge to produce tunnel vision. Most individuals also develop a blurred central vision and become legally blind by adolescence or early adulthood (over 90% of cases).
- Extra finger next to the pinky (postaxial polydactyly)
- Kidney problems (polycystic kidneys)
- Obesity that develops around two to three years of age
- Abnormalities of the genitalia and infertility due to hypogonadism
- Learning disorders

Bardet-Biedl syndrome may also be associated with other features, including:

- Diabetes

- High blood pressure
- Heart defects
- Bowel disease (Hirschsprung disease)
- Neurological problems resulting in gait and coordination impairment
- Speech and language problems
- Behavioral disorders
- Distinctive facial appearance
- Dental abnormalities

INHERITANCE OF BARDET-BIEDL SYNDROME

Bardet-Biedl syndrome has an autosomal recessive pattern of inheritance. This means that to have the syndrome, a person must have a mutation in both copies of the responsible gene in each cell. People with BBS inherit one mutated copy of the gene from each parent, who is referred to as a carrier. Carriers of an autosomal recessive condition typically do not have any signs or symptoms (they are unaffected). When two carriers of an autosomal recessive condition have children, each child has a:

- 25 percent chance to be affected
- 50 percent chance to be an unaffected carrier like each parent
- 25 percent chance to be unaffected and not a carrier

Some cases of BBS (fewer than 10%) appear to require the presence of at least three mutations for a person to have features of the condition. This is known as "triallelic inheritance." In these cases, in addition to inheriting a mutation in the same gene from each parent, a child also needs to have at least one more mutation in another gene to be affected.

TREATMENT OF BARDET-BIEDL SYNDROME

There is no cure for BBS. Treatment generally focuses on the specific signs and symptoms in each individual:

- While there is no therapy for progressive vision loss, early evaluation by a specialist can help to provide

visual aids and mobility training. Additionally, education of affected children should include planning for future blindness.
- Management of obesity may include education, diet, exercise, and behavioral therapies beginning at an early age. Complications of obesity such as abnormally high cholesterol and diabetes mellitus are usually treated as they are in the general population.
- Management of intellectual disability includes early intervention, special education and speech therapy as needed. Many affected adults are able to develop independent living skills.
- Although kidney transplants have been successful, the immunosuppressants used after a transplant may contribute to obesity. Affected individuals may also need surgery for polydactyly (extra fingers and/or toes) or genital abnormalities.
- As children approach puberty, hormone levels should be monitored to determine if hormone replacement therapy is necessary. Additionally, it should not be assumed that affected individuals are infertile—so contraception advice should be offered.

Section 39.5 | **Ocular Albinism**

This section contains text excerpted from the following sources: Text in this section begins with excerpts from "Ocular Albinism," Genetics Home Reference (GHR), National Institutes of Health (NIH), March 17, 2020; Text under the heading "Treatment of Ocular Albinism" is excerpted from "Ocular Albinism Type 1," National Heart, Lung, and Blood Institute (NHLBI), August 10, 2015. Reviewed March 2020.

Ocular albinism is a genetic condition that primarily affects the eyes. This condition reduces the coloring (pigmentation) of the iris, which is the colored part of the eye, and the retina, which is the light-sensitive tissue at the back of the eye. Pigmentation in the eye is essential for normal vision.

Ocular albinism is characterized by severely impaired sharpness of vision (visual acuity) and problems with combining vision from both eyes to perceive depth (stereoscopic vision). Although the vision loss is permanent, it does not worsen over time. Other eye abnormalities associated with this condition include rapid, involuntary eye movements (nystagmus), eyes that do not look in the same direction (strabismus), and increased sensitivity to light (photophobia). Many affected individuals also have abnormalities involving the optic nerves, which carry visual information from the eye to the brain.

Unlike some other forms of albinism, ocular albinism does not significantly affect the color of the skin and hair. People with this condition may have a somewhat lighter complexion than other members of their family, but these differences are usually minor.

The most common form of ocular albinism is known as the "Nettleship-Falls type" or "type 1." Other forms of ocular albinism, such as hearing loss are much rarer and may be associated with additional signs and symptoms.

FREQUENCY OF OCULAR ALBINISM

The most common form of this disorder, ocular albinism type 1, affects at least 1 in 60,000 males. The classic signs and symptoms of this condition are much less common in females.

CAUSES OF OCULAR ALBINISM

Ocular albinism type 1 results from mutations in the *GPR143* gene. This gene provides instructions for making a protein that plays a role in pigmentation of the eyes and skin. It helps control the growth of melanosomes, which are cellular structures that produce and store a pigment called "melanin." Melanin is the substance that gives skin, hair, and eyes their color. In the retina, this pigment also plays a role in normal vision.

Most mutations in the *GPR143* gene alter the size or shape of the *GPR143* protein. Many of these genetic changes prevent the protein from reaching melanosomes to control their growth. In other cases, the protein reaches melanosomes normally but mutations disrupt the protein's function. As a result of these changes, melanosomes in skin cells and the retina can grow abnormally large. Researchers are uncertain how these giant melanosomes are related to vision loss and other eye abnormalities in people with ocular albinism.

Rare cases of ocular albinism are not caused by mutations in the *GPR143* gene. In these cases, the genetic cause of the condition is often unknown.

TREATMENT OF OCULAR ALBINISM

Hypersensitivity to light often called "photo aversion," "photophobia," or "photodysphoria," is the most incapacitating symptom in some people with ocular albinism type 1 (OA1). This symptom may be relieved by sunglasses, transition lenses, or special filter glasses, although many prefer not to wear them because of the reduction in vision from the dark lenses when indoors.

Refractive errors should be detected and treated as early as possible with appropriate spectacle correction. Abnormal head posture may be treated with prismatic spectacle correction.

Strabismus surgery is usually not necessary but may be performed for cosmetic purposes, particularly if the strabismus or the face turn is marked or fixed.

Appropriate education on sunscreens and clothing (preferably by an informed dermatologic consultant) is recommended to moderate the lifelong effects of sun exposure.

Children with ocular albinism who are younger than 16 years of age should have an annual ophthalmologic exam (including assessment of refractive error and the need for filter glasses), as well as psychosocial and educational support. Affected adults should have ophthalmologic exams when needed, typically every 2 to 3 years.

Section 39.6 | **Stargardt Disease**

This section includes text excerpted from "Stargardt Disease," National Eye Institute (NEI), July 10, 2019.

WHAT IS STARGARDT DISEASE?

Stargardt disease is an inherited disorder of the retina—the tissue at the back of the eye that senses light. The disease typically causes vision loss during childhood or adolescence, although in some forms, vision loss may not be noticed until later in adulthood. It is rare for people with the disease to become completely blind. For most people, vision loss progresses slowly over time to 20/200 or worse. (Normal vision is 20/20.)

Stargardt disease is also called "Stargardt macular dystrophy," "juvenile macular degeneration," or "fundus flavimaculatus." The disease causes progressive damage—or degeneration—of the macula, which is a small area in the center of the retina that is responsible for sharp, straight-ahead vision. Stargardt disease is one of several genetic disorders that cause macular degeneration. Experts estimate that 1 in 8 to 10 thousand people have Stargardt disease.

WHAT ARE THE SYMPTOMS OF STARGARDT DISEASE?

The most common symptom of Stargardt disease is variable, often there is a slow loss of central vision in both eyes. People with the disease might notice gray, black, or hazy spots in the center of their vision, or that it takes longer than usual for their eyes to adjust when moving from light to dark environments. Their eyes may be more sensitive to bright light. Some people also develop color blindness later in the disease.

The progression of symptoms in Stargardt disease is different for each person. People with an earlier onset of disease tend to have more rapid vision loss. Vision loss may decrease slowly at first, then worsen rapidly until it levels off. Most people with Stargardt disease will end up with 20/200 vision or worse. People with Stargardt disease may also begin to lose some of their peripheral (side) vision as they get older.

WHAT CAUSES STARGARDT DISEASE

The retina contains light-sensing cells called "photoreceptors." There are two types of photoreceptors: rods and cones. Together, rod and cones detect light and convert it into electrical signals, which are then "seen" by the brain. Rods are found in the outer retina and help us see in dim and dark lighting. Cones are found in the macula and help us see fine visual detail and color. Both cones and rods die away in Stargardt disease, but for unclear reasons, cones are more strongly affected in most cases.

You may have heard about the importance of vitamin A-rich foods in maintaining healthy vision. That is because vitamin A is needed to make key light-sensitive molecules inside photoreceptors. Unfortunately, this manufacturing process can lead to harmful vitamin A byproducts, which turn out to play a key role in Stargardt disease.

Mutations in a gene called "*ABCA4*" are the most common cause of Stargardt disease. This gene makes a protein that normally clears away vitamin A byproducts inside photoreceptors. Cells that lack the *ABCA4* protein accumulate clumps of lipofuscin, a fatty substance that forms yellowish flecks. As the clumps of lipofuscin increase in and around the macula, central vision becomes impaired. Eventually, these fatty deposits lead to the death of photoreceptors and vision becomes further impaired.

Mutations in the *ABCA4* gene are also associated with other retinal dystrophies including cone dystrophy, cone-rod dystrophy, and retinitis pigmentosa, a severe form of retinal degeneration.

How Is Stargardt Disease Inherited?

Genes are bundled together on structures called "chromosomes." One copy of each chromosome is passed by a parent at conception through egg and sperm cells. The X and Y chromosomes, known as "sex chromosomes," determine whether a person is born female (XX) or male (XY) and also carries other nonsex traits.

In autosomal recessive inheritance, it takes two copies of the mutant gene to give rise to the disease. An individual who has one copy of a recessive gene mutation is known as a "carrier." When two carriers have a child, there is a:

- One in four chance of having a child with the disease
- One in two chance of having a child who is a carrier
- One in four chance of having a child who neither has the disease nor is a carrier

In autosomal dominant inheritance, it takes just one copy of the mutant gene to bring about the disease. When an affected parent with one dominant gene mutation has a child, there is a one in two chance that a child will inherit the disease.

Autosomal recessive mutations in the *ABCA4* gene account for about 95 percent of Stargardt disease. The other five percent of cases are caused by rarer mutations in different genes that play a role in lipofuscin function. Some of these mutations are autosomal dominant.

HOW WILL AN EYE DOCTOR CHECK FOR STARGARDT DISEASE?

An eye-care professional can make a positive diagnosis of Stargardt disease by examining the retina. Lipofuscin deposits can be seen as yellowish flecks in the macula. The flecks are irregular in shape and usually extend outward from the macula in a ring-like pattern. The number, size, color, and appearance of these flecks are widely variable.

A standard eye chart and other tests may be used to assess symptoms of vision loss in Stargardt disease, including:

- **Visual field testing.** Visual field testing attempts to measure the distribution and sensitivity of the field of vision. Multiple methods are available for testing; none is painful and most share a requirement for the patient to indicate the ability to see a stimulus/target. This process results in a map of the person's visual field and can point to a loss of central vision or peripheral vision.
- **Color testing.** There are several tests that can be used to detect loss of color vision, which can occur late in Stargardt disease. Three tests are often used to get additional information: fundus photography combined with autofluorescence, electroretinography (ERG), and optical coherence tomography (OCT).

- **A fundus photo** is a picture of the retina. These photos may reveal the presence of lipofuscin deposits. In fundus autofluorescence (FAF), a special filter is used to detect lipofuscin. Lipofuscin is naturally fluorescent (it glows in the dark) when a specific wavelength of light is shined into the eye. This test can detect lipofuscin that might not be visible with standard fundus photography, making it possible to diagnose Stargardt disease earlier.
- **Electroretinography** measures the electrical response of rods and cones to light. During the test, an electrode is placed on the cornea and light is flashed into the eye. The electrical responses are viewed and recorded on a monitor. Abnormal patterns of light response suggest the presence of Stargardt disease or other diseases that involve retinal degeneration.
- **Optical coherence tomography** is a scanning device that works similar to an ultrasound. While ultrasound captures images by bouncing sound waves off of living tissues, OCT does it with light waves. The patient places her or his head on a chin rest while invisible, near-infrared light is focused on the retina. Because the eye is designed to allow light in, it is possible to get detailed pictures deep within the retina. These pictures are then analyzed for any abnormalities in the thickness of the retinal layers, which could indicate retinal degeneration. OCT is sometimes combined with infrared scanning laser ophthalmoscope (ISLO) to provide additional surface images of the retina.

WHAT IS THE TREATMENT FOR STARGARDT DISEASE?

Currently, there is no treatment for Stargardt disease. Some ophthalmologists encourage people with Stargardt disease to wear dark glasses and hats when out in bright light to reduce the buildup of lipofuscin. Cigarette smoking and secondhand smoke should be avoided. Animal studies suggest that high-dose vitamin A may increase lipofuscin accumulation and potentially accelerate vision loss. Therefore, supplements containing more than the recommended daily allowance of vitamin A should be avoided, or taken only under a doctor's supervision. There is no need to worry about getting too much vitamin A through food.

A number of services and devices can help people with Stargardt disease carry out daily activities and maintain their independence. Low-vision aids can be helpful for many daily tasks and range from simple hand-held lenses to electronic devices such as electronic reading machines or closed circuit video magnification systems. Because many people with Stargardt disease will become visually disabled by their 20s, the disease can have a significant emotional impact. Work, socializing, driving and other activities that may have come easily in the past are likely to become challenging. So counseling and occupational therapies often need to be part of the treatment plan.

RESEARCH ON STARGARDT DISEASE

Over the past several decades, researchers have identified hundreds of genes that contribute to inherited eye diseases, including Stargardt disease. This information has led to better diagnostic tests and is providing insight into possible treatments.

Scientists are also working to find new mutations in the *ABCA4* gene, and in other genes, that might contribute to Stargardt disease.

Many studies continue to explore the biology and genetics of Stargardt disease, and of macular degeneration more generally. For example, the National Eye Institute (NEI) is conducting a natural history study of Stargardt and other *ABCA4*-related diseases. The study is following 45 individuals with *ABCA4* mutations for 5 years. The main goals are to better understand the natural course of the disease, to make contact with people who may be interested in future clinical trials, and to collect blood, skin, and DNA samples from those people. These samples can be studied in the lab to explore the mechanisms of Stargardt disease.

Such mechanistic studies can lead to new treatment strategies. One strategy currently under study is to reduce the buildup of lipofuscin and other toxic byproducts in the retina. A National Eye Institute (NEI)-funded group based at Columbia University is working with a synthetic form of vitamin A, called "ALK-001," that is not readily converted into lipofuscin. In mice and larger animal models, an oral form of ALK-001 slows the formation of lipofuscin deposits. ALK-001 is being tested for safety in healthy volunteers before testing begins on people with Stargardt disease.

A group based at Case Western Reserve University (CWRU) and supported by the NEI Translational Research Program (TRP) on therapy for visual disorders is taking another approach. The group has tested a panel of drugs already deemed safe by the U.S. Food and Drug Administration (FDA) in a mouse model of Stargardt. They found that some FDA-approved drugs can reduce retinal damage in the mice. They are now evaluating chemical compounds with a similar structure to FDA-approved drugs and exploring different modes of drug delivery.

Gene therapy—that is, repairing or replacing the defective *ABCA4* gene—also holds promise for treating Stargardt disease. Gene replacement therapy requires a method for delivering the gene of interest into cells, and for some diseases, the solution has been to package the gene inside a small, harmless virus called the "adeno-associated virus" (AAV). The *ABCA4* gene is too large to fit within this virus. Researchers funded by NEI, therefore, modified a larger virus from the lentivirus family and engineered it to carry ABCA4. Tests in the Stargardt mouse model showed that this approach can reduce lipofuscin accumulation. Oxford Biomedica has refined this technology and licensed it under the name StarGen. The human safety trials of StarGen began in 2011.

Stem cell-based therapies are showing promise for Stargardt disease in clinical trials. Stem cells are immature cells that can generate many mature cell types in the body, including the photoreceptors that die off in Stargardt disease. Human stem cells can be derived from embryonic or adult tissues. Both kinds of cells are being tested in patients with Stargardt disease and age-related macular degeneration (AMD), which is a leading cause of vision loss in the United States.

A U.S. company called "Advanced Cell Technology" (ACT) is conducting a trial of retinal pigment epithelium (RPE) cells for AMD and Stargardt disease. These cells provide support and nourishment to the retina. The RPE cells understudy in the ACT trial is derived from human embryonic stem cells.

Other clinical and laboratory studies are making use of adult cells that have been reprogrammed into stem cells, called "induced pluripotent" or "iPS cells." In 2014, Japanese scientists launched the first clinical trial of iPS cells to treat AMD, and indeed the first trial ever of iPS cells. The goal is to coax the iPS cells into making RPE cells. NEI scientists are planning a similar trial and going a step further—by seeding the RPE cells onto a scaffold so that they form a sheet, similar to how they arrange themselves in the eye. NEI scientists also plan to make iPS cells from the skin cells collected in the Stargardt natural history study. These iPS cells could be used to make photoreceptors and RPE cells—for use in potential cell therapies and as a research tool to study how potential drugs will affect these cell types.

Section 39.7 | **Usher Syndrome**

This section includes text excerpted from "Usher Syndrome," National Eye Institute (NEI), July 11, 2019.

WHAT IS USHER SYNDROME?

Usher syndrome is the most common condition that affects both hearing and vision; sometimes it also affects balance. The major symptoms of Usher syndrome are deafness or hearing loss and an eye disease called "retinitis pigmentosa" (RP).

Deafness or hearing loss in Usher syndrome is caused by abnormal development of hair cells (sound receptor cells) in the inner ear. Most children with Usher syndrome are born with moderate to profound hearing loss, depending on the type. Less commonly, hearing loss from Usher syndrome appears during adolescence or later. Usher syndrome can also cause severe balance problems due to abnormal development of the vestibular hair cells, sensory cells that detect gravity and head movement.

Retinitis pigmentosa initially causes night blindness and a loss of peripheral (side) vision through the progressive degeneration of cells in the retina. The retina is the light-sensitive tissue at the back of the eye and is crucial for vision. As RP progresses, the field of vision narrows until only central vision remains, a condition called "tunnel vision." Macular holes (small breaks in the macula, the central part of the retina) and cataracts (clouding of the lens) can sometimes cause an early decline in central vision in people with Usher syndrome.

Who Is Affected by Usher Syndrome?

Usher syndrome affects approximately 4 to 17 per 100,000 people and accounts for about 50 percent of all hereditary deaf-blindness cases. The condition is thought to account for 3 to 6 percent of all children who are deaf, and another 3 to 6 percent of children who are hard-of-hearing.

WHAT CAUSES USHER SYNDROME

Usher syndrome is inherited, which means that it is passed from parents to a child through genes. Each person inherits two copies of a gene, one from each parent. Sometimes genes are altered, or mutated. Mutated genes may cause cells to develop or act abnormally.

Usher syndrome is inherited as an autosomal recessive disorder. "Autosomal" means that men and women are equally likely to have the disorder and equally likely to pass it on to a child of either sex. "Recessive" means that the condition occurs only when a child inherits two copies of the same faulty gene, one from each parent. A person with one abnormal Usher gene does not have the disorder but is a carrier who has a 50 percent chance of passing on the abnormal gene to each child. When two carriers with the same mutated Usher syndrome gene have a child together, each birth has a:

- One in four chance of having a child who neither has Usher syndrome nor is a carrier
- Two in four chance of having a child who is an unaffected carrier
- One in four chance of having Usher syndrome

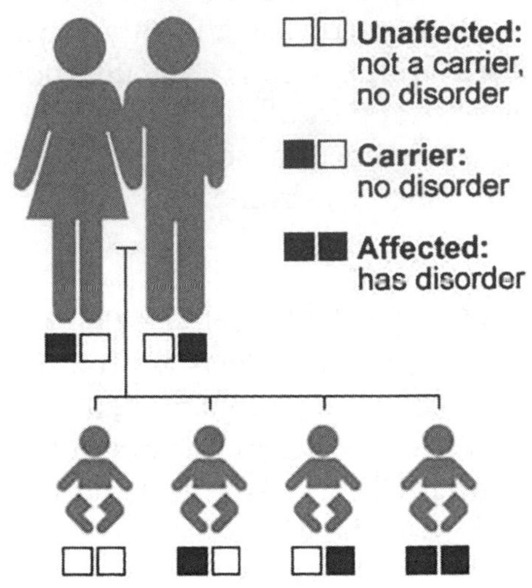

Figure 39.1. Causes of Usher Syndrome

The hearing, balance, and vision of carriers with one mutant Usher gene are typically normal. Carriers are often unaware of their carrier status.

WHAT ARE THE TYPES OF USHER SYNDROME?

There are three types of Usher syndrome. In the United States, types 1 and 2 are the most common. Together, they account for up to 95 percent of Usher syndrome cases.

Type 1. Children with type 1 Usher syndrome have profound hearing loss or deafness at birth and have severe balance problems. Many obtain little or no benefit from hearing aids but may be candidates for a cochlear implant—an electronic device that can provide a sense of sound to people with severe hearing loss or deafness. Parents should consult with their child's doctor and other hearing health professionals early to determine communication options for their child. Intervention should begin promptly, when the brain is most receptive to learning language, whether spoken or signed.

Table 39.1. Types of Usher Syndrome

	Type 1	Type 2	Type 3
Hearing	Profound hearing loss or deafness at birth.	Moderate to severe hearing loss at birth.	Progressive loss in childhood or early teens.
Vision	Decreased night vision by age 10, progressing to severe vision loss by midlife.	Decreased night vision by adolescence, progressing to severe vision loss by midlife.	Varies in severity and age of onset; night vision problems often begin in teens and progress to severe vision loss by midlife.
Balance (vestibular function)	Balance problems from birth.	Normal balance.	Normal to near-normal balance in childhood; chance of later problems.

Balance problems associated with type 1 Usher syndrome delay sitting up without support. Walking rarely occurs prior to 18 months. Vision problems with type 1 Usher syndrome usually begin before age 10, starting with difficulty seeing at night and progressing to severe vision loss over several decades.

Type 2. Children with type 2 Usher syndrome are born with moderate to severe hearing loss but normal balance. Although the severity of hearing loss varies, most children with type 2 Usher syndrome can communicate orally and benefit from hearing aids. RP is usually diagnosed during late adolescence in people with type 2 Usher syndrome.

Type 3. Children with type 3 Usher syndrome have normal hearing at birth. Most have normal to near-normal balance; however, some develop balance problems with age. The decline in hearing and vision varies. Children with type 3 Usher syndrome often develop hearing loss by adolescence, requiring hearing aids by mid-to-late adulthood. Night blindness also usually begins during adolescence. Blind spots appear by the late teens to the early twenties. Legal blindness often occurs by midlife.

HOW DOES THE DOCTOR CHECK FOR USHER SYNDROME?

Diagnosis of Usher syndrome involves asking questions about the patient's medical history and testing of hearing, balance, and vision. Early diagnosis is important, as it improves the likelihood of treatment success. An eye-care specialist can use dilating drops to examine the retina for signs of RP. Visual field testing measures side vision. An electroretinogram measures the electrical response of the eye's light-sensitive cells in the retina. Optical coherence tomography may be helpful to assess macular cystic changes. Videonystagmography measures involuntary eye movements that might signify a balance problem. Audiology testing determines hearing sensitivity at a range of frequencies.

Genetic testing may help diagnose Usher syndrome. So far, researchers have found nine genes that cause Usher syndrome. Genetic testing is available for all of them:

- Type 1 Usher syndrome: *MY07a, USH1C, CDH23, PCHD15, USH1G*
- Type 2 Usher syndrome: *USH2A, GPR98, DFNB31*
- Type 3 Usher syndrome: *CLRN1*

WHAT IS THE TREATMENT FOR USHER SYNDROME?

Presently, there is no cure for Usher syndrome. Treatment involves managing hearing, vision, and balance problems. Early diagnosis helps tailor educational programs that consider the severity of hearing and vision loss and a child's age and ability. Treatment may include hearing aids, assistive listening devices, and cochlear implants. It may also include communication methods such as American Sign Language (ASL) and orientation and mobility training for balance problems. Communication services and independent living training may include Braille instruction, low-vision services, or auditory (hearing) training.

Vitamin A may slow the progression of RP, according to results from a long-term clinical trial supported by the National Eye Institute (NEI) and the Foundation Fighting Blindness. Based on the study, adults with a common form of RP may benefit from a daily supplement of 15,000 IU (international units) of the palmitate form of vitamin A. Patients should discuss this treatment option with their healthcare provider before proceeding. Because people with type 1 Usher syndrome did not take part in the study, high-dose vitamin A is not recommended for these patients.

General precautions for vitamin A supplementation:

- Do not substitute vitamin A palmitate with a beta-carotene supplement.
- Do not take vitamin A supplements greater than the recommended dose of 15,000 IU or modify your diet to select foods with high levels of vitamin A.
- Pregnant women should not take high-dose vitamin A supplements due to the increased risk of birth defects. Women considering pregnancy should stop taking high-dose vitamin A supplements for six months before trying to conceive.

RESEARCH ON USHER SYNDROME

Researchers are trying to identify additional genes that cause Usher syndrome. Efforts will lead to improved genetic counseling and earlier diagnosis, and may eventually expand treatment options.

Scientists are also developing mouse models with characteristics similar to Usher syndrome. Research using mouse models will help determine the function of Usher genes and will inform potential treatments.

Other areas of study include new methods for early identification of children with Usher syndrome, improving treatment strategies for children who use hearing aids and cochlear implants for hearing loss and testing innovative intervention strategies to help slow or stop the progression of RP. Clinical researchers are also characterizing variability in balance among individuals with various types of Usher syndrome.

Section 39.8 | **Wagner Syndrome**

This section includes text excerpted from "Wagner Syndrome," Genetic and Rare Diseases Information Center (GARD), National Center for Advancing Translational Sciences (NCATS), January 23, 2017.

WHAT IS WAGNER SYNDROME?

Wagner syndrome is a hereditary eye disorder that leads to progressive vision loss. It is characterized by changes to the thick, clear gel that fills the eyeball (the vitreous), in which it becomes thin and watery and appears empty. The first signs and symptoms usually appear in childhood, but onset may be as early as two years of age. Signs and symptoms may include: thinning of the light-sensitive tissue that lines the back of the eye (retinal detachment), abnormalities of the blood vessels within the retina (known as the "choroid"), and degeneration of the retina and choroid. Wagner syndrome is caused by mutations in the *VCAN* gene and is inherited in an autosomal dominant manner. Treatment varies depending on the signs and symptoms in each individual and may include the use of glasses or contact lenses and vitreoretinal surgery.

WHAT ARE THE SIGNS AND SYMPTOMS OF WAGNER SYNDROME?

The signs and symptoms of Wagner syndrome vary from person to person. The most distinctive feature affects the vitreous. In individuals with Wagner syndrome, the vitreous appears to be empty with just a concentration of vitreous around the inside of the eyeball, which is often lined with cord-like structures. This unusual finding can be found even in young children. This primary symptom can lead to many secondary features which include:

- Early cataracts (before 40 years of age)
- Degeneration and atrophy of the retina, the underlying retinal pigment epithelium (RPE), and the choroid
- Retinal detachment
- Nearsightedness (myopia)
- Night blindness
- Visual field restriction

WHAT CAUSES WAGNER SYNDROME

Wagner syndrome is caused by mutations in the *VCAN* gene. This gene provides instructions for a protein called "versican," which is a major component of the extracellular matrix (the material that surrounds and supports cells). The versican protein is involved in cell adhesion, proliferation, migration (movement), and angiogenesis (the formation of new blood vessels). It plays a central role in tissue morphogenesis and maintenance. Within the eye, versican interacts with other proteins to maintain the structure and gel-like consistency of the vitreous.

VCAN gene mutations that cause Wagner syndrome are thought to lead to insufficient levels of versican in the vitreous and structural instability. This lack of stability in the vitreous affects other areas of the eye and contributes to the vision problems that occur in people with Wagner syndrome.

HOW IS WAGNER SYNDROME DIAGNOSED?

The diagnosis of Wagner syndrome is based on typical clinical findings and family history of the condition. Genetic testing of the *VCAN* gene is available and can be used to confirm the diagnosis.

HOW MIGHT WAGNER SYNDROME BE TREATED?

There is no cure for Wagner syndrome, but there may be ways to manage the symptoms. Refractive errors (such as myopia) can be corrected by glasses or contact lenses. Cataracts should be removed via standard protocols by an experienced eye-care professional. Retinal breaks can be treated with laser retinopexy (gas bubble placement) or cryotherapy (use of subzero temperatures to treat tissue damage). All individuals with Wagner syndrome should see a vitreoretinal specialist for ophthalmologic evaluation once a year.

Chapter 40 | **Other Congenital Disorders Affecting Vision**

Chapter Contents

Section 40.1 | Anophthalmia and Microphthalmia

This section includes text excerpted from "Facts about Anophthalmia/Microphthalmia," Centers for Disease Control and Prevention (CDC), December 5, 2019.

WHAT IS ANOPHTHALMIA/MICROPHTHALMIA?

Anophthalmia and microphthalmia are birth defects of a baby's eyes. Anophthalmia is a birth defect where a baby is born without one or both eyes. And microphthalmia is a birth defect in which one or both eyes did not develop fully, so they are small. Anophthalmia and microphthalmia develop during pregnancy and can occur alone, with other birth defects, or as part of a syndrome. Anophthalmia and microphthalmia often result in blindness or limited vision.

HOW MANY BABIES ARE BORN WITH ANOPHTHALMIA/MICROPHTHALMIA?

Researchers estimate that about 1 in every 5,200 babies is born with anophthalmia/microphthalmia in the United States.

CAUSES AND RISK FACTORS OF ANOPHTHALMIA/MICROPHTHALMIA

The causes of anophthalmia and microphthalmia among most infants are unknown. Some babies have anophthalmia or microphthalmia because of a change in their genes or chromosomes. Anophthalmia and microphthalmia can also be caused by taking certain medicines, such as isotretinoin (Accutane®) or thalidomide, during pregnancy. These medicines can lead to a pattern of birth defects, which can include anophthalmia or microphthalmia. These defects might also be caused by a combination of genes and other factors, such as the things the mother comes in contact with, in the environment, or what the mother eats or drinks, or certain medicines she uses during pregnancy.

DIAGNOSIS OF ANOPHTHALMIA/MICROPHTHALMIA

Anophthalmia and microphthalmia can either be diagnosed during pregnancy or after birth. During pregnancy, doctors can often identify anophthalmia and microphthalmia through an ultrasound or a computed tomography (CT) scan (special x-ray test) and sometimes with certain genetic testing. After birth, a doctor can identify anophthalmia and microphthalmia by examining the baby. A doctor will also perform a thorough physical exam to look for any other birth defects that may be present.

TREATMENT OF ANOPHTHALMIA/MICROPHTHALMIA

There is no treatment available that will create a new eye or that will restore complete vision for those affected by anophthalmia or microphthalmia. A baby born with one of these conditions should be seen by a team of eye specialists:

- An ophthalmologist, a doctor specially trained to care for eyes
- An ocularist, a healthcare provider who is specially trained in making and fitting prosthetic eyes
- An oculoplastic surgeon, a doctor who specializes in surgery for the eye, and eye socket

The eye sockets are critical for a baby's face to grow and develop properly. If a baby has one of these conditions, the bones that shape the eye socket may not grow properly. Babies can be fitted with a plastic structure called a "conformer" that can help the eye socket and bones to grow properly. As babies get older, these devices will need to be enlarged to help expand the eye socket. Also, as children age, they can be fitted for an artificial eye.

A team of eye specialists should frequently monitor children with these conditions early in life. If other conditions arise, such as a cataract or detached retina, children might need surgery to repair these other conditions. If anophthalmia or microphthalmia affects only one eye, the ophthalmologist can suggest ways to protect and preserve sight in the healthy eye. Depending on the severity of anophthalmia and microphthalmia, children might need surgery. It is important to talk to their team of eye specialists to determine the best plan of action.

Babies born with these conditions can often benefit from early intervention and therapy to help their development and mobility.

Section 40.2 | Bietti Crystalline Dystrophy

This section includes text excerpted from "Bietti's Crystalline Dystrophy," National Eye Institute (NEI), July 2, 2019.

Bietti crystalline dystrophy (BCD) is an inherited eye disease named after Dr. G.B. Bietti, an Italian ophthalmologist, who described three patients with similar symptoms in 1937.

This disease is also known as "Bietti crystalline chorioretinal dystrophy."

WHAT CAUSES BIETTI CRYSTALLINE DYSTROPHY

From family studies, it has been found that BCD is inherited primarily in an autosomal recessive fashion. This means that an affected person receives one nonworking gene from each of her or his parents. A person who inherits a nonworking gene from only one parent will be a carrier, but will not develop the disease. A person with BCD syndrome will pass on one gene to each of her or his children. However, unless the person has children with another carrier of BCD genes, the individual's children are not at risk for developing the disease.

In March 2004, the National Eye Institute (NEI) researchers identified the BCD gene, now named *CYP4V2*. Researchers believe that this gene has a role in fatty acid and steroid metabolism. This is consistent with findings from biochemical studies of patients with BCD.

WHAT ARE THE SYMPTOMS OF BIETTI CRYSTALLINE DYSTROPHY?

The symptoms of BCD include crystals in the cornea (the clear covering of the eye), yellow, shiny deposits on the retina, and progressive atrophy of the retina, choriocapillaris, and choroid (the back layers of the eye). This tends to lead to progressive night blindness and visual field constriction. BCD is a rare disease and appears to be more common in people with Asian ancestry.

People with BCD have crystals in some of their white blood cells (WBCs) (lymphocytes) that can be seen by using an electron

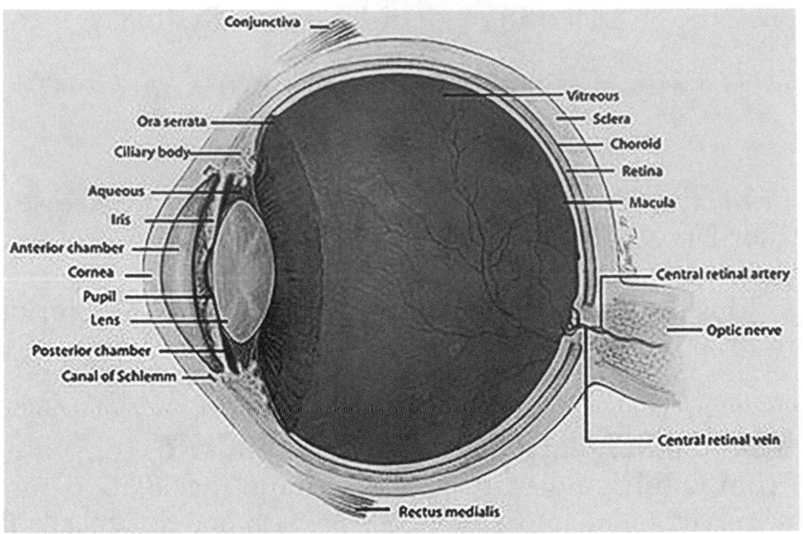

Figure 40.1. Bietti Crystalline Dystrophy

microscope. Researchers have been unable to determine exactly what substance makes up these crystalline deposits. Their presence does not appear to harm the patient in any other way except to affect vision.

WHAT IS THE TREATMENT FOR BIETTI CRYSTALLINE DYSTROPHY?

At this time, there is no treatment for BCD. Scientists hope that findings from gene research will be helpful in finding treatments for patients with BCD.

Section 40.3 | Color Blindness

This section includes text excerpted from "Color Blindness," National Eye Institute (NEI), July 3, 2019.

WHAT IS COLOR BLINDNESS?

If you have color blindness, it means you see colors differently than most people. Most of the time, color blindness makes it hard to tell the difference between certain colors.

Usually, color blindness runs in families. There is no cure, but special glasses and contact lenses can help. Most people who are color blind are able to adjust and do not have problems with everyday activities.

WHAT ARE THE TYPES OF COLOR BLINDNESS?

The most common type of color blindness makes it hard to tell the difference between red and green. Another type makes it hard to tell the difference between blue and yellow. People who are completely color blind do not see color at all, but that is not very common.

WHAT ARE THE SYMPTOMS OF COLOR BLINDNESS?

The main symptom of color blindness is not seeing colors the way most people do. If you are color blind, you may have trouble seeing:

- The difference between colors
- How bright colors are
- Different shades of colors

Symptoms of color blindness are often so mild that you may not notice them. And since a person gets used to the way they see colors, many with color blindness do not know they have it.

People with very serious cases of color blindness might have other symptoms, too—such as quick side-to-side eye movements (nystagmus), or sensitivity to light.

WHO IS AT RISK FOR COLOR BLINDNESS?

Men have a much higher risk than women for color blindness. You are also more likely to have color blindness if you:

- Have a family history of color blindness
- Have certain eye diseases, such as glaucoma or age-related macular degeneration (AMD)
- Have certain health problems, such as diabetes, Alzheimer disease (AD), or multiple sclerosis (MS)
- Take certain medicines
- Are white

If you think you may have color blindness, talk to your doctor about getting checked.

WHAT CAUSES COLOR BLINDNESS

The most common kinds of color blindness are genetic, meaning they are passed down from parents.

Color blindness can also happen because of damage to your eye or your brain. And color vision may get worse as you get older—often because of cataracts (cloudy areas in the lens of the eye).

HOW TO FIND OUT IF YOU HAVE COLOR BLINDNESS

Your eye doctor can usually use a simple test to tell you if you are color blind.

During the test, your eye doctor will show you a circle made of many different colored dots. The circle has a shape inside it that is made out of dots—such as a number, a letter, or a squiggly line. This shape is easy to see if you do not have color blindness, but people who are color blind have a hard time seeing it.

WHAT IS THE TREATMENT FOR COLOR BLINDNESS?

There is no cure for color blindness that is passed down in families, but most people find ways to adjust to it. Children with color blindness may need help with some classroom activities, and adults with color blindness may not be able to do certain jobs, such as being a pilot or graphic designer. Keep in mind that most of the time, color blindness does not cause serious problems.

If your color blindness is happening because of another health problem, your doctor will treat the condition that is causing the problem. If you are taking a medicine that causes color blindness, your doctor may adjust how much you take or suggest you switch to a different medicine.

If color blindness is causing problems with everyday tasks, there are devices and technology that can help, including:

- **Glasses and contacts.** Special contact lenses and glasses may help people who are color blind tell the difference between colors.
- **Visual aids.** You can use visual aids, apps, and other technology to help you live with color blindness. For example, you can use an app to take a photo with your phone or tablet and then tap on part of the photo to find out the color of that area.

Discuss your options with your eye doctor. Remember these tips:

- Ask your doctor about visual aids and technology that can help you with everyday tasks.
- Encourage family members to get checked for color blindness, since it can run in families.

Section 40.4 | **Duane Syndrome**

This section includes text excerpted from "About Duane Syndrome," National Human Genome Research Institute (NHGRI), June 29, 2017.

WHAT IS DUANE SYNDROME?

Duane syndrome (DS) is a miswiring of the eye muscles, causing some eye muscles to contract when they should not and other eye muscles not to contract when they should. People with DS have a limited (and sometimes absent) ability to move the eye outward toward the ear (abduction) and, in most cases, a limited ability to move the eye inward toward the nose (adduction). Other names for this condition include Duane retraction syndrome (or DR syndrome), eye retraction syndrome, retraction syndrome, congenital retraction syndrome, and Stilling-Turk-Duane syndrome.

Often, when the eye moves toward the nose, the eyeball also pulls into the socket (retraction), the eye-opening narrows and, in some cases, the eye will move upward or downward. Many patients with DS develop a face turn to maintain binocular vision and compensate for the improper turning of the eyes.

In about 80 percent of cases of DS, only one eye is affected, most often the left. However, in some cases, both eyes are affected, with one eye usually more affected than the other.

In 70 percent of DS cases, this is the only disorder the individual has. However, other conditions and syndromes have been found in association with DS. These include malformation of the skeleton, ears, eyes, kidneys and nervous system, as well as:

- Okihiro syndrome, an association of DS with forearm malformation and hearing loss
- Wildervanck syndrome (WS), a fusion of neck vertebrae and hearing loss
- Holt-Oram syndrome (HOS), abnormalities of the upper limbs and heart
- Morning Glory syndrome (MGS), abnormalities of the optic disc or "blind spot"
- Goldenhar syndrome, malformation of the jaw, cheek, and ear, usually on one side of the face

WHAT ARE THE SYMPTOMS OF DUANE SYNDROME?

Clinically, DS is often subdivided into three types, each with associated symptoms.

Type 1. The affected eye, or eyes, has limited ability to move outward toward the ear, but the ability to move inward toward the nose is normal or nearly so. The eye-opening narrows and the eyeball pull in when looking inward toward the nose, however, the reverse occurs when looking outward toward the ear. About 78 percent of all DS cases are Type 1.

Type 2. The affected eye, or eyes, has limited ability to move inward toward the nose, but the ability to move outward toward the ear is normal or nearly so. The eye-opening narrows and the eyeball pull in when looking inward toward the nose. About seven percent of all DS cases are Type 2.

Type 3. The affected eye, or eyes, has limited ability to move both inward toward the nose and outward toward the ears. The eye-opening narrows and the eyeball pull in when looking inward toward the nose. About 15 percent of all DS cases are Type 3.

Each of these three types can be further classified into three subgroups, depending on where the eyes are when the individual looks straight (the primary gaze):

- **Subgroup A.** The affected eye is turned inward toward the nose (esotropia).
- **Subgroup B.** The affected eye is turned outward toward the ear (exotropia).
- **Subgroup C.** The eyes are in a straight, primary position.

WHAT CAUSES DUANE SYNDROME

Common thought is that DS is a miswiring of the medial and the lateral rectus muscles, the muscles that move the eyes. Also, patients with DS lack the abducens nerve, the sixth cranial nerve, which is involved in eye movement. However, the etiology or origin of these malfunctions is, at present, a mystery.

Many researchers believe that DS results from a disturbance—either by genetic or environmental factors—during embryonic development. Since the cranial nerves and ocular muscles are developing between the third and eighth week of pregnancy, this is most likely when the disturbance happens.

Presently, it appears that several factors may be involved in causing DS. Therefore, it is doubtful that a single mechanism is responsible for this condition.

HOW IS DUANE SYNDROME DIAGNOSED?

The diagnosis of DS is based on clinical findings. Mutations in the *CHN1* gene are associated with familial isolated Duane syndrome. Direct sequencing of the *CHN1* gene is available as a clinical test and has to date detected missense mutations in seven patients and affected family members. The *CHN1* mutations have not been found to be a common cause of simplex Duane Retraction syndrome.

HEREDITY AND DUANE SYNDROME

Both genetic and environmental factors most likely play a role in the development of DS. For those cases that show evidence of having a genetic cause, both dominant and recessive forms of DS have been found. (When a gene is dominant, only one gene from one parent is needed for the individual to express it physically. However, when a gene is recessive, a copy of the gene from both parents is needed for expression.)

The chromosomal location of the proposed gene for this syndrome is currently unknown. Some research shows that more than one gene may be involved. There is evidence that a gene involved in the development of DS is located on chromosome 2. Also, deletions of chromosomal material from chromosomes 4 and 8, as well as the presence of an extra marker chromosome thought to be derived from chromosome 22, have been linked to DS.

Section 40.5 | **Horner Syndrome**

This section includes text excerpted from "Horner's syndrome," Genetic and Rare Diseases Information Center (GARD), National Center for Advancing Translational Sciences (NCATS), January 3, 2017.

Horner syndrome (HS) is a rare condition characterized by miosis (constriction of the pupil), ptosis (drooping of the upper eyelid), and anhidrosis (absence of sweating of the face). It is caused by damage to the sympathetic nerves of the face. The underlying causes of HS vary greatly and may include a tumor, stroke, injury, or underlying disease affecting the areas surrounding the sympathetic nerves. In rare cases, HS is congenital (present from birth) and may be associated with a lack of pigmentation of the iris (colored part of the eye). Treatment of HS depends on the underlying cause.

SYMPTOMS OF HORNER SYNDROME

Symptoms of HS typically include drooping of the upper eyelid (ptosis), constriction of the pupil (miosis), sinking of the eyeball into the face, and decreased sweating on the affected side of the face (anhidrosis). These symptoms may vary and other symptoms may occur depending on the underlying cause of the condition. Other symptoms that may be seen include, the inability to completely close or open the eyelid, facial flushing, headaches, and pain.

Heterochromia iridium (i.e., a relative deficiency of pigment in the iris of the affected side of the face) is usually present when the syndrome is congenital or caused by a lesion that has occurred before the age of one to two years of age.

For most diseases, symptoms will vary from person to person. People with the same disease may not have all the symptoms listed. This information comes from a database called the "Human Phenotype Ontology" (HPO). The HPO collects information on symptoms that have been described in medical resources. The HPO is updated regularly.

CAUSES OF HORNER SYNDROME

There are many potential causes of HS. It can be caused by any interruption in the function of sympathetic nerve fibers, which start in the hypothalamus and run via the upper spinal cord, near the carotid artery, to the face. The nerve function may be impaired due to factors, such as injury, compression, or a disease process. Examples of causes of HS include:

- Birth trauma to the neck and shoulder
- A stroke in the brainstem
- Injury, blood clot, or dissection of the carotid artery
- Trauma or surgery involving the neck, upper spinal cord, or chest
- A tumor in the brainstem, hypothalamus, upper spinal cord, neck, eye, abdomen, or chest cavity—particularly neuroblastoma or a tumor of the upper part of the lung (Pancoast tumor). Neuroblastoma is one of the most common causes of HS in children.
- Migraines or cluster headaches

- Diseases that cause damage to the protective covering that surrounds nerve fibers (demyelinating diseases)
- Development of a fluid-filled cavity or cyst within the spinal cord (syringomyelia)
- Arnold-Chiari malformation
- Inflammation or growths that affect the lymph nodes of the neck

DIAGNOSIS OF HORNER SYNDROME

An ophthalmologist may confirm the diagnosis by special eye tests. In addition, a careful neurological exam may be necessary to find the cause by determining which, if any, other parts of the nervous system are affected. Tests may include:

- Magnetic resonance imaging (MRI) of the head
- Carotid ultrasound
- Chest x-ray
- Computed tomography (CT) scan of the chest
- Blood tests
- Angiogram
- Eye drop tests

TREATMENT OF HORNER SYNDROME

Treatment depends on the underlying cause. There is no specific treatment for HS itself. In many cases, no effective treatment is known.

Section 40.6 | **WAGR Syndrome**

This section includes text excerpted from "About WAGR Syndrome," National Human Genome Research Institute (NHGRI), May 14, 2014. Reviewed March 2020.

WHAT IS WAGR SYNDROME?

WAGR syndrome is a rare genetic condition that can affect both boys and girls. Babies born with WAGR syndrome often have eye problems and are at high risk for developing certain types of cancer, and mental retardation. The term “WAGR” stands for the first letters of the physical and mental problems associated with the condition:

- (W)ilms’ Tumor, the most common form of kidney cancer in children.
- (A)niridia, some or complete absence of the colored part of the eye, called the “iris” (singular), or “irises/irides” (plural).
- (G)enitourinary problems, such as testicles that are not descended or hypospadias (abnormal location of the opening for urination) in boys, or genital or urinary problems inside the body in girls.
- Mental (R)etardation

Most people who have WAGR syndrome have two or more of these conditions. Also, people can have WAGR syndrome, but not have all of the above conditions.

Other names for WAGR syndrome that are used are:

- WAGR complex
- Wilms’ Tumor-Aniridia-Genitourinary Anomalies-mental retardation syndrome
- Wilms’ Tumor-Aniridia-Gonadoblastoma-mental retardation syndrome
- Chromosome 11p deletion syndrome
- 11p deletion syndrome

The cause of WAGR syndrome is the deletion of a group of genes located on chromosome number 11 (11p13 where the “p13” refers to the specific place on chromosome 11 that is affected). Chromosomes are packages of genetic characteristics. There are 22 pairs of chromosomes that are the same in males and females. The 23rd pair determines a person’s sex with males having an X and Y chromosome and females having two X chromosomes.

WHAT ARE THE SYMPTOMS OF WAGR SYNDROME?

WAGR is called a “genetic syndrome.” The symptoms of WAGR syndrome are usually seen after the baby is born. The mother’s pregnancy and the baby's birth history are not unusual. Enlargement of the baby's kidneys may be seen on a prenatal ultrasound. The eye problems (aniridia) are usually noticed in the newborn period, and for infant boys, the problems with the genitals and urinary systems are also usually obvious in the newborn period.

Individuals born with WAGR syndrome are at higher risk for developing other problems during infancy, childhood, and adulthood. These problems can affect the kidneys, eyes, testes or ovaries. The specific symptoms that happen in a person who has WAGR syndrome depend on the combination of disorders that are present.

Aniridia

In infants who are born with aniridia that is associated with WAGR syndrome, the irises of the eyes fail to develop normally before birth. This causes partial or complete absence of the round colored part of the eye (iris). Aniridia is almost always present in babies born with WAGR syndrome. Other eye problems are often present or can develop as the child grows older. These include the clouding of the lens of the eye (cataract), rapid, involuntary movements of the eye (nystagmus), and all or partial loss of vision due to the high pressure of the fluid in the eye (glaucoma).

HOW IS WAGR SYNDROME DIAGNOSED?

Symptoms that suggest WAGR syndrome, such as aniridia, are usually noted shortly after birth, and genetic testing for the 11p13 deletion is done. A genetic test called a "chromosome analysis" or "karyotype" is done to look for the deleted area (11p13) on chromosome number 11. A more specific genetic test called "fluorescent in situ hybridization" (FISH) is sometimes done to look for the deletion of specific genes on chromosome number 11.

HOW IS WAGR SYNDROME TREATED?

Treatment of WAGR syndrome is aimed at the specific symptoms present in the individual. Monitoring to look for problems is also important to catch problems early so that treatment can be given as soon as possible.

Aniridia

The treatment of aniridia is aimed at keeping the person's vision. Drugs or surgery may help when there is glaucoma or cataracts. Contact lenses can harm the cornea and should be avoided.

IS WAGR SYNDROME INHERITED?

WAGR syndrome is called a "contiguous gene deletion syndrome." This means that it is caused by the loss of a section of genes on chromosome 11 (11p13). Most of the time the changes on chromosome 11p13 happen by chance when the egg or sperm is being formed or during the very early stages of the baby's development in the womb. More rarely, the gene changes are inherited because one of the parents carries a rearrangement (called a "translocation") between two chromosomes that can cause the loss of some genes when she or he has a baby. A baby can also have a mixture of normal cells and cells that have the 11p13 changes in her or his body. This is called "mosaic WAGR syndrome."

Genetic counseling is helpful for determining whether there may be an increased risk of having another child with WAGR syndrome.

Chapter 41 | Infectious Diseases Affecting Vision

Chapter Contents

Section 41.1 | Histoplasmosis

This section includes text excerpted from "Facts About Histoplasmosis," National Eye Institute (NEI), August 2009. Reviewed March 2020.

Histoplasmosis is a disease caused when airborne spores of the fungus *Histoplasma capsulatum* are inhaled into the lungs, the primary infection site. This microscopic fungus, which is found throughout the world in river valleys and soil where bird or bat droppings accumulate, is released into the air when soil is disturbed by plowing fields, sweeping chicken coops, or digging holes. Histoplasmosis is often so mild that it produces no apparent symptoms.

However, histoplasmosis, even mild cases, can later cause a serious eye disease called "ocular histoplasmosis syndrome (OHS)," a leading cause of vision loss in Americans ages 20 to 40.

CAUSES OF OCULAR HISTOPLASMOSIS SYNDROME

Scientists believe that *Histoplasma capsulatum* (histo) spores spread from the lungs to the eye, lodging in the choroid, a layer of blood vessels that provides blood and nutrients to the retina.

How Does Ocular Histoplasmosis Syndrome Develop?

Ocular histoplasmosis syndrome develops when fragile, abnormal blood vessels grow underneath the retina. These abnormal blood vessels form a lesion known as "choroidal neovascularization (CNV)." If left untreated, the CNV lesion can turn into scar tissue and replace the normal retinal tissue in the macula.

SYMPTOMS OF OCULAR HISTOPLASMOSIS SYNDROME

Ocular histoplasmosis syndrome usually has no symptoms in its early stages; the initial OHS infection usually subsides without the need for treatment. This is true for other histo infections; in fact, often the only evidence that the inflammation ever occurred are tiny scars called "histo spots," which remain at the infection sites.

In later stages, OHS symptoms may appear if the abnormal blood vessels cause changes in vision. For example, straight lines may appear crooked or wavy, or a blind spot may appear in the field of vision. Because these symptoms indicate that OHS has already progressed enough to affect vision, anyone who has been exposed to histoplasmosis and perceives even slight changes in vision should consult an eye-care professional.

DIAGNOSIS OF OCULAR HISTOPLASMOSIS SYNDROME

An eye-care professional will usually diagnose OHS if a careful eye examination reveals two conditions:

1. The presence of histo spots, which indicate previous exposure to the histo fungus spores; and
2. Swelling of the retina, which signals the growth of new, abnormal blood vessels.

If fluid, blood, or abnormal blood vessels are present, an eye-care professional may want to perform a diagnostic procedure called "fluorescein angiography."

TREATMENT OF OCULAR HISTOPLASMOSIS SYNDROME

How Is Ocular Histoplasmosis Syndrome Treated?

The only proven treatment for OHS is a form of laser surgery called "photocoagulation." A small, powerful beam of light destroys the fragile, abnormal blood vessels, as well as a small amount of the overlying retinal tissue.

How Effective Is Laser Surgery?

Controlled clinical trials, sponsored by the National Eye Institute, have shown that photocoagulation can reduce future vision loss from OHS by more than half. The treatment is most effective when:

- The CNV has not grown into the center of the fovea, where it can affect vision.
- The eye-care professional is able to identify and destroy the entire area of CNV.

Does Laser Surgery Restore Lost Vision?

Laser photocoagulation usually does not restore lost vision. However, it does reduce the chance of further CNV growth and any resulting vision loss.

Does Laser Surgery Cure Ocular Histoplasmosis Syndrome?

No. OHS cannot be cured. Once contracted, OHS remains a threat to a person's sight for their lifetime.

Is There a Simple Way to Check for Signs of Ocular Histoplasmosis Syndrome Damage to the Macula?

Yes. A person can check for signs of damage to the macula by looking at a printed pattern called an "Amsler grid." If the macula has been damaged, the vertical and horizontal lines of the grid may appear curved, or a blank spot may seem to appear.

Many eye-care professionals advise patients who have received treatment for OHS, as well as those with histo spots, to check their vision daily with the Amsler grid one eye at a time. Patients with OHS in one eye are likely to develop it in the other.

Section 41.2 | **Toxoplasmosis**

This section contains text excerpted from the following sources: Text in this section begins with excerpts from "Toxoplasmosis," MedlinePlus, National Institutes of Health (NIH), October 11, 2019; Text under the heading "Persons with Ocular Disease" is excerpted from "Parasites–Toxoplasmosis (Toxoplasma Infection)—Disease," Centers for Disease Control and Prevention (CDC), September 5, 2018.

Toxoplasmosis is a disease caused by the parasite *Toxoplasma gondii*. More than 60 million people in the United States have the parasite. Most of them do not get sick. But, the parasite causes serious problems for some people. These include people with weak immune systems and babies whose mothers become infected for the first time during pregnancy. Problems can include damage to the brain, eyes, and other organs.

You can get toxoplasmosis from:

- Waste from an infected cat

- Eating contaminated meat that is raw or not well cooked
- Using utensils or cutting boards after they have had contact with contaminated raw meat
- Drinking infected water
- Receiving an infected organ transplant or blood transfusion

Most people with toxoplasmosis do not need treatment. There are drugs to treat it for pregnant women and people with weak immune systems.

PERSONS WITH OCULAR DISEASE

Eye disease (most frequently retinochoroiditis) from Toxoplasma infection can result from congenital infection or infection after birth by any of the modes of transmission. Eye lesions from congenital infection are often not identified at birth but occur in 20 to 80 percent of congenitally infected persons by adulthood. However, in the United States, lesser than two percent of persons infected after birth develop eye lesions. Eye infection leads to an acute inflammatory lesion of the retina, which resolves to leave retinochoroidal scarring. Symptoms of the ocular disease include:

- Eye pain
- Sensitivity to light (photophobia)
- Tearing of the eyes
- Blurred vision

The eye disease can reactivate months or years later, each time causing more damage to the retina. If the central structures of the retina are involved there will be a progressive loss of vision that can lead to blindness.

Section 41.3 | **Trachoma**

This section includes text excerpted from "Hygiene-Related Diseases," Centers for Disease Control and Prevention (CDC), August 2, 2016. Reviewed March 2020.

Trachoma is the world's leading cause of preventable blindness of infectious origin. Caused by the bacterium *Chlamydia trachomatis*, trachoma is easily spread through direct personal contact, shared towels and cloths, and flies that have come in contact with the eyes or nose of an infected person. If left untreated, repeated trachoma infections can cause severe scarring of the inside of the eyelid and can cause the eyelashes to scratch the cornea (trichiasis). In addition to causing pain, trichiasis permanently damages the cornea and can lead to irreversible blindness. Trachoma, which spreads in areas that lack adequate access to water and sanitation, affects the most marginalized communities in the world. Globally, almost eight million people are visually impaired by trachoma; 500 million are at risk of blindness from the disease throughout 57 endemic countries.

The World Health Organization (WHO) has targeted trachoma for elimination by 2020 through an innovative, multi-faceted public health strategy known as "S.A.F.E.":

- Surgery to correct the advanced, blinding stage of the disease (trichiasis)
- Antibiotics to treat an active infection
- Facial cleanliness
- Environmental improvements in the areas of water and sanitation to reduce disease transmission

The comprehensive SAFE strategy combines measures for the treatment of active infection and trichiasis (S&A) with preventive measures to reduce disease transmission (F&E). Implementation of the full SAFE strategy in endemic areas increases the effectiveness of trachoma programs. The F and E components of SAFE, which reduce disease transmission, are particularly critical to achieving sustainable elimination of trachoma.

The "F" in the SAFE strategy refers to facial cleanliness. Because trachoma is transmitted through close personal contact, it tends to occur in clusters, often infecting entire families and communities. Children, who are more likely to touch their eyes and have unclean faces that attract eye-seeking flies, are especially vulnerable to infection, as are women, the traditional caretakers of the home. Therefore, the promotion of good hygiene practices, such as handwashing, and the washing of children's faces at least once a day with water, is a key step in breaking the cycle of trachoma transmission.

The "E" in the SAFE strategy refers to environmental change. Improvements in community and household sanitation, such as the provision of household latrines, help control fly populations and breeding grounds. Increased access to water facilitates good hygiene practices and is vital to achieving sustainable elimination of the disease. Separation of animal quarters from human living space, as well as safe handling of food and drinking water, are also important environmental measures that affected communities can take within a trachoma control program.

Chapter 42 | **Fungal Infections Affecting Vision**

ABOUT FUNGAL EYE INFECTIONS

Eye infections can be caused by many different organisms, including bacteria, viruses, ameba, and fungi. Eye infections caused by fungi are extremely rare, but they can be very serious.

Types of Fungal Eye Infections

Fungal infections can affect different parts of the eye.

- **Keratitis** is an infection of the clear, front layer of the eye (the cornea).
- **Endophthalmitis** is an infection of the inside of the eye (the vitreous and/or aqueous humor). There are two types of endophthalmitis: exogenous and endogenous. Exogenous fungal endophthalmitis occurs after fungal spores enter the eye from an external source. Endogenous endophthalmitis occurs when a bloodstream infection (for example, candidemia) spreads to one or both eyes.

Types of Fungi That Cause Eye Infections

Many different types of fungi can cause eye infections. Common types include:

- ***Fusarium***—a fungus that lives in the environment, especially in soil and on plants.

This chapter includes text excerpted from "About Fungal Eye Infections," Centers for Disease Control and Prevention (CDC), January 27, 2017.

- *Aspergillus*—a common fungus that lives in indoor and outdoor environments.
- *Candida*—a type of yeast that normally lives on human skin and on the protective lining inside the body called the "mucous membrane."

SYMPTOMS OF FUNGAL EYE INFECTIONS

In people who have had exposures that put them at risk for fungal eye infections, the symptoms of a fungal eye infection can appear anywhere from several days to several weeks after the fungi enter the eye. The symptoms of a fungal eye infection are similar to thc symptoms of other types of eye infections (such as those caused by bacteria) and can include:

- Eye pain
- Eye redness
- Blurred vision
- Sensitivity to light
- Excessive tearing
- Eye discharge

If you have any of these symptoms, call your eye doctor right away. If you wear contact lenses, remove them immediately. Fungal eye infections are very rare, but if they are not treated, they can become serious and result in permanent vision loss or blindness.

FUNGAL EYE INFECTIONS RISK AND PREVENTION

Who Gets Fungal Eye Infections

Anyone can get a fungal eye infection. These infections usually are linked to one of these situations:

- Eye injury, particularly with plant material (for example, thorns or sticks)
- Eye surgery (such as corneal transplant surgery or cataract surgery)
- Chronic eye disease involving the surface of the eye
- Wearing contact lenses

- Exposure to contaminated medical products that come in contact with the eye
- Fungal bloodstream infection (such as candidemia)

Also, people who have diabetes, a weakened immune system, or use corticosteroids may be more likely to develop fungal eye infections than other people.

HOW TO PREVENT A FUNGAL EYE INFECTION

- If you are a farmworker or work often with plant materials, wear protective eyewear to help prevent an eye injury.
- People who wear contact lenses should care for their lenses properly.

SOURCES OF FUNGAL EYE INFECTIONS

What Causes Fungal Eye Infections

EYE INJURIES

The most common way for someone to get a fungal eye infection is because of an eye injury, particularly if plant material, such as a stick or a thorn caused the injury. Some fungi that cause eye infections, such as *Fusarium*, live in the environment and are often associated with plant material. Fungi can enter the eye and cause infection after an injury.

EYE SURGERY

Less often, an infection can occur after eye surgery, such as corneal transplant surgery or cataract surgery.

People who have had surgery to replace their corneas (the clear, front layer of the eye) are at higher risk of fungal eye infections. Each year, about 50,000 Americans have a corneal transplant to replace injured or diseased corneas. A small number of people who have this surgery (about 4 to 7 for every 10,000 transplants) develop a fungal eye infection.

From 2007 to 2014, endophthalmitis, or infection of the interior of the eye, became more than twice as common for people with recent corneal transplant surgery. In the past, this type of endophthalmitis was most commonly caused by bacteria. However, now, fungi (most often the *Candida* species) cause about two-thirds of infections.

INVASIVE EYE PROCEDURE

Fungal eye infections could happen after an invasive eye procedure such as an injection. Some infections have been traced to contaminated medical products, such as contact lens solution, irrigation solution, and dye used during eye surgery, or corticosteroids injected directly into the eye.

FUNGAL BLOODSTREAM INFECTION

Rarely, fungal eye infections can happen after a fungal bloodstream infection, such as candidemia spreads to the eye.

FUNGAL EYE INFECTION DIAGNOSIS AND TESTING

To diagnose a fungal eye infection, your eye doctor will examine your eye and might take a small sample of tissue or fluid from your eye. The sample will be sent to a laboratory to be examined under a microscope or cultured. Polymerase chain reaction (PCR) and confocal microscopy are also being used as newer, faster forms of diagnosis; however, culture is the standard method for the definitive diagnosis of a fungal eye infection.

TREATMENT OF FUNGAL EYE INFECTIONS

The treatment for a fungal eye infection depends on:

- The type of fungus
- The severity of the infection
- The parts of the eye affected

Possible forms of treatment for fungal eye infections include:

- Antifungal eye drops
- Antifungal medication, given as a pill or through a vein
- Antifungal medication injected directly into the eye
- Eye surgery

All types of fungal eye infections must be treated with prescription antifungal medication, usually for several weeks to months. Natamycin is a topical (meaning it is given in the form of eye drops) antifungal medication that works well for fungal infections involving the outer layer of the eye, particularly those caused by fungi, such as *Aspergillus* and *Fusarium*. However, infections that are deeper and more severe may require treatment with antifungal medication, such as amphotericin B, fluconazole, or voriconazole. These medications can be given by mouth, through a vein, or injected directly into the eye. Patients whose infections do not get better after using antifungal medications may need surgery, including corneal transplantation, removal of the vitreous gel from the interior of the eye (vitrectomy), or, in extreme cases, removal of the eye (enucleation).

FUNGAL EYE INFECTION STATISTICS

Fungal Keratitis

The exact incidence of fungal keratitis in the general population is unknown, but it is thought to be more common in warmer climates where the fungi that cause these infections are likely more common in the environment.

Exogenous Fungal Endophthalmitis

Endophthalmitis is a very rare complication of eye injury or eye surgery; in the United States, it occurs as a postsurgical complication in approximately 0.1 percent of all cataract surgeries. Here the fungi enter the eye from outside the body. Furthermore, only a small percentage of these infections are caused by fungi; bacterial endophthalmitis is more common.

Endogenous Fungal Endophthalmitis

Endogenous endophthalmitis is extremely rare and is less common than exogenous endophthalmitis; studies have estimated that only 2 to 15 percent of all endophthalmitis cases are endogenous. Here the fungi enter the eye as a result of an existing bloodstream infection. *Candida* species are the most common cause of endogenous fungal endophthalmitis. An estimated one percent of patients with candidemia develop *Candida* endophthalmitis.

Public-Health Surveillance for Fungal Eye Infections

Fungal eye infections are not reportable, which means that healthcare providers are not required to regularly report cases to public-health authorities. However, healthcare providers who are concerned about an unusual number of new cases of fungal eye infections should contact their state or local health department.

Outbreaks of Fungal Eye Infections

In 2012, the Centers for Disease Control and Prevention (CDC), state and local health departments, and the U.S. Food and Drug Administration (FDA) investigated a multistate outbreak of *Fusarium incarnatum-equiseti* species complex endophthalmitis associated with Brilliant Blue-G, a type of dye used during eye surgery, and Bipolaris endophthalmitis associated with eye injections of a steroid called "triamcinolone." Both contaminated products came from the same compounding pharmacy. In 2006, the CDC, state and local health departments, and the FDA investigated a large, multistate outbreak of *Fusarium* keratitis associated with a specific type of contact lens solution, which was later withdrawn from the market.

Chapter 43 | Stroke and Vision Impairment

A stroke occurs when a part of the brain does not get sufficient amount of oxygen. Vision impairment can occur after a stroke since the vision of an individual depends on two factors:

- Healthy eyes to receive visual information
- Healthy visual processing centers in the brain to understand and process the information

Since stroke affects certain parts of the brain, it can also affect the sight of a person.

TYPES OF VISION IMPAIRMENTS CAUSED BY STROKE

The effects of stroke on vision can vary as it depends on the location and severity of the stroke. There are five major types of vision loss that occur after stroke:

Central Vision Loss

Normally, this can affect either one or both the eyes. However, stroke affects both the eyes. It causes partial or complete vision loss making it difficult to see anything in the center of the vision. Depending on how much the eyes are affected, a person may have a peripheral vision alone or nothing at all. Retinal stroke can also cause central vision loss as this type of stroke is caused by blockage of blood vessels in the eye that affect the eyes rather than the brain. Retinal stroke usually affects one eye with symptoms such as blurry vision and blackouts before the stroke.

Visual Field Loss

Unlike central vision loss, visual field loss affects a person's ability to see objects that are right or left to the central line of eyesight. The side of the vision that is affected depends on where the stroke happened in the brain. In most cases, the stroke occurs toward the back of the brain, which causes visual impairment in one half of the eye. Other impairments include:

- Black patches in the vision
- Loss of upper or lower field of vision (in one or both the eyes)
- A quarter of loss of visual field (in one or both the eyes)

Eye Movement Issues

This results when the nerves that control the eyes are damaged. Impaired eye movements can be noticed such as difficulty in following a moving object or looking from one object to another. There might be difficulties in moving the eyes up and down or one eye may move while the other does not. Additionally, control of the eyes might be lost as they constantly move or twitch causing blurriness and dizziness.

Due to impairment in perception of depth, judging the distance of an object can be hard.

Visual Processing Issues

After a stroke, the ability to process or make sense of what an individual sees might be reduced. The most common visual processing issue is visual neglect, which affects a person's perception of things around them, such as trouble differentiating faces or shades of colors. The sense of peripheral vision might also be affected. Additionally, some experience visual hallucinations after a stroke, which can be very stressful for the individual and those around them.

Cortical Blindness

A stroke can cause complete vision loss in one eye, and rarely in both the eyes. The complete vision impairment in one eye is caused due to the blockage of one of the arteries called the "retinal artery," which supplies blood to the eyes. When the occipital lobe (part of the brain that processes optical data received) is affected, vision in both the eyes is lost, a condition called "cortical blindness," meaning the person's eyes still react to light (the pupils get smaller) but the person will be unable to see as the brain cannot perceive the visual message.

Apart from these issues, there can be other eye conditions such as dry eye and sensitivity to light.

TREATMENTS FOR VISION IMPAIRMENTS AFTER A STROKE

There are various treatment methods used to help deal with the visual effects of a stroke. They depend on how serious the eyes are affected by the stroke.

Some experience improvement in their vision in the first six months following the stroke but the recovery depends on the extent of the damage to the brain, the type of stroke suffered, and other existing health issues.

For those affected with a loss of visual field, the vision loss may be permanent. However, there are treatments that involve the following therapies in any combination:

Optical Therapy

This form of therapy uses mirrors and prisms to help position an image in a way that they are in the line of sight of the individual. Prisms can also help improve double vision, depth perception, and other visual impairments due to stroke.

Eye Movement Therapy

Therapy that focuses on the eye movement of a person can help train their eyes and adjust to their new visual scope. This makes it easier for them to read and see the objects within their visual range. This therapy also helps strengthen and train the eye muscles increasing a person's eye movement control.

Visual Restoration Therapy

Visual restoration therapy (VRT) focuses on using light to stimulate the blind spots in a person's visual field. The neurons in the brain affected by the stroke can be sparked by blinking or moving the lights.

COPING WITH VISUAL DIFFICULTIES AFTER A STROKE

Though the quality of the eyesight prior to the stroke cannot be restored, it is possible to improve muscle control and vision. Specific therapies as mentioned earlier can also help adapt to the new eyesight by retraining the brain and eye muscles. At home, eye exercises can be practiced to help gain more control over eye movements. Learning new techniques to focus on using the eyes in different ways can help open up a wide range of possibilities to make the most of the vision.

Vision impairment caused by a stroke can make daily chores more challenging. It is necessary to evaluate a person immediately after the stroke to learn the extent of damage, and continue to closely monitor their improvements to develop a strategy to get that person return to their normal routine at the earliest.

References

1. "Vision Changes Caused by Stroke," Moawad, Heidi. Verywell Health, April 11, 2019.
2. "Stroke-Related Eye Conditions," Royal National Institute of Blind People (RNIB), January 24, 2009.
3. "Vision Problems after Stroke: Understanding & Overcoming Them," Hoffman, Henry. Saebo, June 13th, 2018.

Chapter 44 | Diabetes and Eye Problems

Chapter Contents

Section 44.1 | Diabetic Eye Disease

This section includes text excerpted from "Diabetic Eye Disease," National Institute of Diabetes and Digestive and Kidney Diseases (NIDDK), May 2017.

WHAT IS DIABETIC EYE DISEASE?

Diabetic eye disease is a group of eye problems that can affect people with diabetes. These conditions include diabetic retinopathy, diabetic macular edema, cataracts, and glaucoma.

Over time, diabetes can cause damage to your eyes that can lead to poor vision or even blindness. But, you can take steps to prevent diabetic eye disease, or keep it from getting worse, by taking care of your diabetes.

The best ways to manage your diabetes and keep your eyes healthy are to:

- Manage your blood glucose, blood pressure, and cholesterol sometimes called the "diabetes ABCs"
- If you smoke, get help to quit smoking
- Have a dilated eye exam once a year

Often, there are no warning signs of diabetic eye disease or vision loss when damage first develops. A full, dilated eye exam helps your doctor find and treat eye problems early—often before much vision loss can occur.

HOW DOES DIABETES AFFECT THE EYES?

Diabetes affects your eyes when your blood glucose, also called "blood sugar," is too high.

In the short-term, you are not likely to have vision loss from high blood glucose. People sometimes have blurry vision for a few days or weeks when they are changing their diabetes care plan or medicines. High glucose can change fluid levels or cause swelling in the tissues of your eyes that help you to focus, causing blurred vision. This type of blurry vision is temporary and goes away when your glucose level gets closer to normal.

If your blood glucose stays high over time, it can damage the tiny blood vessels in the back of your eyes. This damage can begin during prediabetes when blood glucose is higher than normal, but not high enough for you to be diagnosed with diabetes. Damaged blood vessels may leak fluid and cause swelling. New, weak blood vessels, may also begin to grow. These blood vessels can bleed into the middle part of the eye, lead to scarring, or cause dangerously high pressure inside your eye.

Most serious diabetic eye diseases begin with blood vessel problems. The four eye diseases that can threaten your sight are:

Diabetic Retinopathy

The retina is the inner lining at the back of each eye. The retina senses light and turns it into signals that your brain decodes, so you can see the world around you. Damaged blood vessels can harm the retina, causing a disease called "diabetic retinopathy."

In early diabetic retinopathy, blood vessels can weaken, bulge, or leak into the retina. This stage is called "nonproliferative diabetic retinopathy" (NPDR).

If the disease gets worse, some blood vessels close off, which causes new blood vessels to grow or proliferate, on the surface of the retina. This stage is called "proliferative diabetic retinopathy." These abnormal new blood vessels can lead to serious vision problems.

Diabetic Macular Edema

The part of your retina that you need for reading, driving, and seeing faces is called the "macula." Diabetes can lead to swelling in the macula, which is called "diabetic macular edema." Over time, this disease can destroy the sharp vision in this part of the eye, leading to partial vision loss or blindness. Macular edema usually develops in people who already have other signs of diabetic retinopathy.

Glaucoma

Glaucoma is a group of eye diseases that can damage the optic nerve—the bundle of nerves that connects the eye to the brain. Diabetes doubles the chances of having glaucoma, which can lead to vision loss and blindness if not treated early.

Symptoms depend on which type of glaucoma you have.

Cataracts

The lenses within the eyes are clear structures that help provide sharp vision—but they tend to become cloudy as you age. People with diabetes are more likely to develop cloudy lenses, called "cataracts." People with diabetes can develop cataracts at an earlier age than people without diabetes. Researchers think that high glucose levels cause deposits to build up in the lenses of your eyes.

HOW COMMON IS DIABETIC EYE DISEASE?

Diabetic Retinopathy

About one in three people with diabetes who are older than age 40, already have some signs of diabetic retinopathy. Diabetic retinopathy is the most common cause of vision loss in people with diabetes. Each person's outlook for the future, however, depends in large part on regular care. Finding and treating diabetic retinopathy early can reduce the risk of blindness by 95 percent.

Glaucoma and Cataracts

Your chances of developing glaucoma or cataracts are about twice that of someone without diabetes.

WHO IS MORE LIKELY TO DEVELOP DIABETIC EYE DISEASE?

Anyone with diabetes can develop diabetic eye disease. Your risk is greater with:

- High blood glucose that is not treated
- High blood pressure that is not treated

High blood cholesterol and smoking may also raise your risk for diabetic eye disease.

Some groups are affected more than others. African Americans, American Indians and Alaska Natives, Hispanics/Latinx, Pacific Islanders, and older adults are at greater risk of losing vision or going blind from diabetes.

If you have diabetes and become pregnant, you can develop eye problems very quickly during your pregnancy. If you already have some diabetic retinopathy, it can get worse during pregnancy. Changes that help your body support a growing baby may put stress on the blood vessels in your eyes. Your healthcare team will suggest regular eye exams during pregnancy to catch and treat problems early and protect your vision.

Diabetes that occurs only during pregnancy, called "gestational diabetes," does not usually cause eye problems. Researchers are not sure why this is the case.

Your chances of developing diabetic eye disease increase the longer you have diabetes.

WHAT ARE THE SYMPTOMS OF DIABETIC EYE DISEASE?

Often there are no early symptoms of diabetic eye disease. You may have no pain and no change in your vision as damage begins to grow inside your eyes, particularly with diabetic retinopathy.

When symptoms do occur, they may include:

- Blurry or wavy vision
- Frequently changing vision—sometimes from day-to-day
- Dark areas or vision loss
- Poor color vision
- Spots or dark strings (also called "floaters")
- Flashes of light

Talk with your eye doctor if you have any of these symptoms.

WHEN TO SEE A DOCTOR

Call a doctor right away if you notice sudden changes to your vision, including flashes of light or many more spots (floaters) than usual. You also should see a doctor right away if it looks like a curtain is pulled over your eyes. These changes in your sight can be symptoms of a detached retina, which is a medical emergency.

HOW DO DOCTORS DIAGNOSE EYE PROBLEMS FROM DIABETES?

Having a full, dilated eye exam is the best way to check for eye problems from diabetes. Your doctor will place drops in your eyes to widen your pupils. This allows the doctor to examine a larger area at the back of each eye, using a special magnifying lens. Your vision will be blurry for a few hours after a dilated exam.

Your doctor will also:

- Test your vision
- Measure the pressure in your eyes

Your doctor may suggest other tests, too, depending on your health history.

Most people with diabetes should see an eye-care professional once a year for a complete eye exam. Your own healthcare team may suggest a different plan, based on your type of diabetes and the time since you were first diagnosed.

HOW DO DOCTORS TREAT DIABETIC EYE DISEASE?

Your doctor may recommend having eye exams more often than once a year, along with the management of your diabetes. This means managing your diabetes ABCs, which include your A1c, blood pressure, and cholesterol; and quitting smoking. Ask your healthcare team what you can do to reach your goals.

Doctors may treat advanced eye problems with medicine, laser treatments, surgery, or a combination of these options.

Medicine

Your doctor may treat your eyes with antivascular endothelial growth factors (VEGF) medicine, such as aflibercept, bevacizumab, or ranibizumab. These medicines block the growth of abnormal blood vessels in the eye. Anti-VEGF medicines can also stop fluid leaks, which can help treat diabetic macular edema.

The doctor will inject an anti-VEGF medicine into your eyes during office visits. You will have several treatments during the first few months, then fewer treatments after you finish the first round of therapy. Your doctor will use medicine to numb your eyes so you do not feel pain. The needle is about the thickness of a human hair.

Anti-VEGF treatments can stop further vision loss and may improve vision in some people.

Laser Treatment

Laser treatment also called "photocoagulation" creates tiny burns inside the eye with a beam of light. This method treats leaky blood vessels and extra fluid, called "edema." Your doctor usually provides this treatment during several office visits, using medicine to numb your eyes. Laser treatment can keep eye disease from getting worse, which is important to prevent vision loss or blindness. But, laser treatment is less likely to bring back vision you have already lost compared with anti-VEGF medicines.

There are two types of laser treatment:

- Focal/grid laser treatment works on a small area of the retina to treat diabetic macular edema.
- Scatter laser treatment, also called "panretinal photocoagulation" (PRP), covers a larger area of the retina. This method treats the growth of abnormal blood vessels, called "proliferative diabetic retinopathy."

Vitrectomy

Vitrectomy is a surgery to remove the clear gel that fills the center of the eye, called the "vitreous gel." The procedure treats problems with severe bleeding or scar tissue caused by proliferative diabetic retinopathy. Scar tissue can force the retina to peel away from the tissue beneath it, like wallpaper peeling away from a wall. A retina that comes completely loose, or detaches, can cause blindness.

During vitrectomy, a clear salt solution is gently pumped into the eye to maintain eye pressure during surgery and to replace the removed vitreous. Vitrectomy is done in a surgery center or hospital with pain medicine.

Cataract Lens Surgery

In a surgery center or hospital visit, your doctor can remove the cloudy lens in your eye, where the cataract has grown, and replace it with an artificial lens. People who have cataract surgery generally have better vision afterward. After your eye heals, you may need a new prescription for your glasses. Your vision following cataract surgery may also depend on treating any damage from diabetic retinopathy or macular edema.

WHAT TO DO TO PROTECT THE EYES

To prevent diabetic eye disease, or to keep it from getting worse, manage your diabetes ABCs: your A1C, blood pressure, and cholesterol; and quit smoking if you smoke.

Also, have a dilated eye exam at least once a year—or more often if recommended by your eye-care professional. These actions are powerful ways to protect the health of your eyes—and can prevent blindness.

WHAT IF YOU ALREADY HAVE SOME VISION LOSS FROM DIABETES?

Ask your eye-care professional to help you find a low vision and rehabilitation clinic. Special eye-care professionals can help you manage vision loss that cannot be corrected with glasses, contact lenses, medicine, or surgery. Special devices and training may help you make the most of your remaining vision so that you can continue to be active, enjoy hobbies, visit friends and family members, and live without help from others.

Section 44.2 | **Diabetic Retinopathy and Diabetic Macular Edema**

This section contains text excerpted from the following sources: Text beginning with the heading "What Is Diabetic Retinopathy?" is excerpted from "Diabetic Retinopathy," National Eye Institute (NEI), August 3, 2019; Text beginning with the heading "What Is Macular Edema?" is excerpted from "Macular Edema," National Eye Institute (NEI), July 8, 2019.

WHAT IS DIABETIC RETINOPATHY?

Diabetic retinopathy is an eye condition that can cause vision loss and blindness in people who have diabetes. It affects blood vessels in the retina (the light-sensitive layer of tissue in the back of your eye).

If you have diabetes, it is important for you to get a comprehensive dilated eye exam at least once a year. Diabetic retinopathy may not have any symptoms at first—but finding it early can help you take steps to protect your vision.

Managing your diabetes—by staying physically active, eating healthy, and taking your medicine—can also help you prevent or delay vision loss.

WHAT ARE THE SYMPTOMS OF DIABETIC RETINOPATHY?

The early stages of diabetic retinopathy usually do not have any symptoms. Some people notice changes in their vision, such as trouble reading, or seeing faraway objects. These changes may come and go.

In later stages of the disease, blood vessels in the retina start to bleed into the vitreous (gel-like fluid in the center of the eye). If this happens, you may see dark, floating spots or streaks that look like cobwebs. Sometimes, the spots clear up on their own—but it is important to get treatment right away. Without treatment, the bleeding can happen again, get worse, or cause scarring.

WHAT OTHER PROBLEMS CAN DIABETIC RETINOPATHY CAUSE?

Diabetic retinopathy can lead to other serious eye conditions:

- **Diabetic macular edema (DME).** Over time, about half of people with diabetic retinopathy will develop DME. DME happens when blood vessels in the retina leak fluid, causing swelling in the macula (a part of the retina). If you have DME, your vision will become blurry because of the extra fluid in your macula.

- **Neovascular glaucoma.** Diabetic retinopathy can cause abnormal blood vessels to grow out of the retina and block fluid from draining out of the eye. This causes a type of glaucoma.
- **Retinal detachment.** Diabetic retinopathy can cause scars to form in the back of your eye. When the scars pull your retina away from the back of your eye, it is called "tractional retinal detachment."

WHO IS AT RISK FOR DIABETIC RETINOPATHY?

Anyone with any kind of diabetes can get diabetic retinopathy—including people with type 1, type 2, and gestational diabetes (diabetes that can develop during pregnancy).

Your risk increases the longer you have diabetes. More than 2 in 5 Americans with diabetes have some stage of diabetic retinopathy. The good news is that you can lower your risk of developing diabetic retinopathy by controlling your diabetes.

Women with diabetes who become pregnant—or women who develop gestational diabetes—are at high risk of getting diabetic retinopathy. If you have diabetes and are pregnant, have a comprehensive dilated eye exam as soon as possible. Ask your doctor if you will need additional eye exams during your pregnancy.

WHAT CAUSES DIABETIC RETINOPATHY

Diabetic retinopathy is caused by high blood sugar due to diabetes. Over time, having too much sugar in your blood can damage your retina—the part of your eye that detects light and sends signals to your brain through a nerve in the back of your eye (optic nerve).

Diabetes damages blood vessels all over the body. The damage to your eyes starts when sugar blocks the tiny blood vessels that go to your retina, causing them to leak fluid or bleed. To make up for these blocked blood vessels, your eyes then grow new blood vessels that do not work well. These new blood vessels can leak or bleed easily.

HOW WILL THE EYE DOCTOR CHECK FOR DIABETIC RETINOPATHY?

Eye doctors can check for diabetic retinopathy as part of a dilated eye exam. The exam is simple and painless—your doctor will give you some eye drops to dilate (widen) your pupil and then check your eyes for diabetic retinopathy and other eye problems.

If you do develop diabetic retinopathy, early treatment can stop the damage and prevent blindness.

If your eye doctor thinks you may have severe diabetic retinopathy or DME, they may do a test called a "fluorescein angiogram" (FA). This test lets the doctor see pictures of the blood vessels in your retina.

WHAT TO DO TO PREVENT DIABETIC RETINOPATHY?

Managing your diabetes is the best way to lower your risk of diabetic retinopathy. That means keeping your blood sugar levels as close to normal as possible. You can do this by getting regular physical activity, eating healthy, and carefully following your doctor's instructions for your insulin or other diabetes medicines.

To help control your blood sugar, you will need a special test called an "A1C test." This test shows your average blood sugar level over a three-month period. Talk with your doctor about lowering your A1c level to help prevent or manage diabetic retinopathy.

Having high blood pressure or high cholesterol along with diabetes increases your risk for diabetic retinopathy. So controlling your blood pressure and cholesterol can also help lower your risk for vision loss.

WHAT IS THE TREATMENT FOR DIABETIC RETINOPATHY AND DIABETIC MACULAR EDEMA?

In the early stages of diabetic retinopathy, your eye doctor will probably just keep track of how your eyes are doing. Some people with diabetic retinopathy may need a comprehensive dilated eye exam as often as every two to four months.

In later stages, it is important to start treatment right away—especially if you experience changes in your vision. While it would not undo any damage to your vision, treatment can stop your vision from getting worse. It is also important to take steps to control your diabetes, blood pressure, and cholesterol.

- **Injections.** Medicines called "anti-VEGF drugs" can slow down or reverse diabetic retinopathy. Other medicines, called "corticosteroids," can also help.
- **Laser treatment.** To reduce swelling in your retina, eye doctors can use lasers to make the blood vessels shrink and stop leaking.
- **Eye surgery.** If your retina is bleeding a lot or you have a lot of scars in your eye, your eye doctor may recommend a type of surgery called a "vitrectomy."

WHAT IS MACULAR EDEMA?

Macular edema is the build-up of fluid in the macula, an area in the center of the retina. The retina is the light-sensitive tissue at the back of the eye and the macula is the part of the retina responsible for sharp, straight-ahead vision. Fluid build-up causes the macula to swell and thicken, which distorts vision.

WHAT ARE THE SYMPTOMS OF MACULAR EDEMA?

The primary symptom of macular edema is blurry or wavy vision near or in the center of your field of vision. Colors might also appear washed out or faded. Most people with macular edema will have symptoms that range from slightly blurry vision to noticeable vision loss. If only one eye is affected, you may not notice your vision is blurry until the condition is well-advanced.

WHAT CAUSES MACULAR EDEMA

Macular edema occurs when there is abnormal leakage, and accumulation of fluid, in the macula from damaged blood vessels in the nearby retina. A common cause of macular edema is diabetic retinopathy, a disease that can happen to people with diabetes. Macular edema can also occur after eye surgery, in association with age-related macular degeneration (AMD), or as a consequence of inflammatory diseases that affect the eye. Any disease that damages blood vessels in the retina can cause macular edema.

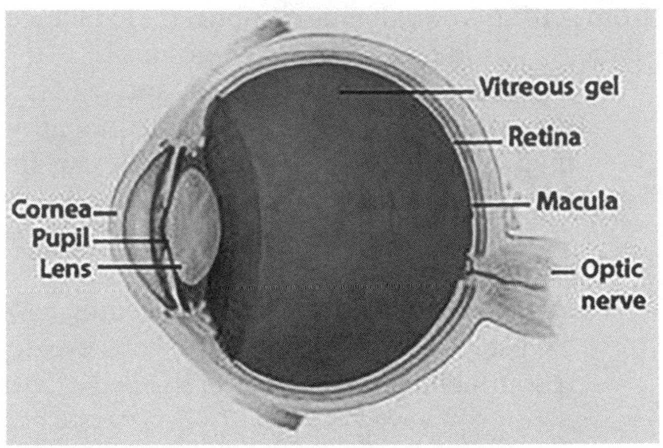

Figure 44.1. Macular Edema

Diabetic Macular Edema

Diabetic macular edema (DME) is caused by a complication of diabetes called "diabetic retinopathy." Diabetic retinopathy is the most common diabetic eye disease and the leading cause of irreversible blindness in working-age Americans. Diabetic retinopathy usually affects both eyes.

Diabetic retinopathy is caused by ongoing damage to the small blood vessels of the retina. The leakage of fluid into the retina may lead to swelling of the surrounding tissue, including the macula.

DME is the most common cause of vision loss in people with diabetic retinopathy. Poor blood sugar control and additional medical conditions, such as high blood pressure, increase the risk of blindness for people with DME. DME can occur at any stage of diabetic retinopathy, although it is more likely to occur later as the disease goes on.

Experts estimate that approximately 7.7 million Americans have diabetic retinopathy and of those, about 750,000 also have DME. A study suggests that non-Hispanic African Americans are three times more likely to develop DME than non-Hispanic Whites, most likely due to the higher incidence of diabetes in the African American population.

Eye surgery

Macular edema may develop after any type of surgery that is performed inside the eye, including surgery for cataract, glaucoma, or retinal disease. A small number of people who have cataract surgery (experts estimate only 1 to 3 percent) may develop macular edema within a few weeks after surgery. If one eye is affected, there is a 50 percent chance that the other eye will also be affected. Macular edema after eye surgery is usually mild, short-lasting, and responds well to eye drops that treat inflammation.

Age-Related Macular Degeneration

Age-related macular degeneration (AMD) is a disease characterized by deterioration or breakdown of the macula, which is responsible for sharp, central vision. In neovascular AMD, also called "wet" AMD, blood vessels begin to grow up from the choroid (the bed of blood vessels below the retina) and into the retina. These new and abnormal blood vessels leak fluid into the macula and cause macular edema.

Blockage of Retinal Blood Vessels

When retinal veins are blocked (retinal vein occlusion), blood does not drain properly and it leaks into the retina. If it leaks into the macula, this produces macular edema. Leakage is worsened by the severity of the blockage, how many veins are involved, and the pressure inside them. Retinal vein occlusion is most often associated with age-related atherosclerosis, diabetes, high blood pressure, and eye conditions, such as glaucoma or inflammation.

Inflammatory Diseases That Affect the Retina

Uveitis describes a group of inflammatory diseases that cause swelling in the eye and destroy eye tissues. The term "uveitis" is used because the diseases most often affect a part of the eye called the "uvea." However, uveitis is not limited to the uvea. Uveitis can affect the cornea, iris, lens, vitreous, retina, optic nerve, and the white of the eye (sclera). Inflammatory diseases and disorders of the immune system may also affect the eye and cause swelling and breakdown of tissue in the macula. These disorders include cytomegalovirus infection, retinal necrosis, sarcoidosis, Behçet syndrome, toxoplasmosis, Eales' disease, and Vogt-Koyanagi-Harada syndrome.

HOW WILL THE EYE DOCTOR CHECK FOR MACULAR EDEMA?

To diagnose macular edema, your eye-care professional will conduct a thorough eye exam and look for abnormalities in the retina. The following tests may be done to determine the location and extent of the disease:

Visual acuity (VA) test. A visual acuity test is a common way to identify vision loss and can help to diagnose vision loss as a result of macular edema. This test uses a standardized chart or card with rows of letters that decrease in size from top to bottom. Covering one eye, you will be asked to read out loud the smallest line of letters that you can see. When done, you will test the other eye.

Dilated eye exam. A dilated eye exam is used to more thoroughly examine the retina. It gives additional information about the condition of the macula and helps detect the presence of blood vessel leakage or cysts. Drops are placed in your eyes to widen, or dilate, your pupils. Your eye-care professional then examines your retina for signs of damage or disease.

Fluorescein angiogram. If earlier tests indicate you could have macular edema, your eye-care professional may perform a fluorescein angiogram. In this test, a special dye is injected into your arm and a camera takes photos of the retina as the dye travels through the blood vessels. This test helps your ophthalmologist identify the amount of damage to the macula.

Optical coherence tomography (OCT). This is a test that uses a special light and a camera for detailed views of the cell layers inside the retina. It detects the thickness of the retina and so it is useful in determining the amount of swelling in the macula. Your eye-care professional may also use optical coherence tomography after your treatment to track how well you are healing.

The Amsler grid. The Amsler grid provides an easy way to test whether or not your central vision has changed. It can recognize even small changes in your vision.

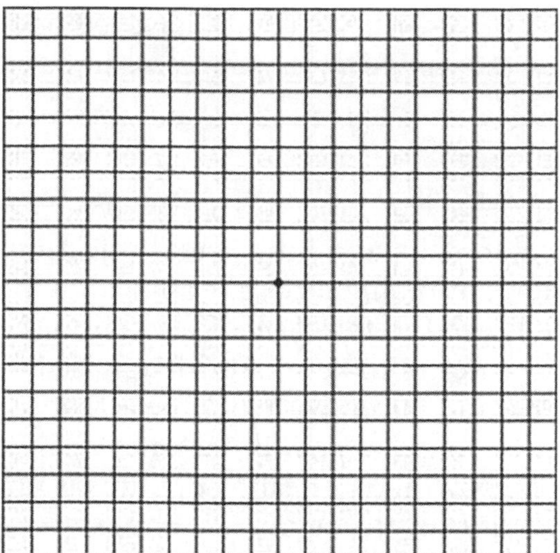

Figure 44.2. Amsler Grid

If you need reading glasses, wear them when you look at the Amsler grid. The grid should be at the same distance from your eyes as your usual reading material—about 14 inches. Test both eyes, one at a time, to see if any parts of the grid look distorted, missing, or dark. Mark the areas of the chart that you are not seeing properly and bring it with you to your next eye exam.

WHAT IS THE TREATMENT FOR MACULAR EDEMA?

Treatment for macular edema is determined by the type of macular edema you have. The most effective treatment strategies first aim at the underlying cause of macular edema, such as diabetes or high blood pressure, and then directly treat the damage in the retina.

Treatments for diabetic macular edema and macular edema caused by other conditions are often the same. However, some cases of macular edema may need additional treatments to address associated conditions.

The standard treatment for macular edema was focal laser photocoagulation, which uses the heat from a laser to seal leaking blood vessels in the retina. However, clinical trials, many of which are supported by the National Eye Institute (NEI), have led doctors to move away from laser therapy to drug treatments injected directly into the eye.

Anti-VEGF Injections

The standard care for macular edema is intravitreal injection. During this painless procedure, numbing drops are applied to the eye, and a short thin needle is used to inject medication into the vitreous gel (the fluid in the center of the eye). The drugs used in this treatment—Avastin, Eylea, and Lucentis—block the activity of a substance called "vascular endothelial growth factor" (VEGF). VEGF promotes blood vessel growth. In a healthy eye, this is not a problem. But, in some conditions, the retina becomes starved for blood and VEGF becomes overactive. This causes the growth of fragile blood vessels which can rupture and leak blood into the retina and macula, causing macular edema. Anti-VEGF treatment blocks the activity of VEGF and slows the progress of macular edema.

The anti-VEGF drugs all work in similar ways to block vessel formation and prevent leakage in the retina. An NEI-supported clinical trial that directly compared the effectiveness of the three drugs for DME found that the drugs performed similarly for patients with mild vision problems. However, Eylea performed better for those with more serious vision loss (20/50 or worse). Your eye-care professional will discuss which drug treatment is the best option for you.

Anti-Inflammatory Treatments

Corticosteroid (steroid) treatments, which reduce inflammation, are the primary treatment for macular edema caused by inflammatory eye diseases. These anti-inflammatory drugs are usually administered via eye drops, pills, or injections of sustained-release corticosteroids into or around the eye. Clinicians have these three options. The U.S. Food and Drug Administration (FDA)-approved sustained-release corticosteroid implants for more serious or longer-lasting conditions:

- **Ozurdex** is an implant that delivers an extended-release dose of dexamethasone. It is approved for DME, macular edema following retinal vein occlusion and (noninfectious) uveitis.
- **Retisert** is an implant that delivers an extended-release dose of fluocinolone acetonide. It is approved for the treatment of uveitis, as well as DME that does not respond to corticosteroids.
- **Iluvien** is an implant that releases small doses of fluocinolone acetonide over the course of several years. The FDA has approved it for treating DME.

Nonsteroidal anti-inflammatory drugs (NSAIDs), in the form of eye drops, are sometimes used either before or after cataract surgery to prevent the development of macular edema. Because they are chemically different from corticosteroids, NSAIDs may be used when the eye does not respond to steroid treatment or to avoid the side effects of steroid use in the eye.

Vitrectomy

Some cases of macular edema are caused when the vitreous (the gel that fills the area between the lens and the retina) pulls on the macula. Surgery to remove the vitreous gel, called a "vitrectomy," relieves the pulling on the macula. Vitrectomy also may be required to remove blood that has collected in the vitreous or to correct vision when other treatments for macular edema are unsuccessful. Most vitrectomy surgeries are performed as outpatient surgery.

WHAT IS THE LATEST RESEARCH ON MACULAR EDEMA?

The NEI-supported researchers are working in laboratories and clinics across the country to better understand why people get macular edema and to develop treatments that are more effective and easier to administer. Ultimately, researchers hope to develop treatments that could reverse, or even prevent, the development of macular edema. For example:

- The NEI-supported Studies of Comparative Treatments for Retinal Vein Occlusion (SCORE) is a Phase III clinical trial to compare treatment protocols for macular edema associated with central retinal vein occlusion. The trial will test two anti-VEGF treatments—Avastin and Eylea—to compare their effectiveness. Because there is a significant difference in cost per dose between the two drugs, it is important for patients and doctors to have information about which drug might work best in specific cases.
- Anti-VEGF therapy has become the standard of care for DME, but not all patients respond to the treatment. In fact, close to half of those treated do not improve. In addition to VEGF, a number of inflammatory factors also influence macular edema. NEI-supported researchers are looking at how growth factors like VEGF interact with inflammatory factors to contribute to macular edema. Their findings could lead to combined treatment approaches that would target both growth and inflammatory factors and be a more effective treatment for people with DME.
- Anti-VEGF drugs have additional limitations. Repeated injections are required and other cell types in the eye may be impacted. The drugs also do not address other factors that may influence the development of macular edema, including inflammation. The NEI-supported researchers are investigating a novel nanoparticle delivery platform that uses micro-ribonucleic acid's (RNA), parts of the genome that influence gene expression, to determine if they can be used to shut down genes associated with the development of macular edema.
- The NEI-supported researchers are investigating the potential to regenerate tissue that is destroyed or damaged in retinal diseases such as macular edema. The researchers are studying how cells in the retina respond when the retina is stressed from lack of blood. The goal is to understand how interactions between different cell types—including nerve cells and the

cells that make blood vessels—can lead to abnormal blood vessel growth. This could potentially lead to the development of drugs to discourage abnormal vessel growth.

Section 44.3 | Stay on TRACK to Prevent Blindness from Diabetes

This section includes text excerpted from "Stay on TRACK to Prevent Blindness From Diabetes," National Eye Institute (NEI), September 9, 2019.

ELEVEN MILLION PEOPLE TO BE AT RISK BY 2030

You cannot feel it. You cannot see it—until it is too late. Diabetic retinopathy, the most common form of diabetic eye disease, is the leading cause of blindness in adults age 20 to 74. It occurs when diabetes damages blood vessels in the retina.

Diabetic retinopathy affects 7.7 million Americans, and that number is projected to increase to more than 11 million people by 2030.

Dr. Paul Sieving, director of the National Eye Institute (NEI), says, "Only about half of all people with diabetes get an annual comprehensive dilated eye exam, which is essential for detecting diabetic eye disease early, when it is most treatable."

With no early symptoms, diabetic eye disease—a group of conditions including cataract, glaucoma, and diabetic retinopathy—can affect anyone with type 1 or type 2 diabetes. African Americans, American Indians/Alaska Natives, and Hispanics/Latinx are at higher risk for losing vision or going blind from diabetes. The longer a person has diabetes, the greater the risk for diabetic eye disease. Once the vision is lost, it often cannot be restored.

Keeping diabetes under control is key to slowing the progression of vision complications such as diabetic retinopathy. There are important steps people with diabetes can take to keep their health on TRACK:

- Take your medications as prescribed by your doctor.

- **R**each and maintain a healthy weight.
- **A**dd physical activity to your daily routine.
- **C**ontrol your ABC's—A1C, blood pressure, and cholesterol levels.
- **K**ick the smoking habit.

Additionally, people with diabetes should have annual comprehensive dilated eye exams to help protect their sight. Early detection, timely treatment, and appropriate follow-up care can reduce a person's risk for severe vision loss from diabetic eye disease by 95 percent.

"More than ever, it is important for people with diabetes to have a comprehensive dilated eye exam at least once a year. New treatments are being developed all the time, and researchers are learning that different treatments may work best for different patients. What has not changed is that early treatment is always better," says Dr. Suber Huang, chair of the Diabetic Eye Disease Subcommittee for the NEI's National Eye Health Education Program (NEHEP) and member of the NEI-funded Diabetic Retinopathy Clinical Research Network (DRCR.net). "There has never been a more hopeful time in the treatment of diabetic retinopathy," he adds.

DID YOU KNOW?

- Diabetes affects more than nine percent of the U.S. population.
- More than one in three people have prediabetes.
- Everyone with diabetes is at risk for diabetic retinopathy—the number one cause of vision loss and blindness in working-age adults.

Remember, if you have diabetes, make annual comprehensive dilated eye exams part of your self-management routine. Living with diabetes can be challenging, but you do not have to lose your vision or go blind because of it.

Chapter 45 | **Other Disorders with Eye-Related Complications**

Chapter Contents

Section 45.1 | Behçet Disease

This section includes text excerpted from "Behçet Disease," Genetic and Rare Diseases Information Center (GARD), National Center for Advancing Translational Sciences (NCATS), May 3, 2018.

Behçet disease is a chronic multisystem inflammatory disorder characterized by ulcers affecting the mouth and genitals, various skin lesions, and abnormalities affecting the eyes. In some people, the disease also results in arthritis (swollen, painful, stiff joints), skin problems, and inflammation of the digestive tract, brain, and spinal cord. Although it can happen at any age, symptoms generally begin when individuals are in their 20s or 30s. The disease is common in Japan, Turkey and Israel, and less common in the United States. The exact cause of Behçet disease is still unknown, but it is thought that it is an autoimmune disease, where the abnormal immune activity is triggered by exposure to an environmental agent (such as an infection) in people with a genetic predisposition to develop the disease. Research shows that people with Behçet disease, especially those of Middle Eastern and Asian descent, have an increased frequency of certain "human leukocyte antigens" (HLAs), specifically HLA-B51, than the general population, which may increase the risk (predispose) to have the disease.

Treatment is symptomatic and supportive. Research is being conducted on the use of interferon-alpha and with agents that inhibit tumor necrosis factor (TNF) for the treatment of Behçet disease. Behçet disease is a lifelong disorder that comes and goes. Spontaneous remission over time is common for individuals with Behçet disease but permanent remission of symptoms has not been reported.

SYMPTOMS OF BEHÇET DISEASE

The signs and symptoms of Behçet disease include recurrent ulcers in the mouth and on the genitals, and eye inflammation (uveitis). It usually begins when people are in their 20s or 30s, although it can happen at any age. It tends to occur more often in men than in women. Behçet disease is a multi-system disease and it may involve all organs of the body. Signs and symptoms may include:

- **Sores inside the mouth or genitals.** The earliest symptom of Behçet disease is usually painful canker round or oval sores with reddish borders on the mucous membranes that line the mouth (aphthous stomatitis) or in the skin of the genitalia. They may be shallow or deep and may be single or multiple lesions that typically heal within a few days, up to a week or more, without scarring, but frequently recur.
- **Eye problems.** Symptoms may include inflammation of the back of the eye ((posterior uveitis), inflammation of the anterior chamber (anterior uveitis or iridocyclitis), inflammation of the iris accompanied by pain, tearing (lacrimation), and accumulation of pus (hypopyon iritis). The retina may become inflamed resulting in blurred vision, abnormal sensitivity to light (photophobia), and/or inflammation of the thin membranous layer of blood vessels behind the retina (chorioretinitis). Repeated recurrences may result in partial loss of vision (decreased visual acuity) or complete blindness if the disease is uncontrolled. In some cases, eye abnormalities may be the first symptom of Behçet disease or they may not develop until several years after the sores of the mouth.
- **Pus-filled lesions and other problems on the skin.** Some affected individuals, especially females, may develop lesions that resemble those of erythema nodosum, a skin disorder characterized by the formation of tender, reddish, inflammatory nodules on the front of the legs. These nodules disappear on their own (spontaneously) sometimes leaving faint scars or discoloration (pigmentation). Some people with Behçet disease may develop small eruptions that resemble acne (acneiform eruptions) and/or inflammation that mistakenly appear to affect the hair follicles on the skin (pseudofolliculitis).
- **Pain in the joints (50% of cases).** Affected individuals have pain (arthralgia) and swelling in various joints

(knees, wrists, elbows, and ankles), before, during, or after the onset of the other symptoms.

- **Recurring ulcers in the digestive tract.** Symptoms vary from mild abdominal discomfort to severe inflammation of the large intestine and rectum accompanied by diarrhea or bleeding.
- **Problems of the central nervous system (CNS) (10 to 20% of the cases).** These symptoms usually appear months or years after the initial symptoms of Behçet disease. Recurring attacks of inflammation involving the brain (parenchymal Neuro-Behçet) or the membranes that surround the brain or spinal cord (meningitis) can result in neurological damage. Symptoms may include headache, cranial nerve palsies, the inability to coordinate voluntary movement (cerebellar ataxia), impaired muscle movements of the face and throat, stroke, memory loss and/or, rarely, seizures.
- **Inflammation of the blood vessels (vasculitis).** The involvement of small vessels is thought to drive many of the problems that the disorder causes. In some instances, inflammation of the large veins, particularly those in the legs may occur along with the formation of blood clots (thrombophlebitis). The walls of an involved artery may bulge forming a sac (aneurysm). In very rare cases, blood clots from the veins travel to the lungs (pulmonary emboli (PE)) resulting in episodes of chest pain, coughing, difficult or labored breathing (dyspnea), and coughing up blood (hemoptysis).

It is especially important to identify Behçet disease when there is ocular, CNS or large blood vessel involvement because these as manifestations are usually the most serious.

CAUSES OF BEHÇET DISEASE

The exact cause of Behçet disease is unknown. Most symptoms of the disease are caused by inflammation of the blood vessels (vasculitis). Inflammation is a characteristic reaction of the body to injury or disease and is marked by four signs: swelling, redness, heat, and pain. Doctors think that an autoimmune reaction may cause the blood vessels to become inflamed, but they do not know what triggers this reaction. Under normal conditions, the immune system protects the body from diseases and infections by killing harmful "foreign" substances, such as germs, that enter the body. In an autoimmune reaction, the immune system mistakenly attacks and harms the body's own tissues. Behçet disease is not contagious; it does not spread from one person to another.

Researchers think that two factors are important for a person to develop Behçet disease:

- First, it is believed that abnormalities of the immune system make some people susceptible to the disease. Scientists think that this susceptibility may be inherited; that is, it may be due to one or more specific genes. People with the disease are more likely to have certain "human leukocyte antigens" (HLAs) in the blood, especially HLA-B51, than the general population. Other genetic markers and their role in the development of Behçet disease are being studied.
- Second, something in the environment, possibly a bacterium (such as *Helicobacter pylori* (*H. pylori*)) or virus (such as herpes simplex virus (HSV), and parvovirus B19) or exposition to certain substances (such as heavy metals), might trigger or activate the disease in susceptible people.

TREATMENT OF BEHÇET DISEASE

Although there is no cure for Behçet disease, people can usually control symptoms with proper medication, rest, exercise, and a healthy lifestyle. The goal of treatment is to reduce discomfort and prevent serious complications, such as disability from arthritis or blindness. The type of medicine and the length of treatment depend on the person's symptoms and their severity. It is likely that a combination of treatments will be needed to relieve specific symptoms.

Patients should tell each of their doctors about all of the medicines they are taking so that the doctors can coordinate treatment.

Topical medicine is applied directly to the sores to relieve pain and discomfort. For example, doctors prescribe rinses, gels, or ointments. Creams are used to treat skin and genital sores. The medicine usually contains corticosteroids (which reduce inflammation), other anti-inflammatory drugs, or an anesthetic, which relieves pain.

Doctors also prescribe medicines taken by mouth to reduce inflammation throughout the body, suppress the overactive immune system, and relieve symptoms. Doctors may prescribe one or more of the medicines listed below to treat the various symptoms of Behçet disease:

- Corticosteroids
- Immunosuppressive drugs (Azathioprine, Chlorambucil or Cyclophosphamide, Cyclosporine, Colchicine, or a combination of these treatments)
- Methotrexate

Interferon-alfa, azathioprine, and TNF-α blockers may be tried in rare cases of patients with resistant, prolonged, and disabling attacks.

The European League Against Rheumatism (EULAR) has recommendations for the management of Behçet disease.

For ocular disease, azathioprine is the first medication that should be used. For severe eye disease (such as drop-in visual acuity, retinal vasculitis, or macular involvement), either cyclosporine A or infliximab may be used in combination with azathioprine and corticosteroids. Interferon-alfa, alone or in combination with corticosteroids, appears to be the second choice in this eye disease.

PROGNOSIS OF BEHÇET DISEASE

Most people with Behçet disease can lead productive lives and control symptoms with proper medicine, rest, and exercise. Doctors can use many medicines to relieve pain, treat symptoms, and prevent complications. When treatment is effective, flares usually become less frequent. Many patients eventually enter a period of remission (a disappearance of symptoms). In some people, treatment does not relieve symptoms, and gradually more serious symptoms, such as eye disease may occur. Serious symptoms may appear months or years after the first signs of Behçet disease.

Section 45.2 | **Cytomegalovirus**

This section includes text excerpted from "HIV-Related Conditions: Entire Lesson," U.S. Department of Veterans Affairs (VA), December 27, 2019.

WHAT IS CYTOMEGALOVIRUS?

Cytomegalovirus (CMV) is transmitted by close contact through sex and through saliva, urine, and other body fluids. It can be passed from mother to child during pregnancy and by breast-feeding. If you are not infected, using condoms during sex may help prevent infection.

Many people are infected with this virus, though they have no symptoms. In people with human immunodeficiency viruses (HIV) who have low CD4 (cluster of differentiation 4) counts, the infection can be extremely serious.

SYMPTOMS OF CYTOMEGALOVIRUS

Symptoms can include:

- Blind spots in vision, loss of peripheral vision
- Headache, difficulty concentrating, sleepiness
- Mouth ulcers
- Pain in the abdomen, bloody diarrhea
- Fever, fatigue, weight loss
- Shortness of breath
- Lower back pain
- Confusion, apathy, withdrawal, personality changes

MEDICATIONS FOR CYTOMEGALOVIRUS

Drugs are available to keep symptoms of the infection under control. HIV drugs can improve the condition, too. If you have CMV and have not started taking drugs for HIV, it may be best to wait until you have been on treatment for CMV for a few weeks.

Treatment can prevent further loss of vision but cannot reverse existing damage. If you experience any vision problems, tell your healthcare provider immediately.

Section 45.3 | **Graves Ophthalmopathy**

This section includes text excerpted from "Graves' Ophthalmopathy," National Center for Biotechnology Information (NCBI), January 25, 2014. Reviewed March 2020.

Graves ophthalmopathy, also called "Graves orbitopathy," is a potentially sight-threatening ocular disease that has puzzled physicians and scientists for nearly two centuries. Generally occurring in patients with hyperthyroidism or a history of hyperthyroidism due to Graves disease, Graves ophthalmopathy is also known as "thyroid-associated ophthalmopathy" or "thyroid eye disease," because it sometimes occurs in patients with euthyroid or hypothyroid chronic autoimmune thyroiditis. The condition has an annual adjusted incidence rate of 16 women and 3 men per 100,000 population.

The close clinical and temporal relationships between hyperthyroidism, Graves ophthalmopathy, and thyroid dermopathy suggest that these conditions evolve from a single underlying systemic process with variable expression in the thyroid, eyes, and skin. Bilateral ocular symptoms and hyperthyroidism most often occur simultaneously or within 18 months of each other, although occasionally Graves ophthalmopathy precedes or follows the onset of hyperthyroidism by many years.

Almost half of the patients with Graves hyperthyroidism report symptoms of Graves ophthalmopathy, including a dry and gritty ocular sensation, photophobia, excessive tearing, double vision, and a pressure sensation behind the eyes. The most common clinical features of Graves ophthalmopathy are upper eyelid retraction, edema, and erythema of the periorbital tissues and conjunctivae, and proptosis.

Approximately 3 to 5 percent of patients with Graves ophthalmopathy have severe disease with intense pain, inflammation, and sight-threatening corneal ulceration or compressive optic neuropathy (CON). Subclinical eye involvement is common: in nearly 70 percent of adult patients with Graves hyperthyroidism, magnetic resonance imaging (MRI) or computed tomographic (CT) scanning reveals extraocular-muscle enlargement (EOME). Although clinically unilateral Graves ophthalmopathy occurs occasionally, orbital imaging generally confirms the presence of asymmetric bilateral disease.

Cigarette smoking is the strongest modifiable risk factor for Graves ophthalmopathy, and the risk is proportional to the number of cigarettes smoked daily. In smokers with Graves ophthalmopathy, as compared with nonsmokers, severe disease is more likely to develop and is more likely to respond less well to immunosuppressive therapies.

Many clinical signs and symptoms of Graves ophthalmopathy arise from soft-tissue enlargement in the orbit, leading to increased pressure within the bony cavity. Most patients have enlargement of both extraocular muscle and adipose tissue, with a predominance of one or the other in some. Patients under 40 years of age tend to have fat expansion, whereas patients over 60 years of age have more extraocular-muscle swelling.

The quality of life (QOL) is markedly decreased in patients with Graves ophthalmopathy. Unraveling the Graves ophthalmopathy conundrum would enable the design of effective means of prevention or treatment.

Section 45.4 | **Holmes-Adie Syndrome**

This section contains text excerpted from the following sources: Text in this section begins with excerpts from "Adie Syndrome," Genetic and Rare Diseases Information Center (GARD), National Center for Advancing Translational Sciences (NCATS), February 16, 2016. Reviewed March 2020; Text beginning with the heading "Treatment of Holmes-Adie Syndrome" is excerpted from "Holmes-Adie Syndrome Information Page," National Institute of Neurological Disorders and Stroke (NINDS), March 27, 2019.

Holmes-Adie syndrome is a neurological disorder affecting the pupil of the eye and the autonomic nervous system. It is characterized by one eye with a pupil that is larger than normal that constricts slowly in bright light (tonic pupil), along with the absence of deep tendon reflexes, usually in the Achilles tendon.

In most cases, the cause of Adie syndrome is unknown. Some cases may result from trauma, surgery, lack of blood flow, or infection.

Treatment may not be necessary. Glasses and eye drops may help when treatment is needed.

The term "Adie syndrome" is used when both the pupil and deep tendon reflexes are affected. When only the pupil is affected, the disorder may be referred to as "Adie's pupil."

SYMPTOMS OF HOLMES-ADIE SYNDROME

Adie syndrome is characterized by one eye with a pupil that is larger than normal that constricts slowly in bright light (tonic pupil), along with the absence of deep tendon reflexes, usually in the Achilles tendon. It typically begins gradually in one eye and often progresses to involve the other eye. At first, it may only cause the loss of deep tendon reflexes on one side of the body but then progress to the other side. The eye and reflex symptoms may not appear at the same time. People with Adie syndrome may also sweat excessively, sometimes only on one side of the body. The combination of these three symptoms—abnormal pupil size, loss of deep tendon reflexes, and excessive sweating—is usually called "Ross syndrome," although some doctors will still diagnose the condition as a variant of Adie syndrome. Some individuals will also have cardiovascular abnormalities. The symptoms of Adie syndrome can appear on their own, or in association with other diseases of the nervous system, such as Sjogren syndrome or migraine.

CAUSES OF HOLMES-ADIE SYNDROME

In most cases, the cause of Adie syndrome is unknown (idiopathic). The tonic pupil in Adie syndrome is believed to result from inflammation or damage to the ciliary ganglion (a cluster of nerve cells found behind the eye) or damage to the postganglionic nerves. The ciliary ganglion is part of the parasympathetic nervous system, a component of the autonomic nervous system. It helps control the pupil's response to light and other stimuli. In most cases, damage to the ciliary ganglion or postganglionic nerves is caused by an infection. Damage may also result from autoimmune processes, tumors, trauma, and complications of surgery.

The loss of deep tendon reflexes in Adie syndrome is believed to be caused by damage to the dorsal root ganglion, a cluster of nerve cells in the root of the spinal nerves.

In rare cases, Adie syndrome may be inherited. In these cases, it appears to follow an autosomal dominant pattern of inheritance.

TREATMENT OF HOLMES-ADIE SYNDROME

Doctors may prescribe reading glasses to compensate for impaired vision in the affected eye, and pilocarpine drops to be applied three times daily to constrict the dilated pupil. Thoracic sympathectomy, which severs the involved sympathetic nerve, is the definitive treatment for excessive sweating.

PROGNOSIS OF HOLMES-ADIE SYNDROME

Holmes-Adie syndrome is not life-threatening or disabling. The loss of deep tendon reflexes is permanent. Some symptoms of the disorder may progress. For most individuals, pilocarpine drops and glasses will improve vision.

Section 45.5 | **Idiopathic Intracranial Hypertension**

This section includes text excerpted from "Idiopathic Intracranial Hypertension," National Eye Institute (NEI), July 5, 2019.

WHAT IS IDIOPATHIC INTRACRANIAL HYPERTENSION?

Idiopathic intracranial hypertension is a condition due to high pressure within the spaces that surround the brain and spinal cord. These spaces are filled with cerebrospinal fluid (CSF), which cushions the brain from mechanical injury, provides nourishment, and carries away waste.

WHAT ARE THE SYMPTOMS OF IDIOPATHIC INTRACRANIAL HYPERTENSION?

The most common symptoms of idiopathic intracranial hypertension are headaches and visual loss, including blind spots, poor peripheral (side) vision, double vision, and short temporary episodes of blindness. Many patients experience permanent vision loss. Other common symptoms include pulsatile tinnitus (ringing in the ears) and neck and shoulder pain.

WHAT ARE THE TYPES OF IDIOPATHIC INTRACRANIAL HYPERTENSION?

Idiopathic intracranial hypertension can be either acute or chronic. In chronic intracranial hypertension, the increased CSF pressure can cause swelling and damage to the optic nerve—a condition called "papilledema."

Chronic intracranial hypertension can be caused by many conditions including certain drugs, such as tetracycline, a blood clot in the brain, excessive intake of vitamin A, or brain tumors. It can also occur without a detectable cause. This is idiopathic intracranial hypertension.

Because the symptoms of idiopathic intracranial hypertension (IIH) can resemble those of a brain tumor, it is sometimes known by the older name "pseudotumor cerebri," which means "false brain tumor."

WHO IS AT RISK FOR IDIOPATHIC INTRACRANIAL HYPERTENSION?

An estimated 100,000 Americans have IIH, and the number is rising as more people become obese or overweight. The disorder is most common in women between the ages of 20 and 50; about 5 percent of those affected are men. Obesity, defined as a body mass index (BMI) greater than 30, is a major risk factor. BMI is a number based on your weight and height. The Centers for Disease Control and Prevention (CDC) offers an online BMI calculator (www.cdc.gov/healthyweight/assessing/bmi/adult_bmi/english_bmi_calculator/bmi_calculator.html). A recent gain of 5 to 15 percent of total body weight is also considered a risk factor for this disorder, even for people with a BMI of less than 30.

HOW WILL THE EYE DOCTOR CHECK FOR IDIOPATHIC INTRACRANIAL HYPERTENSION?

A thorough medical history and physical exam are needed to identify risk factors for IIH and to evaluate for the many potential causes of increased intracranial pressure. A neurological exam will also be performed. In IIH, the exam is normal except for findings related to increased intracranial pressure, including papilledema, visual loss, and possible weakness in the lateral rectus muscles, which are located near your temples and help turn the eyes outward. Weakness in these muscles can cause the eyes to turn inward, toward the nose, producing double vision.

A number of vision tests may also be performed, including a comprehensive dilated eye exam to look for signs of papilledema. Visual field testing is done to evaluate your peripheral vision. This testing measures the area of space you can see at a given instant without moving your head or eyes.

Brain imaging, including computed tomography (CT) and magnetic resonance imaging (MRI) scans, will be performed to look for a brain tumor, injury, or other potential cause for your symptoms. Normal findings on these exams are essential to a diagnosis of IIH.

A lumbar puncture, also known as a "spinal tap," will be performed. In this procedure, a needle is inserted into a CSF-filled sac below the spinal cord in the lower back. The CSF pressure will be measured, and a small amount of CSF will be collected for analysis to look for causes of increased intracranial pressure. The procedure may also cause a temporary reduction in CSF pressure and symptoms.

WHAT IS THE TREATMENT FOR IDIOPATHIC INTRACRANIAL HYPERTENSION?

If a diagnosis of IIH is confirmed, regular visual field tests and comprehensive dilated eye exams are recommended to monitor any changes in vision.

Sustainable weight loss through healthy eating, salt restriction, and exercise is a critical part of treatment for people with IIH who are overweight. Studies show that modest weight loss, around 5 to 10 percent of total body weight, may be sufficient to reduce signs and symptoms. If lifestyle changes are not successful in reducing weight and relieving IIH, weight loss surgery may be recommended for those with a BMI greater than 40.

For many people, weight loss can be difficult to achieve and maintain. And for those who are able to adjust their weight, relief from IIH tends to be gradual. Acetazolamide (Diamox), a drug that decreases CSF production, is therefore often used as an add-on therapy to weight loss. The drug is taken orally. Common side effects include fatigue, nausea, tingling hands and feet, and a metallic taste, usually triggered by carbonated drinks. These can be reversed by lowering the dose or stopping the drug.

It is important to remember that some medications, such as tetracycline, may help trigger IIH, and that stopping them may lead to improvement.

In rapidly progressive cases that do not respond to other treatments, surgery may be needed to relieve pressure on the optic nerve. Therapeutic shunting, which involves surgically inserting a tube to drain CSF from ventricles or inner brain cavities, can be used to remove excess CSF and lower pressure. In a procedure called "optic nerve sheath fenestration," pressure on the optic nerve is relieved by making a small window into the covering that surrounds the nerve just behind the eyeball.

WHAT IS THE PROGNOSIS?

For most people, IIH usually improves with treatment. For others, it progressively worsens with time, or it can resolve and then recur. About 5 to 10 percent of women with IIH experience disabling vision loss. Most patients do not need surgical treatment.

Section 45.6 | **Multiple Sclerosis**

This section includes text excerpted from "Multiple Sclerosis: Hope through Research," National Institute of Neurological Disorders and Stroke (NINDS), January 7, 2020.

WHAT IS MULTIPLE SCLEROSIS?

Multiple sclerosis (MS) is a neuroinflammatory disease that affects myelin, a substance that makes up the membrane (called the "myelin sheath") that wraps around nerve fibers (axons). Myelinated axons are commonly called "white matter." Researchers have learned that MS also damages the nerve cell bodies, which are found in the brain's gray matter, as well as the axons themselves in the brain, spinal cord, and optic nerve (the nerve that transmits visual information from the eye to the brain). As the disease progresses, the brain's cortex shrinks (cortical atrophy).

The term multiple sclerosis refers to the distinctive areas of scar tissue (sclerosis or plaques) that are visible in the white matter of people who have MS. Plaques can be as small as a pinhead or as large as the size of a golf ball. Doctors can see these areas by examining the brain and spinal cord using a type of brain scan called "magnetic resonance imaging" (MRI).

While MS sometimes causes severe disability, it is only rarely fatal and most people with MS have a normal life expectancy.

WHAT ARE THE SIGNS AND SYMPTOMS OF MULTIPLE SCLEROSIS?

The symptoms of MS usually begin over one to several days, but in some forms, they may develop more slowly. They may be mild or severe and may go away quickly or last for months. Sometimes the initial symptoms of MS are overlooked because they disappear in a day or so and normal function returns. Because symptoms come and go in the majority of people with MS, the presence of symptoms is called an "attack," or in medical terms, an "exacerbation." Recovery from symptoms is referred to as remission, while a return of symptoms is called a "relapse." This form of MS is therefore called "relapsing-remitting MS," in contrast to a more slowly developing form called "primary progressive MS." Progressive MS can also be a second stage of the illness that follows years of relapsing-remitting symptoms.

A diagnosis of MS is often delayed as MS shares symptoms with other neurological conditions and diseases.

The first symptoms of MS often include:

- Vision problems, such as blurred or double vision or optic neuritis, which causes pain in the eye and a rapid loss of vision
- Weak, stiff muscles, often with painful muscle spasms
- Tingling or numbness in the arms, legs, trunk of the body, or face
- Clumsiness, particularly difficulty staying balanced when walking
- Bladder control problems, either the inability to control the bladder or urgency
- Dizziness that does not go away

Multiple sclerosis may also cause later symptoms such as:

- Mental or physical fatigue which accompanies the above symptoms during an attack
- Mood changes, such as depression or euphoria
- Changes in the ability to concentrate or to multitask effectively
- Difficulty making decisions, planning, or prioritizing at work or in private life

Some people with MS develop transverse myelitis, a condition caused by inflammation in the spinal cord. Transverse myelitis causes loss of spinal cord function over a period of time lasting from several hours to several weeks. It usually begins as a sudden onset of lower back pain, muscle weakness, or abnormal sensations in the toes and feet, and can rapidly progress to more severe symptoms, including paralysis. In most cases of transverse myelitis, people recover at least some function within the first 12 weeks after an attack begins. Transverse myelitis can also result from viral infections, arteriovenous malformations (AVMs), or neuroinflammatory problems unrelated to MS. In such instances, there are no plaques in the brain that suggest previous MS attacks.

Neuromyelitis optica (NMO) is a disorder associated with transverse myelitis as well as optic nerve inflammation. Patients with this disorder usually have antibodies against a particular protein in their spinal cord, called the "aquaporin channel." These patients respond differently to treatment than most people with MS.

Most individuals with MS have muscle weakness, often in their hands and legs. Muscle stiffness and spasms can also be a problem. These symptoms may be severe enough to affect walking or standing. In some cases, MS leads to partial or complete paralysis. Many people with MS find that weakness and fatigue are worse when they have a fever or when they are exposed to heat. MS exacerbations may occur following common infections.

Tingling and burning sensations are common, as well as the opposite, numbness and loss of sensation. Moving the neck from side to side or flexing it back and forth may cause "Lhermitte's sign," a characteristic sensation of MS that feels like a sharp spike of electricity coursing down the spine.

While it is rare for the pain to be the first sign of MS, pain often occurs with optic neuritis and trigeminal neuralgia, a neurological disorder that affects one of the nerves that runs across the jaw, cheek, and face. Painful spasms of the limbs and sharp pain shooting down the legs or around the abdomen can also be symptoms of MS.

Most individuals with MS experience difficulties with coordination and balance at some time during the course of the disease. Some may have a continuous trembling of the head, limbs, and body, especially during movement, although such trembling is more common with other disorders such as Parkinson disease (PD).

Fatigue is common, especially during exacerbations of MS. A person with MS may be tired all the time or maybe easily fatigued from mental or physical exertion.

Urinary symptoms, including loss of bladder control and sudden attacks of urgency, are common as MS progresses. People with MS sometimes also develop constipation or sexual problems.

Depression is a common feature of MS. A small number of individuals with MS may develop more severe psychiatric disorders, such as bipolar disorder and paranoia, or experience inappropriate episodes of high spirits, known as "euphoria."

People with MS, especially those who have had the disease for a long time, can experience difficulty with thinking, learning, memory, and judgment. The first signs of what doctors call cognitive dysfunction may be subtle. The person may have problems finding the right word to say, or trouble remembering how to do routine tasks on the job or at home. Day-to-day decisions that once came easily may now be made more slowly and show poor judgment. Changes may be so small or happen so slowly that it takes a family member or friend to point them out.

WHAT CAUSES MULTIPLE SCLEROSIS

The ultimate cause of MS is damage to myelin, nerve fibers, and neurons in the brain and spinal cord, which together make up the central nervous system (CNS). But how that happens, and why, are questions that challenge researchers. Evidence appears to show that MS is a disease caused by genetic vulnerabilities combined with environmental factors.

Although there is little doubt that the immune system contributes to the brain and spinal cord tissue destruction of MS, the exact target of the immune system attacks and which immune system cells cause the destruction is not fully understood.

Researchers have several possible explanations for what might be going on. The immune system could be:

- Fighting some kind of infectious agent (for example, a virus) that has components which mimic components of the brain (molecular mimicry)
- Destroying brain cells because they are unhealthy
- Mistakenly identifying normal brain cells as foreign

The last possibility has been the favored explanation for many years. Research now suggests that the first two activities might also play a role in the development of MS. There is a special barrier, called the "blood-brain barrier" (BBB), which separates the brain and spinal cord from the immune system. If there is a break in the barrier, it exposes the brain to the immune system for the first time. When this happens, the immune system may misinterpret the brain as "foreign."

Genetic Susceptibility

Susceptibility to MS may be inherited. Studies of families indicate that relatives of an individual with MS have an increased risk for developing the disease. Experts estimate that about 15 percent of individuals with MS have one or more family members or relatives who also have MS. But even identical twins, whose deoxyribonucleic acid (DNA) is exactly the same, have only a 1 in 3 chance of both having the disease. This suggests that MS is not entirely controlled by genes. Other factors must come into play.

Research suggests that dozens of genes and possibly hundreds of variations in the genetic code (called "gene variants") combine to create vulnerability to MS. Some of these genes have been identified. Most of the genes identified so far are associated with the functions of the immune system. Additionally, many of the known genes are similar to those that have been identified in people with other autoimmune diseases, such as type 1 diabetes, rheumatoid arthritis (RA) or lupus. Researchers continue to look for additional genes and to study how they interact with each other to make an individual vulnerable to developing MS.

Sunlight and Vitamin D

A number of studies have suggested that people who spend more time in the sun and those with relatively high levels of vitamin D are less likely to develop MS. Bright sunlight helps human skin produce vitamin D. Researchers believe that vitamin D may help regulate the immune system in ways that reduce the risk of MS. People from regions near the equator, where there is a great deal of bright sunlight, generally have a much lower risk of MS than people from temperate areas, such as the United States and Canada.

Other studies suggest that people with higher levels of vitamin D generally have less severe MS and fewer relapses.

Smoking

A number of studies have found that people who smoke are more likely to develop MS. People who smoke also tend to have more brain lesions and brain shrinkage than nonsmokers. The reasons for this are currently unclear.

Infectious Factors and Viruses

A number of viruses have been found in people with MS, but the virus most consistently linked to the development of MS is Epstein Barr virus (EBV), the virus that causes mononucleosis.

Only about 5 percent of the population has not been infected by EBV. These individuals are at a lower risk for developing MS than those who have been infected. People who were infected with EBV in adolescence or adulthood and who therefore develop an exaggerated immune response to EBV are at a significantly higher risk for developing MS than those who were infected in early childhood. This suggests that it may be the type of immune response to EBV that predisposes to MS, rather than EBV infection itself. However, there is still no proof that EBV causes MS.

Autoimmune and Inflammatory Processes

Tissue inflammation and antibodies in the blood that fight normal components of the body and tissue in people with MS are similar to those found in other autoimmune diseases. Along with overlapping evidence from genetic studies, these findings suggest that MS results from some kind of disturbed regulation of the immune system.

HOW DO DOCTORS TREAT VISION PROBLEMS CAUSED BY MULTIPLE SCLEROSIS?

Eye and vision problems are common in people with MS but rarely result in permanent blindness. Inflammation of the optic nerve or damage to the myelin that covers the optic nerve and other nerve fibers can cause a number of symptoms, including blurring or graying of vision, blindness in one eye, loss of normal color vision, depth perception, or a dark spot in the center of the visual field (scotoma). Uncontrolled horizontal or vertical eye movements (nystagmus) and "jumping vision" (opsoclonus) are common to MS, and can be either mild or severe enough to impair vision.

Double vision (diplopia) occurs when the two eyes are not perfectly aligned. This occurs commonly in MS when a pair of muscles that control a specific eye movement aren't coordinated due to weakness in one or both muscles. Double vision may increase with fatigue or as the result of spending too much time reading or on the computer. Periodically resting the eyes may be helpful

Section 45.7 | Rosacea

This section includes text excerpted from "Rosacea," National Institute of Arthritis and Musculoskeletal and Skin Diseases (NIAMS), April 2016. Reviewed March 2020.

Rosacea is a long-term disease that causes reddened skin and pimples, usually on the face. It can also make the skin thicker and cause eye problems.

WHO GETS ROSACEA

Anyone can get rosacea, but it is more common among these groups:

- Adults who are 30 to 60 years of age
- Women, especially during menopause
- People with fair skin. Lighter skin also makes the disease more apparent.

WHAT ARE THE SYMPTOMS OF ROSACEA?

Many people who have rosacea get eye problems. These may include:

- Eyes becoming red, dry, itchy, burning or watery. You might feel like you have sand in your eye.
- Eyelids becoming inflamed and swollen
- Eyes becoming sensitive to light
- Blurred vision, or some other kind of vision problem

WHAT CAUSES ROSACEA

Doctors do not know what causes rosacea, but your family history or genes might make you more likely to get the disease.

HOW IS ROSACEA TREATED?

Treatment for eye problems may include:

- Medicines, such as steroid eye drops
- Cleaning your eyelids to reduce infections. Your doctor may recommend scrubbing your eyelids gently with watered-down baby shampoo or an eyelid cleaner and then applying a warm (but not hot) compress a few times a day.

Whatever you do, be sure to talk about treatments and possible side effects with your doctor first.

Part 7 | Vision Impairment Rehabilitation and Recent Research

Chapter 46 | **Defining Vision Impairment**

Chapter Contents

Section 46.1 | What Is Low Vision?

This section includes text excerpted from "Low Vision," National Eye Institute (NEI), July 5, 2019.

Low vision, also known as "vision impairment" or "blindness," is a vision problem that makes it hard to do everyday activities. It cannot be fixed with glasses, contact lenses, or other standard treatments such as medicine or surgery.

You may have low vision if you cannot see well enough to do things such as:

- Read
- Drive
- Recognize people's faces
- Tell colors apart
- See your television or computer screen clearly

WHAT ARE THE TYPES OF LOW VISION?

The type of low vision that you have depends on the disease or condition that caused your low vision. The most common types of low vision are:

- Central vision loss (not being able to see things in the center of your vision)
- Peripheral vision loss (not being able to see things out of the corners of your eyes)
- Night blindness (not being able to see in low light)
- Blurry or hazy vision

WHAT CAUSES LOW VISION

Many different eye conditions can cause low vision, but the most common causes are:

- Age-related macular degeneration (AMD)
- Cataracts
- Diabetic retinopathy (a condition that can cause vision loss in people with diabetes)
- Glaucoma

Low vision is more common in older adults because many of the diseases that can cause it are more common in older adults. Aging does not cause low vision on its own.

Eye and brain injuries and certain genetic disorders can also cause low vision.

HOW DOES THE EYE DOCTOR CHECK FOR LOW VISION?

Your doctor can check for low vision as part of a dilated eye exam. The exam is simple and painless. Your doctor will ask you to read letters that are up close and far away and will check whether you can see things in the center and at the edges of your vision.

Then, they will give you some eye drops to dilate (widen) your pupil and check for other eye problems—including conditions that could cause low vision.

WHAT IS THE TREATMENT FOR LOW VISION?

Unfortunately, low vision is usually permanent. Eyeglasses, medicine, and surgery cannot usually cure low vision—but sometimes they can improve vision, help you do everyday activities more easily, or keep your vision from getting worse.

Treatment options will depend on the specific eye condition that caused your low vision. Ask your doctor if there are any treatments that could improve your vision or help protect your remaining vision.

HOW YOU CAN MAKE THE MOST OF YOUR REMAINING SIGHT

If you have low vision, you can find ways to make the most of your vision and keep doing the things you love to do.

If your vision loss is minor, you may be able to make small changes to help yourself see better. You can do things such as:

- Use brighter lights at home or work
- Wear antiglare sunglasses
- Use a magnifying lens for reading and other up close activities

If your vision loss is getting in the way of everyday activities, ask your eye doctor about vision rehabilitation. A specialist can help you learn how to live with your vision loss. This can include things such as:

- Training on how to use a magnifying device for reading
- Guidance for setting up your home so you can move around easily
- Sharing resources to help you cope with your vision loss

Section 46.2 | What Is Legal Blindness?

"What Is Legal Blindness?" © 2017 Omnigraphics. Reviewed March 2020.

Complete or total blindness is the inability to see light, shapes, or anything at all. But "legal blindness," as defined by government agencies and statutes, has a different meaning. It refers to a specific level of visual impairment that is required by law for a person to qualify for government-funded disability benefits, or for a person to be disqualified from engaging in certain government-regulated activities (such as driving a car). About 1.3 million people in the United States, or about 0.5 percent of the population, are considered legally blind.

DEFINITION OF LEGAL BLINDNESS

The generally accepted definition of legal blindness includes measurements of two aspects of eyesight: central visual acuity, and field of vision. Having a certain level of visual impairment in either measurement—with corrective eyeglasses or contact lenses—meets the definition of legal blindness. The levels of visual impairment required by the Social Security Administration (SSA) and most other U.S. government agencies are as follows:

- Reduced central visual acuity of 20/200 or less in your better eye with the use of the best eyeglass lens or contact lens to correct your eyesight, or

- Limitation of your field of view such that the widest diameter of the visual field in your better eye is no greater than 20°.

Reduced Visual Acuity

Visual acuity is the clarity or sharpness of eyesight. It is measured using a Snellen eye chart, which has rows of letters that gradually decrease in size from top to bottom. The patient typically stands about 20 feet (6 meters) away from the chart, covers one eye, and tries to read the letters on each line. The size of the letters on one of the lines corresponds to normal visual acuity, or what a person with normal eyesight can read from a distance of 20 feet.

Using the Snellen system, a person with normal visual acuity is said to have a 20/20 vision. The numerator (top number) of the Snellen fraction refers to the patient's distance from the eye chart, while the denominator (bottom number) refers to the distance at which a person with normal visual acuity can read that line. Therefore, a person with 20/200 vision standing 20 feet away from the eye chart can only read letters that a person with normal visual acuity can read from 200 feet away. In other words, a legally blind person has a vision that is 10 times worse than that of a normally sighted person.

To be considered legally blind, a person's visual acuity must be 20/200 or less even while they are using the best possible corrective lenses. If wearing eyeglasses or contact lenses improves their vision beyond that measurement—even in just one eye—they do not meet the definition of legal blindness.

Limited Visual Field

The second aspect of eyesight included in the definition of legal blindness is a visual field, also known as "peripheral vision." People with a normal field of vision will be able to see almost 180° laterally (directly to either side) and 135° vertically (up and down) without moving their heads. People who are legally blind due to a restricted visual field can see a maximum of 20° in any direction. Their field of vision may be limited in all directions, creating a condition known as "tunnel vision," or it may be limited in multiple areas by the presence of blind spots. Peripheral vision is vital to personal safety in many everyday activities, such as driving a car or walking across a street. As a result, people with a severely restricted visual field are considered legally blind even if their central visual acuity is 20/20.

CAUSES OF LEGAL BLINDNESS

Some people are born with visual disabilities that affect their sight to the point that they are considered legally blind. Some of the conditions that may lead to a diagnosis of legal blindness include congenital cataracts, infantile glaucoma, and retinopathy of prematurity. Many other people become legally blind later in life due to health conditions that affect the eyes, such as age-related macular degeneration (AMD or ARMD), cataracts, diabetic retinopathy, and glaucoma.

TESTS FOR LEGAL BLINDNESS

Legal blindness must be diagnosed by an eye doctor as part of a comprehensive eye examination. The eye doctor will test the patient's central visual acuity using a Snellen chart while the patient is wearing corrective lenses. If the corrected visual acuity is below 20/200, the patient will be diagnosed as legally blind.

There are several different methods of testing the patient's field of vision. One example is a perimetry test, in which the patient stares at a dot inside a machine. The machine flashes lights at various points around the visual field, and the patient pushes a button each time they see a flash. At the end of the test, the machine prints a report showing gaps or blind spots within the patient's field of vision. If the diameter of the visual field measures less than 20°, the patient will be diagnosed as legally blind.

Upon receiving a diagnosis of legal blindness, a person may become eligible for government-funded disability benefits in the form of financial assistance, tax deductions, educational accommodations, and job training. There are also a number of service organizations that provide training and resources to help people who are legally blind to live independently.

References

1. Hellem, Amy. "What Does 'Legally Blind' Mean?" All About Vision, February 2017.
2. "Legally Blind," Think about Your Eyes, 2016.
3. Wachler, Brian Boxer. "What Does It Mean to Be Legally Blind?" WebMD, 2015.

Chapter 47 | Vision Rehabilitation—An Overview

Chapter Contents

Section 47.1 | **Improving Quality of Life with Vision Rehabilitation**

This section includes text excerpted from "Vision Rehabilitation Maximizes Hope and Independence," National Eye Institute (NEI), January 31, 2017.

As the last of the baby-boom generation approaches the age of 65, the number of cases of visual impairment and blindness is projected to experience a boom of its own in the coming years. According to recent studies funded by the National Eye Institute (NEI) of the National Institutes of Health (NIH), the number of Americans who are visually impaired—including those with low vision—is expected to double to more than 8 million by 2050.

Low vision is when people have difficulty seeing, even with regular glasses, contact lenses, medicine, or surgery. People with low vision may find it challenging to perform everyday activities, such as getting around the neighborhood, reading the mail, shopping, cooking, or watching television.

Most people with low vision are age 65 or older. The leading causes of vision loss in older adults are age-related macular degeneration (AMD), diabetic retinopathy, cataract, and glaucoma. Among younger people, vision loss is most often caused by inherited eye conditions, infectious and autoimmune eye diseases, or trauma.

Because the consequences of vision loss may leave people feeling anxious, helpless, and depressed, it is important to remind them that there is help. "People experiencing vision loss should talk to their eye-care professional and seek a referral to a low vision specialist," advises Paul A. Sieving, M.D., Ph.D., director of NEI, one of the federal government's principal agencies for vision research.

A low vision specialist is an ophthalmologist or optometrist trained to help people who have low vision maximize their remaining sight and continue to live safe, productive, and rewarding lives. This specialist can develop a vision rehabilitation plan that identifies the appropriate strategies and assistive devices for a person's particular needs. "A vision rehabilitation plan helps people reach their true visual potential when nothing more can be done from a medical or surgical standpoint," explains Mark Wilkinson, O.D., a low vision specialist at the University of Iowa Hospitals and Clinics and chair of the low vision subcommittee for the National Eye Health Education Program (NEHEP).

A report from the National Academies of Sciences, Engineering, and Medicine (NASEM) noted that vision rehabilitation is essential to maximizing the independence, functioning, participation, safety, and overall quality of life (QOL) for people with visual impairment. Vision rehabilitation services are provided by a team of professionals, such as occupational therapists, orientation and mobility instructors, low vision therapists, rehabilitation teachers, and adaptive-technology specialists. These specialists work together to teach people with vision loss a variety of skills, including the following:

- Using magnifying and adaptive devices
- Navigating safely around the home and in public
- Performing daily activities, such as cooking, shopping, and reading
- Finding resources and support

Eye diseases and vision loss have become major public-health concerns in the United States. The NEI is committed to finding new ways to improve the lives of people living with visual impairment. In addition to providing information and resources, the NEI has dedicated more than $24 million to low vision research efforts, including learning how the brain adapts to vision loss, finding strategies to improve vision rehabilitation, and developing new technologies that help people with low vision to read, shop, and find their way in unfamiliar places. Research such as this will help people with low vision make the most of their remaining sight and maintain their independence and QOL.

Section 47.2 | Working with Your Vision-Rehabilitation Team

This section includes text excerpted from "Living with Low Vision," National Eye Institute (NEI), September 2016. Reviewed March 2020.

WHAT YOU CAN DO IF YOU HAVE LOW VISION

To cope with vision loss, you must first have an excellent support team. This team should include you, your primary eye-care professional, and an optometrist or ophthalmologist specializing in low vision.

Occupational therapists, orientation and mobility specialists, certified low-vision therapists, counselors, and social workers are also available to help. Together, the low-vision team can help you make the most of your remaining vision and maintain your independence. Second, talk with your eye-care professional about your vision problems. Even though it may be difficult, ask for help. Find out where you can get more information about support services and adaptive devices. Also, find out which services and devices are best for you and which will give you the most independence. Third, ask about vision rehabilitation, even if your eye-care professional says that "nothing more can be done for your vision." Vision-rehabilitation programs offer a wide range of services, including training for magnifying and adaptive devices, ways to complete daily living skills safely and independently, guidance on modifying your home, and information on where to locate resources and support to help you cope with your vision loss.

Medicare may cover part or all of a patient's occupational therapy, but the therapy must be ordered by a doctor and provided by a Medicare-approved healthcare provider. To see if you are eligible for Medicare-funded occupational therapy, call 800-MEDICARE or 800-633-4227.

Finally, be persistent. Remember that you are your best healthcare advocate. Explore your options, learn as much as you can, and keep asking questions about vision rehabilitation. In fact, write down questions to ask your doctor before your exam, and bring along a notepad to jot down answers. There are many resources to help people with low vision, and many of these programs, devices, and technologies can help you maintain your day-to-day life.

WHAT QUESTIONS YOU SHOULD ASK YOUR EYE-CARE TEAM?

An important part of any doctor–patient relationship is effective communication. Here are some questions to ask your eye-care professional or specialist in low vision to jump-start the discussion about vision loss.

Questions to ask your eye-care professional:

- What changes can I expect in my vision?
- Will my vision loss get worse? How much of my vision will I lose?
- Will regular eyeglasses improve my vision?
- What medical or surgical treatments are available for my condition?
- What can I do to protect or prolong my vision?
- Will diet, exercise, or other lifestyle changes help?
- If my vision cannot be corrected, can you refer me to a specialist in low vision?
- Where can I get vision rehabilitation services?

Questions to ask your specialist in low vision:

- How can I continue my normal, routine activities?
- Are there resources to help me in my job?
- Will any special devices help me with daily activities, such as reading, sewing, cooking, or fixing things around the house?
- What training and services are available to help me live better and more safely with low vision?

Chapter 48 | Vision Impairment and Related Functional Limitations

Vision impairment affects approximately 3.22 million persons in the United States and is associated with social isolation, disability, and decreased quality of life (QOL). Cognitive decline is more common in adults with vision impairment. Subjective cognitive decline (SCD), which is the self-reported experience of worsening or more frequent confusion or memory loss within the past 12 months, affects 11.2 percent of adults aged ≥45 years in the United States. One consequence of SCD is the occurrence of functional limitations, especially those related to usual daily activities; however, it is not known whether persons with vision impairment are more likely to have functional limitations related to SCD.

This chapter is based on a report that describes the association of vision impairment and SCD-related functional limitations using the Behavioral Risk Factor Surveillance System (BRFSS) surveys for the years 2015 to 2017. Adjusting for age group, sex, race/ethnicity, education level, health insurance, and smoking status, 18 percent of adults aged ≥45 years who reported vision impairment also reported SCD-related functional limitations, compared with only 4 percent of those without vision impairment. Preventing, reducing, and correcting vision impairments might lead to a decrease in SCD-related functional limitations among adults in the United States.

This chapter includes text excerpted from "Vision Impairment and Subjective Cognitive Decline-Related Functional Limitations—United States, 2015–2017," Centers for Disease Control and Prevention (CDC), May 23, 2019.

Functional limitations have been reported by 50 percent of adults aged ≥45 years with SCD, and vision impairment has been reported by 6 percent. Previous studies have determined that vision impairment and cognitive decline might coocuur and might be causally related. Studies have pointed to changes in the retina as a potential biomarker for dementia, highlighting the link between vision impairment and cognitive decline. However, the association of vision impairment with SCD-related functional limitations has not been well characterized. This report found that among adults aged ≥45 years, SCD-related functional limitations were three-and-a-half times higher among adults with vision impairment than among those with no vision impairment. The number of adults in the United States with vision impairment is projected to double in the next 30 years; therefore, understanding the impact of cooccuring vision impairment and SCD on functional abilities is an important public-health concern.

Vision impairment might lead to decreased QOL, functional limitations, and an increased risk of mortality. Vision impairment might prevent persons from performing instrumental activities of daily living. However, a previous study found that the relationship between vision impairment and cognitive decline might be modified by a tailored vision rehabilitation program. Further work can help to determine whether vision rehabilitation is also an effective strategy to improve functional limitations associated with SCD.

Vision impairment can be caused by treatable forms of vision loss such as cataracts and refractive errors, along with age-related macular degeneration (AMD), diabetic retinopathy, and glaucoma. Measures to prevent vision impairment and vision loss include receiving eye care and a comprehensive eye exam. Additional ways to protect eyes and prevent vision loss include knowing the family history of eye health, eating healthy, maintaining a healthy weight, wearing protective eyewear, quitting or never starting smoking, washing hands before removing contact lens, and practicing workplace eye safety.

The findings in the report referred to, are subject to at least three limitations. First, these results are based on self-reported vision difficulty and SCD-related functional limitations. Objective measures of cognitive and visual functioning were not administered as part of BRFSS. Second, response bias might have affected the response to questions on vision impairment, SCD, and functional limitations. For example, older persons might be less likely to report SCD-related functional limitations if they consider them to be part of the aging process, thus reducing the reported prevalence of these limitations in this population. Finally, BRFSS is only administered to noninstitutionalized adults, thereby excluding those living in long-term care facilities where nearly one-third of residents might have a vision and cognitive impairments. These limitations might have biased these results toward the null hypothesis and might limit their generalizability across all populations. The strength of this analysis is that it includes nearly all states, Puerto Rico, and DC, representing 253 million U.S. adults.

Vision impairment is an important, growing public-health concern in the United States. Adults with vision impairment might have higher levels of difficulties with activities of daily living (e.g., eating and bathing) and instrumental activities of daily living (e.g., managing finances and using a telephone). Having vision impairment might increase the likelihood that persons with SCD report related functional limitations. Addressing vision impairment through prevention or corrective treatment might reduce functional SCD-associated limitations in the adult population.

Chapter 49 | Vision Impairment and Dealing with Associated Mental-Health Issues

It has been found that visual impairment is known to be accompanied by other mental-health issues such as anxiety, depression, posttraumatic stress disorder (PTSD), and suicidal thoughts. For example, the individuals experiencing visual impairment are twice likely to be affected by depression when compared to general population.

EFFECTS OF VISUAL IMPAIRMENT ON MENTAL HEALTH

Following are some of the major effects that visual impairment has on the mental health of an individual:

Depression

Various researches state that poor eyesight is consistently associated with depression. Vision loss remains a substantial cause of depression, after age, gender, financial strain, and social support. This is because vision impairment affects almost every daily activity of an individual. Additionally, it has been observed that people affected with cataract are more likely to be depressed while waiting to receive cataract surgery—the waiting time to receive the surgery may be several months in many developed countries.

Anxiety

Similar to depression, vision impairment can also increase feelings of anxiety in an individual. Psychological or emotional distress and increased level of anxiety are found to be one of the most common reactions to vision impairment. The individual shall feel anxious participating in any social events and may feel embarrassed about any vision-related errors that they might make. Those affected by a mild vision impairment feel anxious about losing their complete eyesight in the course of time.

Isolation

Visual impairment increases social withdrawal and isolation in an individual. Apart from a physiological impairment, loss of vision can extensively impair the day-to-day activities of a person. It may also stop a person from pursuing the activities that were previously of their interest. Visual impairment is more likely to affect the mobility and access to social contacts resulting in social isolation, disengagement, loneliness, and loss of social support.

Social Withdrawal

Social withdrawal can negatively affect the well-being of visually impaired individuals because relationships and social support are the key to recovery from any illness. A sudden visual impairment will undoubtedly prevent an individual from socializing, working, and leading a normal life. One will virtually be home-bound, and social withdrawal can be observed when one lacks opportunities for social interaction and contact.

COPING WITH VISION PROBLEMS AND MENTAL HEALTH

One of the most important ways to cope with vision impairment is mindfulness. It is necessary to pay attention to the signs and symptoms of the individual be it a child or an adult.

Family members, friends, colleagues, and teachers all play a crucial role in recognizing the emotional difficulties that the individual is dealing with due to vision impairment. It is important to note the signs and changes in their behavior such as:

- A loss of appetite
- Continuous exhaustion
- Reduced interest in their favorite activities

Many common vision impairments such as double vision, hyperopia (farsightedness), myopia (nearsightedness), amblyopia (lazy eye), and postconcussion vision are treatable. Treatments for improving the vision include vision correction devices, therapeutic lenses, visual exercises, or special prism glasses. An ophthalmologist can help make a significant impact on treating the eyes and improving the quality of life and reduce mental-health issues.

SELF-AWARENESS ABOUT MENTAL HEALTH

The following are some suggestions to raise self-awareness about good mental health:

- Talk about the mental struggles faced due to vision impairment. Speak to family and friends or find a local support program.
- Develop healthy personal relationships that help improve the mental health since those with good social connections are less likely to feel depressed.
- It is proven that having a pet reduces stress and anxiety and helps eliminate the feeling of loneliness. A guide dog can be very useful for people with visual impairment.
- Vision therapy can be an option for both children and adults.
- Low vision or visual impairment can have a negative impact on an individual's mental health. It is necessary to seek healthcare professional's help and find the best suitable treatment for the individual.

References

1. "What Are the Effects of Poor Eyesight on Your Mental Health?" Green, Kate. Optimax, May 21, 2019.
2. "Vision Loss and Mental Health: The Hidden Connection," Social Work Today, May 3, 2014.
3. "Mental Health and Visual Impairment: Peer Perspectives," VisionAware, May 30, 2017.
4. "Mental Health and Your Vision," Maple Grove Vision Clinic, May 8, 2019.
5. "Module 10: Eye Disease and Mental Health," Unite For Sight, August 23, 2019.

Chapter 50 | **Goals of Vision Rehabilitation**

The chapter offers several definitions of vision impairment. Low vision is defined as a visual impairment severe enough to interfere with the successful performance of activities of daily living (ADL) although some usable vision is retained. The World Health Organization (WHO) offers the following definitions of low vision, using standard measures of visual acuity and field diameter:

- **Moderate visual impairment.** Best-corrected visual acuity is less (worse) than 20/60 (including 20/70 to 20/160).
- **Severe visual impairment.** Best-corrected visual acuity is less than 20/160 (including 20/200 to 20/400) or visual field diameter is 20 or less.
- **Profound visual impairment.** Best-corrected visual acuity is less than 20/400 (including 20/500 to 20/1000) or visual field diameter is 10 or less.

The categorization of visually impaired persons into a legally blind/legally sighted dichotomy may inappropriately limit access to public benefits. Some who fall under the diagnostic category of legally blind could function highly, while others who are categorized as legally sighted could have a greater need for services because of comorbidities or socioeconomic or other factors. Therefore, those

This chapter includes text excerpted from "Vision Rehabilitation," Agency for Healthcare Research and Quality (AHRQ), U.S. Department of Health and Human Services (HHS), October 2002. Reviewed March 2020.

with the greatest need for services may not be eligible for public benefits because they do not meet diagnostic criteria.

Low vision can result from a variety of ophthalmologic and neurologic disorders. The most common causes of low vision in the United States include:

- Age-related macular degeneration (AMD)
- Glaucoma
- Diabetic retinopathy
- Cataracts

In addition, a number of other diseases, such as stroke, head injury, or tumors may result in conditions such as field cuts or visual neglect, in which individuals never see a certain portion of the visual field or in which the brain does not perceive half the visual world (i.e., a person with left visual neglect will not even be aware that they are unable to see the left side of the world).

Vision rehabilitation usually encompasses services, such as adaptive equipment, skills training, and social support for individuals whose visual impairment cannot be satisfactorily addressed through corrective lenses, medication, or surgery. While preventive interventions fall outside the focus of this review, it is important to note that some vision loss can be prevented. Drug therapy and surgical procedures may help in preventing vision loss or stopping the progression of diseases, such as glaucoma, diabetic retinopathy, and AMD.

Early detection and treatment can prevent up to 90 percent of cases of diabetes-related blindness. Treatments for diabetic retinopathy include laser surgery (photocoagulation) and standard surgery (vitrectomy). Treatments to slow the progression of glaucoma are available and include medications, laser surgery, standard surgery, and drainage implant devices. Many people could benefit from laser surgery but do not get it. Medical treatment for glaucoma is available, but drugs are costly, must be taken for life, and have side effects although newer glaucoma drugs are associated with reduced side effects. Glaucoma treatments are only effective when the disease is detected early (through a dilated eye exam). It is estimated that half of Americans with glaucoma are unaware that they have the condition. Although there is no evidence for effective treatments for most individuals with AMD, experimental and investigational treatments are available (e.g., submacular surgery, external-beam radiation therapy, and thalidomide) and basic research is currently being conducted in a number of promising areas (e.g., retinal transplantation, electronic retinal prosthesis, and gene therapy). However, as noted earlier, a vision that is lost cannot be restored with currently available treatments.

The overall goal of vision rehabilitation is to "recapture, strengthen and maintain self-confidence for safe, independent functioning." The American Academy of Ophthalmology (AAO) states that rehabilitation training teaches individuals how to best use their remaining sight and provides patients with practical adaptations for ADLs. AAO states that vision rehabilitation is more effective if it is started as soon as functional difficulties are identified.

One of the more specific goals of vision rehabilitation is improved functional independence through training in orientation and mobility. Areas of orientation and mobility assessment may include indoor travel, public indoor travel, outdoor travel, and public transportation. For example, curricula in orientation and mobility travel skills are determined based on individual needs, abilities, and limitations, but can include the development of orientation skills, development of language skills, concept development, sensory development, development and understanding of functional vision, if any, learning a system for movement, and identification of resources.

Reading is one of the instrumental or basic ADLs that is most affected by vision loss. Because reading is so integral to communication, it is often targeted as a goal of vision rehabilitation. Activities that are commonly affected by low vision include the following:

- Self-care (e.g., grooming and healthcare)
- Meal preparation
- Home management (e.g., housekeeping, car maintenance)
- Financial management
- Functional mobility including driving
- Shopping

- Leisure and community activities
- Recognizing faces

Vision rehabilitation plans are created following a functional assessment of ADL skills. The individualized written rehabilitation plan may specify the client's goals for improving performance, the skills to be addressed, and how long the instruction is expected to take place.

Chapter 51 | Essential Skills for Everyday Living with Vision Impairment

Vision impairment that occurs suddenly can pose special challenges in everyday activities. After relying on the eyesight for the most part of life, the individual has to learn to adapt to how daily life and activities are managed.

ESSENTIAL SKILLS FOR DAILY ACTIVITIES

Vision impairment does not have to prevent an individual from living an active, healthy, and effective life. There are many tips that an individual can learn to achieve their daily activities independently.

Lighting for Reading

For an individual with low vision, it is necessary to find the perfect lighting to make everyday tasks such as reading much easier and comfortable. The individual has to remember that depending on the eye condition, the lighting can also cause a glare that can make it difficult to read. Learning about different lighting can help to choose the one that can best suit an individual's eye condition. Mostly, it is better to use directed lighting (such as a flexible table lamp) that can be adjusted to focus directly on what the person is reading. Some types of lightings are:

SUNLIGHT OR NATURAL LIGHT

Though sunlight is perfect for most of the daily chores it can also pose difficulties as it is not consistent throughout the day and can create glare spots.

INCANDESCENT LIGHT OR BASIC LIGHT BULB

This is closer to sunlight and the incandescent light bulb is very concentrated, making it the best choice for spot illuminating works such as reading, sewing, and crafts.

FLUORESCENT LIGHT AND COMPACT FLUORESCENT LIGHTS (CFLS)

The fluorescent light and compact fluorescent lights are more cost effective than a basic light bulb as they produce less heat and consume less energy. These bulbs are recommended for overall room lighting as they do not create glare spots or shadows.

LIGHT-EMITTING DIODES (LEDS)

The LED bulbs produce minimal heat and consume lesser energy than the CFLs. They are recommended for concentrated lighting in an adjustable lamp with shades that direct the light downward. They do not work well for overall room illumination.

HALOGEN LIGHT

The halogen light can be used for multiple purposes such as lamps, track lighting, ceiling fixtures, and are also available in adjustable lamps.

COMBINATION LIGHTING

A type of lighting that uses a combination of fluorescent light, CFL, and LED. This is mostly recommended for everyday activities as it covers the entire room and closely resembles the sunlight.

Movement and Orientation

With the sudden loss of vision, it becomes hard to navigate both indoor and outdoor. A person might wonder how to do certain tasks such as:

- Locating doorways
- Avoiding obstacle on the way
- Detecting the edge of a turning or steps
- Locating a store or any other building
- Using public transport and crossing the street

These tasks can be done efficiently by using a technique called "nonvisual information," which uses other senses such as hearing, touch, or smell. Following are some examples of using nonvisual information:

USE YOUR HEARING

Everyday sounds such as the hum of the refrigerator, traffic sounds on the street, and people passing on the sidewalk can provide clues about the surrounding.

- One can use the hum of the refrigerator or traffic sound as a landmark to determine the surrounding.
- Use the sense of hearing to understand the direction of the sound and its distance.
- People passing on the sideway can help determine the width of the street, the location of the traffic signal, and the direction in which the person has to face while crossing the road.

USE YOUR SENSE OF TOUCH

- The textures under the feet while indoor or outdoor such as carpet, tiles, grass, or broken concrete.

USE YOUR SENSE OF SMELL

- Use distinctive scent to help determine the surroundings such as entering the bathroom or entering stores such as a pizza shop, shoe shop, or bakery.

Using the Telephone

Common difficulties that people with a vision impairment face while using the telephone are:

- Getting disconnected because it requires more than 10 seconds to locate and dial the next digit.
- Dialing an incorrect number.

The following are some tips, techniques, and suggestions to use the telephone with ease and comfort.

LEARNING TO DIAL BY TOUCH

It is useful to become accustomed to the keypad and get accustomed to dial by using the index, middle, and ring fingers to explore the keypad.

TELEPHONE TECHNOLOGY

With the updated technology it is easier to navigate through a telephone. Some technologies that can be used to simplify the usage of a telephone are:

- Speed dialing
- Voice-activated telephones (allows a person to dial a number by speaking the name of a person that is preprogrammed in the telephone)
- Auto-dial or programmable telephone (the auto-dialer shall scroll through the contact list and automatically dial the number of the person's choice)

ADAPTED AND SPECIALTY TELEPHONES

- Large print telephones
- Amplified large print telephones
- Amplified talking telephones with braille
- Talking caller ID
- Voice-activated phone dialers

Being visually impaired does not necessarily mean loss of independence. These tips, suggestions, and strategies can help an individual to simplify and achieve the daily chore that can make living with a visual impairment a challenge.

References

1. "Essential Skills for Everyday Living With Vision Loss," VisionAware, June 9, 2016.
2. "Skills You Need for Everyday Living," VisionAware, July 4, 2016.

Chapter 52 | Safety Tips for Persons with Low Vision

Try and remember that whether vision loss is sudden or gradual people commonly experience anxiety, depression, confusion, and loss of independence. You, as a spouse or loved one, play a significant role in helping that person adjust to their impairment and their ability to remain independent.

You can help your loved one by following the key points below:

- Encourage independence and self-confidence. Do not assist with daily living tasks that your loved one can complete alone. It is very common to want to help or "take over" certain tasks for your loved one but in reality, this actually makes rehabilitation more difficult for the person who has vision loss.
- Encourage your loved one to ask for help when necessary.
- Discuss openly difficulties and work together to find solutions.
- When communicating with your loved one, remember that communication is both verbal and nonverbal (facial expressions, head nodding, and hand gestures) and your visually impaired loved one may not be able to see these movements. This can pose a challenge when talking to a person that is visually impaired.
- Keep your voice at normal levels unless the visually impaired person is also hearing impaired.

This chapter includes text excerpted from "Helping Your Loved One with Low Vision," U.S. Department of Veterans Affairs (VA), May 7, 2017.

- Keep your home organized so that things can be found easily.
- Do not move household objects or furniture without your loved one's knowledge.
- Keep objects and papers off of the floor as this can pose serious safety issues.
- During a high anxiety situation, such as an eye examination or doctor appointments most people will not remember all of thc information presented and discussed. If possible, be with your loved one (with their permission) to all examinations and rehab appointments. Two sets of ears are better than one.

LIGHTING TIPS FOR LOW VISION PATIENTS

Increase Illumination

Use floor or table lamps, illuminated magnifiers, and flashlights. As we age, we require more light to see well. A visually impaired person may require even more lighting.

Decrease Glare from Lighting

Glare can reduce vision and cause fatigue. You may be prescribed special tints for indoor and outdoor use.

Use Goose-Neck Lamps to Provide Good Illumination

These lamps are adjustable so they do not increase additional glare.

LOW VISION MEDICATION SAFETY TIPS

- Attach a white label with large black print to medication bottles.
- Place your pills on a contrasting color mat so that they will be visible. White pills on a countertop are hard to see.
- Use hand magnifiers to see print.
- Use a talking recorder that is made for medicine bottles, such as Script Talk (provided at a VA pharmacy) that can record your medicine name and dosage.

- Use a medicine organizer. These are available in large print.

LOW VISION SAFETY TIPS FOR THE HOME

- Area rugs can be used to define areas but the edges should be tacked down to prevent tripping and falling.
- Floor coverings can be a help or a hindrance some things to remember:
  - Plain floor covering rather than patterned floor coverings is easier to visualize
  - Thresholds should not be more than ¼ inch high to prevent tripping
- To increase safety and visibility using stairs localized lighting (like in movie theaters) can be helpful.
- Make sure the handrail to the steps is visible in a contrasting color from the wall.
- Most falls happen on the top stair step so this step should be marked with a different color or illuminated to make a contrast. This is also a good idea for the last step as well.
- Use track lighting in the hallway or a chair/guide rail to act as a guide.
- Install a runner in a contrasting color down the center of a hallway to serve as a guide. Be sure to tack down the edges to avoid tripping.
- Use different textures in halls and adjacent rooms to provide tactile cues.
- When purchasing tables, consider using ovals or round tables to avoid hitting sharp corners in the event of a fall.

LOW VISION TIPS FOR THE KITCHEN

Eating

- Use dishes that have a dark side and light side to provide contrast to your food.
- Avoid patterns on dinnerware.
- Use placemats or table clothes to increase contrast.
- Do NOT use clear glasses or dishes as they appear invisible.

- Use a gooseneck lamp directly over your plate.
- Have a system for placing food on the plate, for example, meat at 6:00, potatoes at 9:00 and vegetables at 3:00.
- Eat food inward from the edge to avoid pushing food on the table.

Cooking

- To avoid burns, get in the habit of shutting the burner off before removing food. Know the off position of the stove knobs.
- To judge liquid levels, use pots or containers with a white interior to see dark colored liquids and black interiors with white liquids.
- Attach lights to underside of cabinets to improve illumination. Try not to create glare.
- Organize shelves systematically and in alphabetical order.
- Have a system for locating food in the pantry and refrigerator.
- Do not wear loose clothing that could catch on fire.
- Turn pan handles inward from the stove or counters to avoid spills and burns.
- Use Corel or plastic dishes if you are worried about broken glass.
- Set a timer or turn on a light to remind you that the stove or oven is on.
- Mark dials on the microwave, stove, and refrigerators.
- Use special aids for the kitchen:
  - Large print kitchen timer
  - Cutting board with a black side and a white side to enhance contrast
  - Special measuring cups that enhance contrast
  - Use a knife with an adjustable slicing guide
  - Use an audible liquid level guide when pouring

LOW VISION TIPS FOR THE HOME WORKSHOP

- Use good lighting. Many workshops do not have many windows, and lighting is very important when it comes to making near tasks easier.

- Use a swing arm or goose-neck lamp that can be placed over tools and machines while they are being used.
- Organize tools and mark with larger numbers or bump dots so they are easily located.
- Put contrasting tape on the handles of tools for easy visibility.
- Use a large print measuring tape.
- Make measuring marks with a felt tip pen for heavy black lines that are easier to see.
- Use magnifiers on a goose-neck stand to provide magnification.
- Use safety goggles at all times.

LOW VISION TIPS FOR WATCHING TELEVISION

- To see your television more clearly, adjust the lighting of the room to avoid glare that interferes with the images on the television.
- Sit closer to the television. Sitting one foot in front of the TV will not hurt your eyes.
- Use a large print television remote control or mark your remote control for greater visibility.
- To see your TV more clearly, place it in front of your recliner or buy a larger TV. A high definition television has the most contrast and resolution and may be easier to see.
- Open or close drapes or curtains to adjust for glare. Some people will find that bright illumination is helpful while others find it increases glare problems.

LOW VISION TIPS FOR WRITING

- To make the print easier to see, use a black felt marker (such as a Sharpie) or a gel pen.
- Use special heavy lined paper made specifically for people with vision impairment.
- Place the light-colored paper on a dark surface to help define the edges.

- Use writing templates for envelopes, checks and writing papers.
- Use large print checks or checks with tactile lines.
- Use large print address books to keep track of phone numbers.
- Use large print calendars or voice memo recorders to keep track of appointments or important dates.

Chapter 53 | **Braille Services for Visually Impaired**

Chapter Contents

Section 53.1 | **About Braille**

This section includes text excerpted from "NLS Factsheet: About Braille," U.S. Library of Congress (LOC), October 23, 2010. Reviewed March 2020.

READING BY TOUCH

Braille is a system of touch reading and writing in which raised dots represent the letters of the alphabet and numbers, as well as music notes and symbols. Braille contains symbols for punctuation marks and provides a system of contractions and short-form words to save space, making it an efficient method of tactile reading.

Braille is read by moving one or more fingers along each line. Both hands are usually involved in the reading process, and reading is generally done with the index fingers. Usually, one hand reads the majority of one line while the other hand locates the beginning of the next. Average reading speed is approximately 125 words per minute, but greater speeds of up to 200 words per minute are possible.

By using braille, blind people can review and study the written word. They may become aware of conventions, such as spelling, punctuation, paragraphing, and footnotes. Most important, braille provides blind individuals access to a wide range of reading materials—educational and recreational reading as well as informational manuals. Blind people also are able to pursue hobbies and cultural enrichment with such braille materials as music scores, hymnals, playing cards, and board games.

THE HISTORY OF BRAILLE

The system of embossed writing invented by Louis Braille in 1821 gradually came to be accepted throughout the world as the fundamental form of written communication for blind individuals.

Various methods—many of them raised versions of print letters—had been attempted over the years to enable blind people to read. The braille system has succeeded because it is based on a rational sequence of signs devised for the fingertips, rather than imitating signs devised for the eyes. In addition, braille can be written by blind people and used for any notation that follows an accepted sequence, such as numerals, musical notes, or chemical tables.

Braille has undergone many modifications, particularly the addition of contractions representing groups of letters or whole words that appear frequently in a language. The use of contractions permits faster reading and helps reduce the size of braille books, making them less cumbersome.

Several groups have been established over the past century to modify and standardize the braille code. The major goal is to develop easily understood contractions without making the code too complex.

The official braille code, English Braille, American Edition, was first published in 1932 by what is now the Braille Authority of North America (BANA). This organization represents many agencies and consumer groups and has been responsible for updating and interpreting the basic literary braille code and the specialized codes for music, mathematics, computer braille, and other uses in the United States and Canada. Other countries have similar authorities.

LOUIS BRAILLE: A REMARKABLE INVENTOR

In 1821 a blind twelve-year-old boy took a secret code devised for the military and recognized in it the basis for written communication for blind individuals. Louis Braille, enrolled at the National Institute of the Blind in Paris, spent many years developing and refining the system of raised dots that has come to be known by his name.

The original military code was called night writing and was used by soldiers to communicate after dark. It was based on a twelve-dot cell, two-dots wide by six-dots high. Each dot or combination of dots within the cell stood for a phonetic sound. The problem with the military code was that a single fingertip could not feel all the dots with one touch.

Braille created a reading method based on a cell of six dots. This crucial improvement meant that a fingertip could encompass the entire cell unit with one impression and move rapidly from one cell to the next.

Braille himself was blind from the age of three. He was born in the village of Coupvray near Paris on January 4, 1809. One day he was playing with a sharp tool belonging to his father, a harness maker. The child accidentally injured one eye with the tool and developed an infection that later caused total blindness.

Until 1819, Braille attended the local village school, where his superior mental abilities put him at the head of his class. He received a scholarship to the National Institute of the Blind, where he was the youngest student. Soon afterward, he began the development of the embossed code. In 1829 he published the code in Procédé pour Ecrire les Paroles, la Musique et le Plain-Chant au Moyen de Points, which also contained a braille music code based on the same six-dot cell.

After he developed his system for reading and writing, Braille remained at the institute as an instructor. Eventually, an incessant cough made it impossible for him to lecture. He died at the age of forty-three and was buried in the family plot in the village cemetery in Coupvray. In 1952, on the centennial of his death, his body was ceremoniously transferred to the Pantheon in Paris. A monument to Louis Braille stands in the main square of Coupvray.

THE BRAILLE ALPHABET

The braille cell, an arrangement of six dots, is the basic unit for reading and writing braille. Sixty-three different patterns are possible from these six dots. For purposes of identification and description, these dots are numbered downward 1-2-3 on the left and 4-5-6 on the right:

The first ten letters of the alphabet (a–j) use only the dots in the upper two rows of the cell.

The next ten letters of the alphabet (k–t) are formed by adding dot 3 to each of the first ten letters.

The remaining letters, except for w, are formed by adding dots 3 and 6 to each of the first five letters.

The letter "w" is an exception because the French alphabet did not contain a "w" when the code was created; the symbol for "w" was added later.

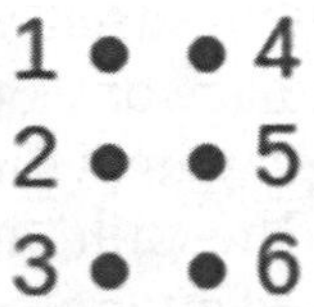

1 ● ● 4
2 ● ● 5
3 ● ● 6

Figure 53.1. Braille Dot in the Six-Dot Configuration

(Note: As shown here, the "?" symbol represents a raised braille dot in the six-dot configuration. The " " symbol represents a position in the cell where no braille dot occurs.)

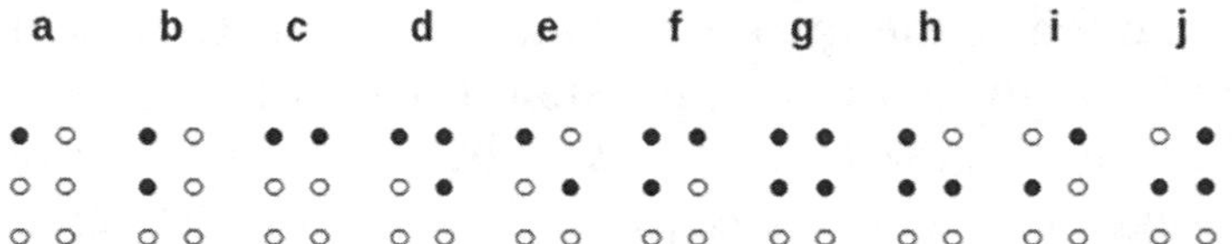

Figure 53.2. Braille Dot (a–j)

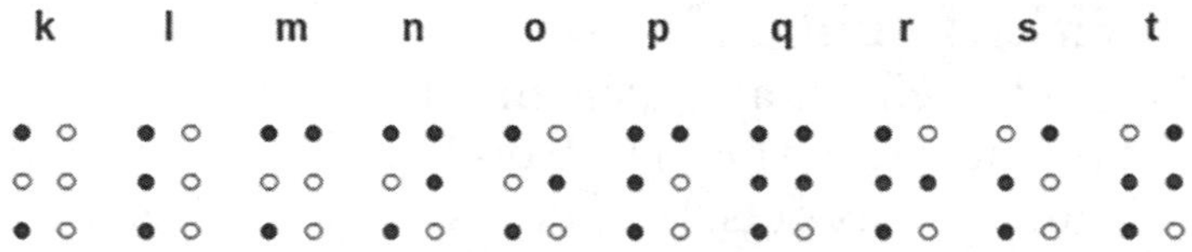

k l m n o p q r s t

Figure 53.3. Braille Dot (k–t)

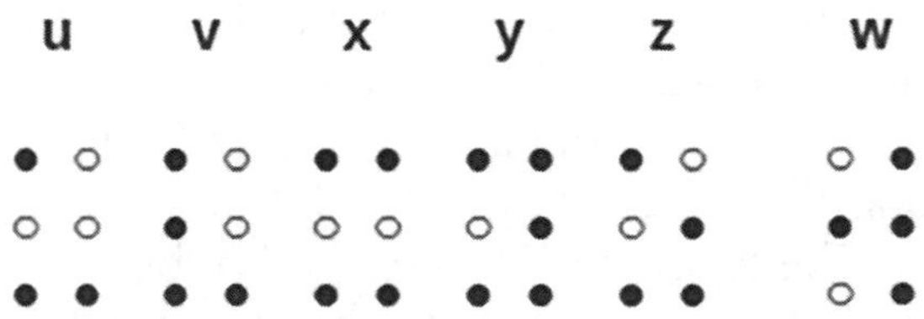

u v x y z w

Figure 53.4. Braille Dot (u–z except w)

BRAILLE AND ADVANCES IN TECHNOLOGY

Access to information in braille has evolved considerably in recent years. Braille can now be translated and formatted with a computer. Braille characters can be entered directly into a computer with six keys on the computer's keyboard. In addition, text that is entered into a computer via scanning or typing can be put into braille by using special software programs. Braille embossers can take output from a computer and produce single- or double-sided braille materials in a fraction of the time it took to create braille by hand. While this process represents a major advance in braille production, computer-assisted braille translation is not perfect and materials must always be checked by a qualified braille proofreader.

Blind individuals use devices with refreshable braille displays to take notes, read braille materials, prepare school assignments, and perform many other tasks in braille that were not possible even twenty years ago. These advances in braille technology have had a profound impact on educational and professional opportunities available to blind braille readers.

BRAILLE TRANSCRIBERS AND PROOFREADERS

Throughout the United States, dedicated braille transcribers and proofreaders work, often on a volunteer basis, to produce braille materials. These materials supplement the books and magazines produced in quantity by NLS and other organizations. Sighted and blind individuals may become certified after completing a lengthy, detailed course of braille transcribing, culminating in the award by the Library of Congress of a certificate of proficiency in the appropriate braille code.

Their activities include transcribing print material into braille, duplicating/embossing copies, binding braille books, preparing materials for use with electronic refreshable braille displays, and proofreading.

Many braille transcribers and proofreaders work as volunteers for NLS and its national network of cooperating libraries that distributes books and magazines to blind and physically handicapped readers, state departments of special education, and local school systems.

Many individuals work as volunteers to gain the experience necessary to be hired by braille production agencies and school systems. The National Braille Association (NBA), a professional organization for transcribers, provides transcribers with guidance and professional development opportunities.

Brailling is a skill that requires training, intellectual curiosity, patience, meticulousness, and the ability to work under pressure and to understand and follow directions. Braille transcribers report a great sense of accomplishment in learning a completely new system of reading and writing, and in empowering blind people to independently access the reading materials they need for education, work, and other life activities.

Section 53.2 | **Devices and Aids**

This section includes text excerpted from "Devices and Aids," U.S. Library of Congress (LOC), June 28, 2017.

This section links to information on a variety of assistive technology products, magnifying devices, braille displays, notetakers, and embossers, and the Bureau of Engraving and Printing U.S. Currency Reader Program.

Accessible software applications (Apps) for smartphones and other mobile devices can be used by those who are visually impaired to read books, newspapers, magazines, and other print material. These apps convert digital text to speech or provide braille output to a compatible braille device.

- Accessible Mobile Reading Apps (2019) (www.loc.gov/nls/resources/blindness-and-vision-impairment/devices-aids/accessible-mobile-reading-apps/)
- Accessible Mobile Reading Apps (2019) [ebraille (BRF)]
- GPS and Wayfinding Apps (2020) (www.loc.gov/nls/resources/general-resources-on-disabilities/gps-and-wayfinding-apps/)

Assistive Technology products convert digital text or print into synthetic speech, braille, or enlarged text. Most are available from multiple vendors, which are listed below the entry along with the price points at the time this publication was compiled.

- Assistive Technology Products for Information Access (2019) (www.loc.gov/nls/resources/blindness-and-vision-impairment/devices-aids/assistive-technology-products-information-access/)
- Assistive Technology Products for Information Access (2018) [ebraille (BRF)]

Braille devices are used to access and represent information in braille. The link below provides a list of available models. The section also lists the sources to purchase these items and a selection of references and resources on the subject.

- Braille Displays and Notetakers (2018) (www.loc.gov/nls/resources/blindness-and-vision-impairment/devices-aids/braille-displays-notetakers/)
- Braille Displays and Notetakers (2018) [ebraille (BRF)]

Below are listed braille embossers and the vendors that offer them and details specialized braille paper, braille translation software, and sources to purchase these items.

- Braille Embossers (2018) (www.loc.gov/nls/resources/blindness-and-vision-impairment/devices-aids/braille-embossers/)
- Braille Embossers (2018) [ebraille (BRF)]

The Bureau of Engraving and Printing (BEP) is providing currency readers, free of charge, to eligible blind and visually impaired individuals. For additional questions or comments about the U.S. Currency Reader Program, you may call 844-815-9388 toll-free or E-mail: meaningful.access@bep.gov.

- Bureau of Engraving and Printing U.S. Currency Reader Program (www.bep.gov/uscurrencyreaderpgm.html)

National Library Service (NLS) players are available only to individuals who cannot see to read regular print or handle print materials and who are registered for the free library service. Individuals may choose to purchase commercial digital talking-book players that are also authorized to play NLS produced talking books and magazines.

- Digital Audiobook Players and Braille Book Reader (2018) (www.loc.gov/nls/resources/blindness-and-vision-impairment/devices-aids/digital-audiobook-players-and-braille-book-readers/)
- Digital Audiobook Players (2018) [ebraille (BRF)]

National Library Service patrons who have registered for the Braille and Audio Reading Download (BARD) service may download digital-talking books onto USB drives or customized cartridges. The section below lists sources for customized cartridges that play in the NLS Digital Talking Book Machine (DTBM):

- Sources for cartridges and cables (www.loc.gov/nls/enrollment-equipment/equipment-needed-for-nls-materials/cartridges-cables-for-bard/)

Magnifying devices assist people with low vision to engage more easily in activities such as reading standard print, enjoying a hobby, or viewing a presentation by increasing the size of text and objects. Magnifiers come in many weights and styles.

- Magnifying Devices (2018) (www.loc.gov/nls/resources/blindness-and-vision-impairment/devices-aids/magnifying-devices/)
- Magnifying Devices (2018) [ebraille (BRF)]

Section 53.3 | **Braille Services**

This section includes text excerpted from "BARD Access," U.S. Library of Congress (LOC), June 13, 2017.

Braille and Audio Reading Download (BARD) is a free library service of downloadable braille and audio reading material for residents of the United States and U.S. citizens living abroad who are unable to read or use standard printed material because of visual or physical disabilities. BARD provides access to thousands of special-format books, magazines, and music scores. The site is password-protected. All files are downloadable as compressed audio or formatted ebraille files. BARD is a partnership between NLS and its network of cooperating libraries. NLS maintains the website, uploads titles, and supplies libraries with circulation statistics.

THREE STEPS TO BEGIN USING BARD

- Become an NLS patron
- Register for BARD
- Get a Device

You can get a free talking-book player on long-term loan from your network library, buy a commercial model on your own if there are features you prefer, or download the free app to your smart device. BARD Mobile is available at the App Store for iOS or the Play Store or Amazon Appstore for Android.

FOUR STEPS TO GETTING BOOKS ON BARD MOBILE

- **Sign In**
  Sign In to BARD on your mobile device. You will be asked for your user ID and password. Your user ID is your email address. Your user ID and password are case-sensitive.
  For help with BARD, access the BARD Mobile User Manual for iOS or the BARD Mobile User Manual for Android. You can also access videos on How to Use BARD Mobile or send an email to NLSDownload@loc.gov
- **Find Books**
  You can search through recently added audio books, audio magazines, braille books, and braille magazines. Or you may browse BARD by selecting the author, title, or

subject. You can also search through special collections of music books and scores, foreign-language materials, and magazines. Each magazine in the drop-down list is followed by whether it is braille or audio. Recent upgrades in 2018 include "My previous downloads" and "Most popular books" to Get Books menu.

- **Add to Wish List**
  You can add items to your wish list by selecting "Add to wish list." The wish list stores items you have selected for future download. Once an item is downloaded it will no longer appear on the wish list.
- **Download**
  You can use the download link to download an item on BARD Mobile. You may be charged for data depending on your carrier's plan.

FOUR STEPS TO GETTING BOOKS ON THE DIGITAL TALKING-BOOK PLAYER

- **Sign In**
  Sign In to BARD on a computer
  You will be asked for your user ID and password. Your user ID is your email address. Your user ID and password are case-sensitive. To create a new password, it must 1) be at least eight characters, 2) contain at least one letter and one number, and 3) have no immediately repeated characters. Once your new password is accepted, you will receive an e-mail message confirming that you have changed your password.
  E-mail NLSDownload@loc.gov for help or visit NLS BARD Frequently Asked Questions.
- **Finding books and magazines on BARD**
  The easiest way to find a book is to use the "Search the collection" field on the BARD main page. Enter a word or two that relates to the title, author, or subject. You will receive more targeted results if you put an exact phrase from the title or the exact title in quotes. You can browse

the entire NLS online catalog by author, title, or subject and the links provided.

- **Download**
  Once you download a book to your computer, two places to check for it are your Downloads and Documents folders. If you know how to search your computer for files and folders, you can search DB- to locate audiobooks or BR- to locate braille books.
  Each web browser handles downloads slightly differently. In most cases, unless you set a default location for downloads, you will be asked where you would like to save it each time. Many users choose to create a "My downloads" folder inside their documents folder and use that as the default destination for downloads.
- **Unzip to cartridge or flash drive and play**
  Open the .zip file you downloaded to your computer. There are several popular software packages that handle this function. If you are using Windows XP, Windows Vista, or Mac OS X, this function is built in. Windows 8 and Windows 10 are also operating systems that offer the built-in unzipping software. Once you have copied the files to their destination, insert the cartridge into your player and press the play button.

WHAT IS BARD EXPRESS?

Braille and Audio Reading Download Express provides NLS patrons with an easy way to access BARD. Use BARD Express to browse thousands of audio books and magazines, download them to your Windows-based computer, and transfer them to an NLS cartridge. BARD Express simplifies the process by providing a menu-driven interface, reducing the need to memorize a complex set of keyboard commands. What does this mean? BARD Express can be used with as few as four keys, while providing advanced functionality for the more adventurous user.

FREQUENTLY ASKED QUESTIONS ABOUT BARD EXPRESS

Who Can Use BARD Express?

Braille and Audio Reading Download Express is available for use by eligible NLS patrons. You must have an established BARD account, with a user name and password, to use BARD Express.

What Types of Books and Magazines Are Available for Download?

Braille and Audio Reading Download Express enables users to download audio materials that are available in the BARD collection.

What Type of Computer Do I Need to Run BARD Express?

Braille and Audio Reading Download Express is a Windows-based application that runs on personal computers running Windows XP, Windows Vista, Windows 7, Windows 8 and 8.1, and Windows 10. BARD Express does not run on Apple computers.

Which Screen Readers Work with BARD Express?

Window eyes, NVDA, and JAWS For Windows were tested with BARD Express.

Where Do I Get BARD Express?

You can download BARD Express from the link on the BARD Main Page under the heading Additional Links.

How Do I Access BARD with Bard Express

Use your BARD user name and password to log into BARD Express.

If you do not have a BARD account, contact your regional library, or apply for one here: BARD Individual Application. From this page choose your library from the drop-down list of network libraries and select the Submit button. Fill in all of the information in the application.

Note that the field labeled "Please select the type of player you will be using" is for users of 3rd party talking-book players and/or braille notetakers. You do not need to select anything from this list. Submit your application.

Once your application is processed by your network library, you will be e-mailed a temporary password. You must login to BARD using a web browser and change your password before logging into BARD Express.

Where Can I Get Some Help Using BARD Express?

Braille and Audio Reading Download Express comes with a comprehensive Help system. While running the program, press the F1 key to access the Help system.

A full user guide is available here: [Insert link to full user guide]

The NLS has also produced a set of tutorial videos, called the "BARD Express How-To Series," that describe how to use the functions and features of BARD Express. Select the link below to access the video of your choice.

- An Introduction
- Browsing the BARD Collection
- Transferring Materials to a Cartridge
- Browsing the Recently Added and Most Popular Lists
- Searching the BARD Collection
- Using Your Wish List
- Setting and Changing Preferences
- Managing Devices
- Tips and Tricks

Access the whole series here: BARD Express How-To Series For additional assistance or support contact your local braille and talking-book library.

WHAT IF I FORGET MY BARD PASSWORD?

Option 1: Open the BARD login page using your computer at: nlsbard.loc.gov and choose the link "Reset your BARD password here." Fill out the form to create a new password.

Option 2: Contact your local braille and talking-book library and tell them you would like assistance resetting your BARD password.

Option 3: Send an email to nlsdownload@loc.gov to request assistance resetting your BARD password. After using the temporary password you are provided, reestablish a permanent password on the BARD website, then log into BARD Express with your user name and new password.

Note that BARD Express will remember your login credentials after the first time you log in. If you change your username (e-mail address) or password using the BARD web interface you will need to reset your credentials in BARD Express, or simply log into BARD Express using your new username or password.

How Can I Change My User Id/E-mail Address?

Your user ID is your e-mail address. To change it, log into your BARD account. Choose the link "Update Account Settings," and then the link "Change Your Email Address." On this section, you can enter a new e-mail address. You will need to enter it twice to make sure you have entered it correctly. If the two entries do not match exactly, the new address will not be accepted.

Your new e-mail address becomes your user ID. A new temporary password will be sent to this address, so make sure you use an e-mail address to which you have immediate access.

Any time you update the email address associated with your BARD account, BARD will require you to change your password.

Note that BARD Express will remember your login credentials after the first time you log in. If you change your username (e-mail address) or password using the BARD web interface you will need to reset your credentials in BARD Express, or simply log into BARD Express using your new username or password.

I JUST DOWNLOADED A TITLE USING BARD EXPRESS, WHERE DID IT GO?

All materials you download using BARD Express will be stored on your BARD Express Bookshelf, which is accessed using the Bookshelf button from the main menu.

How Do I Move an Audiobook from the Computer to a Cartridge for Playback in My Digital Talking-Book Player?

After choosing a title from the BARD Express bookshelf, use the Copy To Cartridge button to begin the process of moving your book or magazine to an external storage device connected to your computer, such as an NLS cartridge or USB flash drive. Highlight the drive to which you want to move the book or magazine, and select the Okay button. BARD Express will unzip the file that was downloaded from BARD and copy it to the storage device. Disconnect the device from your computer and enjoy your book!

Chapter 54 | Guide Animals and Mobility Aids

An old adage says a dog is man's best friend, but for members of a guide-dog team, the situation is mutual. Guide-dog schools take great care to match a dog with a compatible human because the dog and handler will navigate the world with each relying on the other.

Guide dogs were first trained in Germany to assist World War I veterans. In 1928, Dorothy Harrison Eustis, an American dog breeder living in Switzerland, published a piece titled "The Seeing Eye" in the Saturday Evening Post describing this new phenomenon. Inspired by her article, Morris Frank, a blind man living in Tennessee, wrote to Eustis about the need for a school to train guide dogs in the United States. She invited him to Switzerland where during a five-week visit she trained him with Buddy, one of her German shepherds. After Morris Frank went home with Buddy and their partnership proved successful, Dorothy Eustis returned to the United States. In 1929, Eustis and Frank collaborated to found the Seeing Eye, the first guide-dog school in this country.

Training usually begins when the dog is a puppy, with the dog raiser working under the supervision of a trainer from a guide-dog school. The program includes socialization, basic commands, and good manners. Later the dogs receive more rigorous training in the how-to guide. They are taught to navigate obstacles, whether on the ground or hanging above, locate specific places, such as restrooms or exits, and practice intelligent disobedience in the presence of a threat that their owner does not detect.

Not every canine is up to the job. Guide dogs have to be large enough to work in a guide harness but small enough to fit in

This chapter includes text excerpted from "Guide Dogs and Service Dogs," U.S. Library of Congress (LOC), July 2017.

confined spaces, as well as calm, confident, and not easily frightened. They also need to have sufficient intelligence to assess a situation and a personality amenable to working as part of a team. The most commonly used breeds are Labrador Retrievers and Golden Retrievers.

Since the 1970s, dogs have been trained to help people in other ways. Service dogs can alert deaf people to important sounds, recognize the beginning of an epileptic seizure, and assist people with posttraumatic stress disorder (PTSD). Therapy dogs are trained to provide comfort for people in schools, hospitals, and nursing homes.

Chapter 55 | **Harnessing New Technologies for Assisting People with Visual Impairment**

February is Low Vision Awareness Month. During this month, the National Eye Institute (NEI), part of the National Institutes of Health (NIH), highlighted new technologies and tools in the works to help the 4.1 million Americans living with low vision or blindness. The innovations are expected to help people with vision loss more easily accomplish daily tasks, from navigating office buildings to crossing a street. Many of the innovations take advantage of computer vision, a technology that enables computers to recognize and interpret the complex assortment of images, objects, and behaviors in the surrounding environment.

Low vision means that even with glasses, contact lenses, medicine, or surgery, people find everyday tasks difficult to do. It can affect many aspects of life, from walking in crowded places to reading or preparing a meal, explained Cheri Wiggs, Ph.D., program director for low vision and blindness rehabilitation at the NEI. The tools needed to stay engaged in everyday activities vary based on the degree and type of vision loss. For example, glaucoma causes loss of peripheral vision, which can make walking or driving, difficult. By contrast, age-related macular degeneration (AMD) affects

This chapter includes text excerpted from "Five Innovations Harness New Technologies for People with Visual Impairment, Blindness," National Eye Institute (NEI), February 3, 2017.

central vision, creating difficulty with tasks such as reading, she said.

Here is a look at a few NEI-funded technologies under development that aim to lessen the impact of low vision and blindness.

COROBOTIC CANE

Navigating indoors can be especially challenging for people with low vision or blindness. While existing GPS-based assistive devices can guide someone to a general location such as a building, GPS is not much help in finding specific rooms, said Cang Ye, Ph.D., of the University of Arkansas at Little Rock. Ye has developed a corobotic cane that provides feedback on a user's surrounding environment.

Ye's prototype cane has a computerized 3-D camera to "see" on behalf of the user. It also has a motorized roller tip that can propel the cane toward the desired location, allowing the user to follow the cane's direction. Along the way, the user can speak into a microphone and a speech recognition system interprets verbal commands and guides the user via a wireless earpiece. The cane's credit card-sized computer stores preloaded floor plans. However, Ye envisions being able to download floor plans via Wi-Fi upon entering a building. The computer analyzes 3-D information in real-time and alerts the user of hallways and stairs. The cane gauges a person's location in the building by measuring the camera's movement using a computer vision method. That method extracts details from a current image captured by the camera and matches them with those from the previous image, thus determining the user's location by comparing the progressively changing views, all relative to a starting point. In addition to receiving NEI support, Ye was awarded a grant from the NIH's Coulter College Commercializing Innovation Program to explore the commercialization of the robotic cane.

ROBOTIC GLOVE

In the process of developing the corobotic cane, Ye realized that closed doorways pose yet another challenge for people with low vision and blindness. "Finding the doorknob or handle and getting the door open slows you way down," he said. To help someone with low vision locate and grasp small objects more quickly, he designed a fingerless glove device.

On the back surface is a camera and a speech recognition system, enabling the user to give the glove voice commands such as "door handle," "mug," "bowl," or "bottle of water." The glove guides the user's hand via tactile prompts to the desired object. "Guiding the person's hand left or right is easy," Ye said. "An actuator on the thumb's surface takes care of that in a very intuitive and natural way." Prompting a user to move her or his hand forward and backward, and getting a feel for how to grasp an object, is more challenging.

Ye's colleague Yantao Shen, Ph.D., University of Nevada, Reno, developed a novel hybrid tactile system that comprises an array of cylindrical pins that send either a mechanical or electrical stimulus. The electric stimulus provides an electro-tactile sensation, meaning that it excites the nerves on the skin of the hand to simulate a sense of touch. Picture four cylindrical pins in alignment down the length of your index finger. One by one, starting with the pin closest to your fingertip, the pins pulse in a pattern indicating that the hand should move backward.

The reverse pattern indicates the need for forward motion. Meanwhile, a larger electro-tactile system on the palm uses a series of cylindrical pins to create a 3-D representation of the object's shape. For example, if your hand is approaching the handle of a mug, you would sense the handle's shape in your palm so that you could adjust the position of your hand accordingly. As your hand moves toward the mug handle, any slight shifts in angle are noted by the camera and the tactile sensation on your palm reflects such changes.

SMARTPHONE CROSSWALK APP

Street crossings can be especially dangerous for people with low vision. James Coughlan, Ph.D., and his colleagues at the Smith-Kettlewell Eye Research Institute have developed a smartphone app that gives auditory prompts to help users identify the safest crossing location and stay within the crosswalk.

The app harnesses three technologies and triangulates them. A global positioning system (GPS) is used to pinpoint the intersection where a user is standing. Computer vision is then used to scan the area for crosswalks and walk lights. That information is integrated with a geographic information system (GIS) database containing a crowd-sourced, detailed inventory about an intersection's quirks, such as the presence of road construction or uneven pavement. The three technologies compensate for each other's weaknesses. For example, while computer vision may lack the depth perception needed to detect a median in the center of the road, such local knowledge would be included in the GIS template. And while GPS can adequately localize the user to an intersection, it cannot identify on which corner a user is standing. Computer vision determines the corner, as well as where the user is in relation to the crosswalk, the status of the walk lights and traffic lights, and the presence of vehicles.

CAMIO SYSTEM

Imagine a system that enables visually impaired biology students to explore a 3-D anatomical model of a heart by touching an area and hearing "aortic arch" in response. The same system could also be used to get an auditory readout of the display on a device such as a glucose monitor. The prototype system, designed with a low-cost camera connected to a laptop computer, can make physical objects—from 2-D maps to digital displays on microwaves—fully accessible to users with low vision or blindness.

The CamIO (short for camera input-output also under development by Coughlan, provides real-time audio feedback as the user explores an object in a natural way, turning it around and touching it. Holding a finger stationary on 3-D or 2-D objects signals the system to provide an audible label of the location in question or an enhanced image on a laptop screen. CamIO was conceived by Joshua Miele, Ph.D., a blind scientist at Smith-Kettlewell who develops and evaluates novel sound/touch interfaces to help people with vision loss. Coughlan plans to develop a smartphone app version of CamIO.

HIGH-POWERED PRISMS, PERISCOPES FOR SEVERE TUNNEL VISION

People with retinitis pigmentosa and glaucoma can lose most of their peripheral vision, making it challenging to walk in crowded places like airports or malls. People with severe peripheral field vision loss can have a residual central island of vision that is as little as 1 to 2 percent of their full visual field. Eli Peli, O.D., of Schepens Eye Research Institute, Boston, has developed lenses constructed of many adjacent one-millimeter wide prisms that expand the visual field while preserving central vision. Peli designed a high-powered prism, called a "multiplexing prism" that expands one's field of view by about 30°. "That's an improvement, but it's not good enough," explained Peli.

In a study, he and his colleagues mathematically modeled people walking in crowded places and found that the risk of collision is highest when other pedestrians are approaching from a 45-degree angle. To reach that degree of peripheral vision, he and his colleagues are employing a periscope-like concept. Periscopes, such as those used to see the ocean surface from a submarine, rely on a pair of parallel mirrors that shift an image, providing a view that would otherwise be out of sight. Applying a similar concept, but with nonparallel mirrors, Peli and colleagues have developed a prototype that achieves a 45-degree visual field. Their next step is to work with optical labs to manufacture a cosmetically acceptable prototype that can be mounted into a pair of glasses. "It would be ideal if we could design magnetic clip-ons spectacles that could be easily mounted and removed," he said.

Chapter 56 | Driving When You Have Macular Degeneration

For most people, driving represents freedom, control, and competence. Driving enables most people to get to the places they want to go and to see the people they want to see when they want. Driving is a complex skill. Our ability to drive safely can be challenged by changes in our physical, emotional, and mental condition. The goal of this chapter is to help you, your family and your healthcare professional talk about how macular degeneration may affect your ability to drive safely.

HOW CAN HAVING MACULAR DEGENERATION AFFECT YOUR DRIVING?

Macular degeneration can distort your central vision and can lead to loss of sharp vision. Macular degeneration also can make it difficult to see road signs, traffic, and people walking, and may affect your ability to drive safely.

CAN YOU STILL DRIVE WITH MACULAR DEGENERATION?

If your eye-care expert has told you that you have macular degeneration, there are certain things that you should know and do to stay a safe driver.

This chapter includes text excerpted from "Driving When You Have Macular Degeneration," National Highway Traffic Safety Administration (NHTSA), June 2003. Reviewed March 2020.

People experience the visual effects of macular degeneration in different ways.

In the early stages of macular degeneration, you may only have small central areas of vision loss or distortion that may not affect your driving. In fact, you may not even notice any change in your eyesight. As macular degeneration progresses, it may become harder for you to see clearly. This may make you worry about your vision and make it harder to drive safely.

WHAT CAN YOU DO WHEN MACULAR DEGENERATION AFFECTS YOUR DRIVING?

If you have a family history of macular degeneration or have any changes in your central vision, you should immediately contact your eye-care expert. After a definitive diagnosis of macular degeneration, how often you visit your eye-care expert depends on your doctor's advice, the type of macular degeneration that you have, and your symptoms.

Although there is not much that can be done to stop the disease from getting worse, the use of antioxidant vitamins may help retard its progression. Additionally, there are surgical procedures that may help if they are done in the early stages of the disease.

Your eye-care expert may refer you to a specialist who can go on a drive with you to see if macular degeneration has affected your driving. The specialist also may offer training to improve your driving skills. Improving your skills could help keep you and others around you safe. To find a specialist near you, call the Association of Driver Rehabilitation Specialists (ADED) at 866-672-9466 or go to their website at www.aded.net. You also can call hospitals and rehabilitation facilities to find an occupational therapist who can help with the driving skills assessment.

WHAT IF YOU HAVE TO GIVE UP AND CUT BACK ON DRIVING?

You can keep your independence even if you have to give up or cut back on your driving. It may take planning ahead on your part, but it will get you to the places you want to go and the people you want to see.

Consider:

- Rides with family and friends
- Taxi cabs
- Shuttle buses or vans
- Public buses, trains, and subways

Also, senior centers, and religious and other local service groups often offer transportation services for older adults in your community.

Chapter 57 | Education for Children with Vision Impairment through IDEA

HOW THE INDIVIDUALS WITH DISABILITIES EDUCATION ACT DEFINES VISUAL IMPAIRMENT

The Individuals with Disabilities Education Act (IDEA) provides the nation with definitions of many disabilities that can make children eligible for special education and related services in schools. Visual impairment is one such disability the law defines—as follows:

Visual impairment including blindness means an impairment in vision that, even with correction, adversely affects a child's educational performance. The term includes both partial sight and blindness.

THE HELP AVAILABLE UNDER IDEA

If you suspect (or know) that your child has a visual impairment, you will be pleased to know there is a lot of help available under IDEA—beginning with a free evaluation of your child. IDEA requires that all children suspected of having a disability be evaluated without cost to their parents to determine if they do have a disability and, because of the disability, need special services under IDEA. Those special services are:

This chapter includes text excerpted from "Visual Impairment, Including Blindness," Center for Parent Information & Resources (CPIR), U.S. Department of Education (ED), March 31, 2017.

- **Early intervention.** A system of services to support infants and toddlers with disabilities (before their 3rd birthday) and their families.
- **Special education and related services.** Services available through the public-school system for school-aged children, including preschoolers (ages 3 to 21).

Visual impairment, including blindness, is one of the disabilities specifically mentioned and defined in IDEA. If a child meets the definition of visual impairment in IDEA as well as the state's criteria (if any), then she or he is eligible to receive early intervention services or special education and related services under IDEA (depending on her or his age).

How to Identify the Early Intervention Program in Your Neighborhood

Ask your child's pediatrician for a referral. You can also call the local hospital's maternity ward or pediatric ward and ask for the contact information of the local early intervention program.

Accessing Special Education and Related Services

If your child is between 3 and 21 years of age, you should get in touch with your local public-school system. Calling the public school in your neighborhood is an excellent place to start. The school should be able to tell you the next steps to having your child evaluated free of charge. If found eligible, your child can begin receiving services specially designed to address her or his educational needs and other needs associated with the disability.

Developing a Written Plan of Services

In both cases—in early intervention for a baby or toddler with a visual impairment and in special education for a school-aged child, parents work together with program professionals to develop a plan of services the child will receive based on her or his needs. In early intervention, that plan is called the "individualized family service plan" (IFSP). In special education, the plan is called the "individualized education program" (IEP). Parents are part of the team that develops their child's IFSP or IEP.

There is a lot to know about early intervention for infants and toddlers with disabilities and about special education and related services for school-aged children. Find out more about these essential services for eligible children with visual impairments, beginning at:

- Early intervention (www.parentcenterhub.org/repository/babies/)
- Special education and related services (www.parentcenterhub.org/repository/schoolage/)

Chapter 58 | **Blindness and Vision Impairments in the Workplace and the Americans with Disabilities Act**

The Americans with Disabilities Act (ADA), which was amended by the Americans with Disabilities Act Amendments Act of 2008 ("Amendments Act" or "ADAAA"), is a federal law that prohibits discrimination against qualified individuals with disabilities. Individuals with disabilities include those who have impairments that substantially limit a major life activity, have a record (or history) of a substantially limiting impairment, or are regarded as having a disability.

Title I of the ADA covers employment by private employers with 15 or more employees as well as state and local government employers. Section 501 of the Rehabilitation Act provides similar protections related to federal employment. In addition, most states have their own laws prohibiting employment discrimination on the basis of disability. Some of these state laws may apply to smaller employers and may provide protections in addition to those available under the ADA.

This chapter includes text excerpted from "Questions and Answers about Blindness and Vision Impairments in the Workplace and the Americans with Disabilities Act (ADA)," U.S. Equal Employment Opportunity Commission (EEOC), September 28, 2009. Reviewed March 2020.

The U.S. Equal Employment Opportunity Commission (EEOC) enforces the employment provisions of the ADA. This chapter explains how the ADA applies to job applicants and employees with vision impairments. In particular, this chapter explains:

- When an employer may ask an applicant or employee questions about his vision impairment and how it should treat voluntary disclosures
- What types of reasonable accommodations employees with visual disabilities may need
- How an employer should handle safety concerns about applicants and employees with visual disabilities
- How an employer can ensure that no employee is harassed because of a visual disability or any other disability

GENERAL INFORMATION ABOUT VISION IMPAIRMENTS

Estimates vary as to the number of Americans who are blind and visually impaired. One reason for the different estimates is that different terminology is used to assess the number of individuals with some degree of vision problems. According to one estimate, approximately 6.6 million people in the United States are blind or visually impaired. Another estimate concluded that there are 10 million blind or visually impaired people in the United States and of these 1.3 million are considered legally blind. The 2011 National Health Interview Survey Preliminary Report estimated that 21.2 million American adults (over 10% of all American adults) reported that they had trouble seeing even when wearing corrective lenses or that they were blind or unable to see. Only 36.8 percent of non-institutionalized working-age adults (21 to 64) with a significant vision loss are employed.

The Centers for Disease Control and Prevention (CDC) define "vision impairment" to mean that a person's eyesight cannot be corrected to a "normal level." Vision impairment may result in a loss of visual acuity, where an individual does not see objects as clearly as the average person, and/or in a loss of visual field, meaning that an individual cannot see as wide an area as the average person without moving the eyes or turning the head. There are varying degrees of vision impairments, and the terms used to describe them are not always consistent. The CDC and the World Health Organization define low vision as a visual acuity between 20/70 and 20/400 with the best possible correction, or a visual field of 20 degrees or less. Blindness is described as visual acuity worse than 20/400 with the best possible correction, or a visual field of 10 degrees or less. In the United States, the term "legally blind," means visual acuity of 20/200 or worse with the best possible correction, or a visual field of 20 degrees or less. Although there are varying degrees of vision impairments, the visual problems an individual faces cannot be described simply by the numbers; some people can see better than others with the same visual acuity.

There are many possible causes for vision impairment, including damage to the eye and the failure of the brain to interpret messages from the eyes correctly. The most common causes of vision impairment in American adults are diabetic retinopathy, age-related macular degeneration (AMD), cataracts, and glaucoma. Additionally, many individuals have monocular vision perfect or nearly perfect vision in one eye, but little or no vision in the other. Vision impairment can occur at any time in life, but adults aged 40 and older are at the greatest risk for eye diseases, such as cataract, diabetic retinopathy, glaucoma, and AMD.

Persons with vision impairments successfully perform a wide range of jobs and can be dependable workers. Yet, many employers still automatically exclude them from certain positions based on generalizations about vision impairments and false assumptions that it would be too expensive, or perhaps even too dangerous, to employ them. Thus, employers may erroneously assume that any accommodation that would allow a person with a vision impairment to do her job would be too costly. Employers also may have liability concerns related to the fear of accidents and/or injuries.

When Does Someone with a Vision Impairment Have a Disability within the Meaning of the Americans with Disabilities Act?

As a result of changes made by the ADAAA, people who are blind should easily be found to have a disability within the meaning of the first part of the ADA's definition of disability because they are substantially limited in the major life activity of seeing. Individuals with a vision impairment other than blindness will meet the first part of the ADA's definition of disability if they can show that they are substantially limited in seeing or another major life activity (e.g., the major bodily function of special sense organs). A determination of disability must ignore the positive effects of any mitigating measure that is used. For example, a mitigating measure may include the use of low vision devices that magnify, enhance, or otherwise augment a visual image. Another type of mitigating measure is the use of learned behavioral modifications (for example, a person with monocular vision may turn his head from side to side to compensate for the lack of peripheral vision). A person with monocular vision, regardless of such compensating behaviors, will be substantially limited in seeing compared to most people in the general population.

Is Everyone Who Wears Glasses a Person with a Disability?

No, not everyone who wears glasses is a person with a disability under the ADA. Although the ADA generally requires that the positive effects of mitigating measures be ignored in assessing whether someone has a disability, the law requires that one consider the positive effects of the use of ordinary eyeglasses or contact lenses (that is, lenses that are intended to fully correct visual acuity or to eliminate refractive error). If the use of ordinary lenses results in no substantial limitation to a major life activity, then the person's vision impairment does not constitute a disability under the first part of the ADA's definition of disability.

Even though individuals who use ordinary eyeglasses or contact lenses that are intended to fully correct their vision will not be covered under the first definition of disability, they are protected from discrimination based on an employer's use of uncorrected vision standards that are not job-related and consistent with business necessity.

Individuals with a history of vision impairment will be covered under the second part of the definition of disability if they have a record of an impairment that substantially limited a major life activity in the past (for example, where surgery corrected a past substantially limiting vision impairment). Finally, an individual is covered under the third ("regarded as") prong of the definition of disability if an employer takes a prohibited action (for example, refuses to hire or terminates the individual) because of a vision impairment or because the employer believes the individual has a vision impairment, other than an impairment that lasts fewer than six months and is minor.

OBTAINING, USING, AND DISCLOSING MEDICAL INFORMATION

Before an Offer of Employment Is Made

MAY AN EMPLOYER ASK A JOB APPLICANT WHETHER SHE OR HE HAS OR HAD A VISION IMPAIRMENT OR ABOUT HER OR HIS TREATMENT RELATED TO ANY VISION IMPAIRMENT PRIOR TO MAKING A JOB OFFER?

No. An employer may not ask questions about an applicant's medical condition or require an applicant to have a medical examination before it makes a conditional job offer. This means that an employer cannot legally ask an applicant such questions as:

- Whether she or he has ever had any medical procedures related to her or his vision (for example, whether the applicant ever had eye surgery)
- Whether she or he use any prescription medications, including medications for conditions related to the eye
- Whether she or he has any condition that may have caused a vision impairment (for example, whether the applicant has diabetes)

An employer may ask questions pertaining to the applicant's ability to perform the essential functions of the position, with or without reasonable accommodation, such as:

- Whether the applicant can read labels on packages that need to be stocked
- Whether the applicant can work the night shift
- Whether the applicant can inspect small electronic components to determine if they have been damaged

DOES THE ADA REQUIRE AN APPLICANT TO DISCLOSE THAT SHE OR HE HAS OR HAD A VISION IMPAIRMENT OR SOME OTHER DISABILITY BEFORE ACCEPTING A JOB OFFER?

No. The ADA does not require applicants to disclose that they have or had a vision impairment or another disability unless they will need a reasonable accommodation for the application process (for example, written application materials to be printed in a larger font). Some individuals with a vision impairment, however, choose to disclose or discuss their condition to dispel myths about vision loss or to ensure that employers do not assume that the impairment means the person is unable to do the job.

Sometimes, the decision to disclose depends on whether an individual will need a reasonable accommodation to perform the job (for example, specialized equipment, removal of a marginal function, or another type of job restructuring). A person with a vision impairment, however, may request an accommodation after becoming an employee even if she did not do so when applying for the job or after receiving the job offer.

MAY AN EMPLOYER ASK QUESTIONS ABOUT AN OBVIOUS VISION IMPAIRMENT OR FOLLOW-UP QUESTIONS IF AN APPLICANT DISCLOSES A NONOBVIOUS VISION IMPAIRMENT?

No. An employer generally may not ask an applicant about obvious impairments. Nor may an employer ask an applicant who has voluntarily disclosed that he has a vision impairment any questions about the nature of the impairment, when it began, or how the individual copes with the impairment. However, if an applicant has an obvious impairment or has voluntarily disclosed the existence of vision impairment and the employer reasonably believes that he will require an accommodation to perform the job because of the impairment, the employer may ask whether the applicant will need an accommodation and what type. The employer must keep any information an applicant discloses about his medical condition confidential.

Example. A woman appears with her guide dog for an interview for a job as a school principal. The position requires significant reading. Because her vision impairment is obvious, the employer may ask her if she will need an accommodation to perform functions that involve reading and, if so, what type.

After an Offer of Employment Is Made

After making a job offer, an employer may ask questions about the applicant's health (including questions about the applicant's disability) and may require a medical examination, as long as all applicants for the same type of job are treated equally (that is, all applicants are asked the same questions and are required to take the same examination). After an employer has obtained basic medical information from all individuals who have received job offers, it may ask specific individuals for more medical information if the request is medically related to the previously obtained medical information. For example, if an employer asks all applicants post-offer about their general physical and mental health, it can ask individuals who disclose a particular illness, disease, or impairment for medical information or require them to have a medical examination related to the condition disclosed.

WHAT MAY AN EMPLOYER DO WHEN IT LEARNS THAT AN APPLICANT HAS OR HAD A VISION IMPAIRMENT AFTER SHE HAS BEEN OFFERED A JOB BUT BEFORE SHE STARTS WORKING?

When an applicant discloses after receiving a conditional job offer that she has or had a vision impairment, an employer may ask the applicant additional questions, such as how long she has had the vision impairment; what, if any, vision the applicant has; what specific visual limitations the individual experiences; and what, if any, reasonable accommodations the applicant may need to perform the job. The employer also may send the applicant for a follow-up vision or medical examination or ask her to submit documentation from her doctor answering questions specifically designed to assess her ability to perform the job's functions safely. Permissible follow-up questions at this stage differ from those at the preoffer stage when an employer only may ask an applicant who voluntarily discloses a disability whether she needs an accommodation to perform the job and what type.

An employer may not withdraw an offer from an applicant with vision impairment if the applicant is able to perform the essential functions of the job, with or without reasonable accommodation, without posing a direct threat (that is, a significant risk of substantial harm) to the health or safety of himself or others that cannot be eliminated or reduced through reasonable accommodation.

Example. A county sheriff with a monocular vision applied for a position with the state police as a criminal investigator. He was highly qualified for the job and was conditionally offered a position pending qualification under the state police department's medical criteria for criminal investigators. The doctor who conducted the medical examination of the applicant determined that because of his monocular vision he did not meet the state's safety standards, and the conditional offer of employment was withdrawn. The state police department did not violate the ADA by requiring the medical exam. However, the department must be prepared to show that the applicant was unable to do the essential functions of the job, with or without reasonable accommodation, or that he would have posed a direct threat to safety that could not be reduced or eliminated by a reasonable accommodation if he had been hired.

Employees

The ADA strictly limits the circumstances under which an employer may ask questions about an employee's medical condition or require the employee to have a medical examination. Once an employee is on the job, his actual performance is the best measure of the ability to do the job.

WHEN MAY AN EMPLOYER ASK AN EMPLOYEE IF A VISION IMPAIRMENT, OR SOME OTHER MEDICAL CONDITION, MAY BE CAUSING HER PERFORMANCE PROBLEMS?

Generally, an employer may ask disability-related questions or require an employee to have a medical examination when it knows about a particular employee's medical condition, has observed performance problems, and reasonably believes that the problems are related to a medical condition. At other times, an employer may ask for medical information when it has observed symptoms, such as difficulties visually focusing, or has received reliable information from someone else (for example, a family member or coworker) indicating that the employee may have a medical condition that is causing performance problems. Often, however, poor job performance is unrelated to a medical condition and generally should be handled in accordance with an employer's existing policies concerning performance.

Example. A data entry clerk has recently been making numerous errors when entering information into the employer's computer system. For example, he seems to be confusing the numbers 1, 7, and 9. The clerk's supervisor also has begun to see the clerk rubbing his eyes frequently and looking more closely at both his computer screen and printed materials. The employer has a reasonable belief based on objective evidence that the clerk's performance problems are related to a medical condition (i.e., an eye problem) and, therefore, may ask for medical information.

Example. A receptionist, with a known degenerative eye condition, has not been answering all the calls that come into the office in her usual friendly manner. The employer may counsel the receptionist about how she answers the phone, but may not ask her questions about her eye condition unless there is evidence that this may be the reason for her changed demeanor.

ARE THERE ANY OTHER INSTANCES WHEN AN EMPLOYER MAY ASK AN EMPLOYEE WITH A VISION IMPAIRMENT ABOUT HER CONDITION?

Yes. An employer also may ask an employee about a vision impairment when it has a reasonable belief that the employee will be unable to safely perform the essential functions of her job because of the vision impairment. In addition, an employer may ask an employee about her vision impairment to the extent the information is necessary:

- To support the employee's request for reasonable accommodation needed because of her vision impairment;
- To verify the employee's use of sick leave related to her vision impairment if the employer requires all

employees to submit a doctor's note to justify their use of sick leave; or
- To enable the employee to participate in a voluntary wellness program.

Example. An employer's leave policy requires all employees who are absent because of a medical appointment to submit a note from their doctor verifying the appointment. Jack, an employee, uses sick leave for an ophthalmological examination. In accordance with its policy, the employer can require Jack to submit a doctor's note for his absence; however, it may not require the note to include any information beyond that which is needed to verify that Jack used his sick leave properly (such as, the results of the examination, or a statement about the employee's diagnosis or any treatment).

Keeping Medical Information Confidential

With limited exceptions, an employer must keep confidential any medical information it learns about an applicant or employee. Under the following circumstances, however, an employer may disclose that an employee has a vision impairment:
- To supervisors and managers, if necessary to provide a reasonable accommodation or meet an employee's work restrictions;
- To first aid and safety personnel if an employee may need emergency treatment or require some other assistance at work;
- To individuals investigating compliance with the ADA and similar state and local laws; and
- Where needed for workers' compensation or insurance purposes (for example, to process a claim).

MAY AN EMPLOYER TELL EMPLOYEES WHO ASK WHY THEIR COWORKER IS ALLOWED TO DO SOMETHING THAT GENERALLY IS NOT PERMITTED (SUCH AS WORKING AT HOME OR WORKING A MODIFIED SCHEDULE) THAT SHE IS RECEIVING A REASONABLE ACCOMMODATION?

No. Telling coworkers that an employee is receiving a reasonable accommodation amounts to a disclosure that the employee has a disability. Rather than disclosing that the employee is receiving a reasonable accommodation, the employer should focus on the importance of maintaining the privacy of all employees and emphasize that its policy is to refrain from discussing the work situation of any employee with coworkers. Employers may be able to avoid many of these kinds of questions by training all employees on the requirements of equal employment laws, including the ADA.

Additionally, an employer will benefit from providing information about reasonable accommodation to all of its employees. This can be done in a number of ways, such as through written reasonable accommodation procedures, employee handbooks, staff meetings, and periodic training. This kind of proactive approach may lead to fewer questions from employees who misperceive coworker accommodations as "special treatment."

Example. Most of the paralegals in a large firm have outdated computer monitors. A paralegal who is on medication for a disability that causes vision problems requests, and is given, a new monitor with a special program that allows her to see the screen better. If the other paralegals ask why she has a new screen and they do not, the employer may not divulge any information about her impairment, including the fact that the monitor is a reasonable accommodation.

Accommodating Employees with Visual Disabilities

The ADA requires employers to provide adjustments or modifications—called reasonable accommodations?—to enable applicants and employees with disabilities to enjoy equal employment opportunities unless doing so would be an undue hardship (that is, a significant difficulty or expense). Accommodations vary depending on the needs of the individual with a disability. Not all employees with a visual disability will need accommodation or require the same accommodations.

WHAT TYPES OF REASONABLE ACCOMMODATIONS MAY EMPLOYEES WITH VISUAL DISABILITIES NEED?

Some employees may need one or more of the following accommodations:

- Assistive technology, including:
    - A closed-circuit television system (CCTV) for reading printed materials
    - An external computer screen magnifier
    - Digital recorders
    - Software that will read the information on the computer screen
    - An optical scanner that can create documents in electronic form from printed ones
    - A refreshable Braille display
    - A Braille embosser
- Written materials in an accessible format, such as in large print, Braille, in a recorded format, or on a computer disk
- Modification of employer policies to allow the use of a guide dog in the workplace
- Modification of an employment test
- A person to read printed materials
- A driver or payment for the cost of transportation to enable the performance of essential functions
- An accessible website
- Permission to work at home
- Modified training or training in the use of assistive technology

Example. An employer has decided to upgrade its computer programs. In order to teach its staff about the new systems, it has set up five "hands-on" training classes in which groups of employees will be shown how to execute various functions using the new software and then will have an opportunity to complete a series of exercises using those functions with guidance from the instructor. Most of the demonstrations and exercises will involve the use of a computer mouse to execute functions. A blind employee who uses a screen reading program is unable to use a computer mouse effectively and will require individualized instruction that will enable her to learn how to perform necessary functions using keyboard commands. The employer must grant this accommodation as long as it would not result in an undue hardship.

A Modified Work Schedule

Example. A blind employee does not have easy access to public transportation and must rely on paratransit service to get to work most mornings. He asks that, on days when his ride to work arrives after the employer's usual 8:30 a.m. start time, he is allowed to work later in the evening to make up the time rather than being required to take annual leave or face discipline for tardiness. The employer must grant this accommodation as long as it would not result in an undue hardship.

Time Off

Time off, in the form of accrued, paid leave or unpaid leave if paid leave has been exhausted or is unavailable.

Example. An employer provides a total of three weeks of leave (sick and annual leave) per employee each year. An employee with a degenerative eye condition has, over time, lost most of her vision and has decided to start using a guide dog. Training the guide dog will require her to attend a six-week residential program. Although the six weeks of leave that are needed exceed the amount of leave provided to each employee, the employer must provide additional unpaid leave as a reasonable accommodation as long as it would not result in an undue hardship. The same rule would apply if the employee needs time off for treatment related to a visual disability.

Reassignment to a Vacant Position

Example. A city police officer is shot and blinded during an attempt to stop a robbery. He no longer is able to perform his job as a police officer, but he is qualified for a vacant 911 emergency operator position. The job pays less than a police officer, but it is the closest vacant position in terms of pay, status, and benefits for which the officer is qualified. The city must reassign the officer to the 911 emergency operator position as a reasonable accommodation as long as it would not result in an undue hardship.

Although these are some examples of the types of accommodations commonly requested by employees with visual disabilities, other employees may need different changes or adjustments. Employers should ask the particular employee requesting accommodation that he needs that will help him do his job. There also are extensive public and private resources to help employers identify reasonable accommodations. For example, the website for the Job Accommodation Network (JAN) (askjan.org) provides information about many types of accommodations for employees with visual disabilities.

HOW DOES AN EMPLOYEE WITH A VISUAL DISABILITY REQUEST A REASONABLE ACCOMMODATION?

There are no "magic words" that a person has to use when requesting a reasonable accommodation. A person simply has to tell the employer that she needs an adjustment or change at work because of her visual impairment. A request for reasonable accommodation also can come from a family member, friend, health professional, or other representatives on behalf of a person with a visual disability. If an employer requires more information about the disability and why an accommodation is needed, it should engage in an "interactive process"—a dialogue with the employee—to obtain information that will help the employer in handling the request.

Example. A blind man calls regarding a job opening he heard advertised on the radio. The employer explains that part of the application process is a written exam and part is an in-person interview. The man says that he will need some help with the exam because of his impairment. This is a request for reasonable accommodation.

Example. While an employee has been out on extended medical leave for her diabetes, her visual disability has gradually gotten worse. When she returns to work, she presents a note from her doctor stating that she will need "some assistance" in order to perform the essential functions of the job. This is a request for reasonable accommodation.

MAY AN EMPLOYER REQUEST DOCUMENTATION WHEN AN EMPLOYEE WHO HAS A VISUAL DISABILITY REQUESTS A REASONABLE ACCOMMODATION?

Sometimes. When a person's vision impairment is not obvious, the employer may ask the person to provide reasonable documentation about how the condition limits major life activities (that is, whether the person has a disability) and why a reasonable accommodation is needed. An employer, however, is entitled only to documentation sufficient to establish that the employee has a visual disability and to explain why an accommodation is needed. A request for an employee's entire medical record, for example, would be inappropriate, as it likely would include information about conditions other than the employee's visual disability.

Example. A customer service representative with a nonobvious vision impairment requests a larger computer monitor. The employee's ophthalmologist provides a letter describing the employee's impairment and its limitations. The letter explains that the employee cannot drive and can read standard-sized print but only very slowly, for short periods of time, and with considerable effort. The condition is not expected to deteriorate further, but no improvement is expected either. The ophthalmologist concludes that providing some kind of magnification device for the computer or a larger monitor would be helpful. The employee has provided sufficient documentation that his eye condition is an ADA disability and that he needs a reasonable accommodation. The employer may not request further documentation, such as the results of all the tests conducted to diagnose the condition.

DOES AN EMPLOYER HAVE TO GRANT EVERY REQUEST FOR A REASONABLE ACCOMMODATION?

No. An employer does not have to provide accommodation if doing so would be an undue hardship. Undue hardship means that providing reasonable accommodation will result in significant difficulty or expense. An employer also does not have to eliminate an essential function of a job as a reasonable accommodation, tolerate performance that does not meet its standards, or excuse violations of conduct rules that are job-related and consistent with business necessity and that the employer applies consistently to all employees (such as rules prohibiting violence, threatening behavior, theft, or destruction of property). Nor do employers have to provide employees with personal use items, such as eyeglasses or other devices that are used both on and off the job.

If more than one accommodation would be effective, the employee's preference should be given primary consideration, although the employer is not required to provide the employee's first choice of reasonable accommodation. If a requested accommodation is too difficult or expensive, an employer may choose to provide easier or less costly accommodation as long as it is effective in meeting the employee's needs.

Example. An editor for a publishing company has a visual disability and needs magnification to read the text. She asks the company to hire a full-time reader for her. The employer is able to purchase a computer program that will magnify text on the screen and speak the words to her. If this is cheaper and easier for the employer to do, and allows the editor to do her work just as effectively, then it may be provided as a reasonable accommodation.

Example. A blind job applicant requests a reader for an employment test. The employer requires the applicant to take the test in Braille instead, although he has told the employer he is not proficient in Braille. In this situation, because providing the test in Braille is not an effective accommodation, the employer must provide a reader unless to do so would be an undue hardship.

MAY AN EMPLOYER BE REQUIRED TO PROVIDE MORE THAN ONE ACCOMMODATION FOR THE SAME EMPLOYEE WITH A VISUAL DISABILITY?

Yes. The duty to provide reasonable accommodation is an ongoing one. Although some employees with visual disabilities may require only one reasonable accommodation, others may need more than one. An employer must consider each request for reasonable accommodation and determine whether it would be effective and whether providing it would pose an undue hardship.

Example. An employee who is blind has assistive technology for his computer that works with the employer's network and enables him to send and receive email messages easily. When the employer upgrades computer equipment for all employees, it must provide new or updated assistive technology so that the blind employee will be integrated into the new networks, absent undue hardship.

Example. An employee with retinitis pigmentosa, a degenerative eye condition that results, over time, in total or near-total blindness, has been able to read printed materials related to her job with a magnifier and some adjustments to the lighting in her work area. When she is no longer able to do this, she asks for a reader. Absent undue hardship, the employer must provide a reader or some other effective accommodation.

WHAT KINDS OF REASONABLE ACCOMMODATIONS ARE RELATED TO THE BENEFITS AND PRIVILEGES OF EMPLOYMENT?

Reasonable accommodations related to the benefits and privileges of employment include accommodations that are necessary to provide individuals with disabilities access to facilities or portions of facilities to which all employees are granted access (for example, employee break rooms and cafeterias), access to information communicated in the workplace, and the opportunity to participate in employer-sponsored training and social events.

Example. An employer offers employees opportunities to accept six-month assignments to jobs outside of their workgroup or department. Temporary assignments are considered valuable training opportunities that can lead to employee advancement. An employee with a visual disability, who has worked successfully in her current position with only slight modifications to her computer equipment, requests a temporary assignment to a position that will involve considerably more reading and asks that a part-time reader be provided. The employer may not deny the temporary assignment because of the need to make reasonable accommodation but must provide a reader or some other effective accommodation if this would not result in an undue hardship.

Example. An employer typically posts job openings on bulletin boards. An employee with a visual disability requests that electronic notices of all job postings be emailed to him so that he will have timely notice of the postings. Unless this would result in undue hardship, the employer must provide this accommodation.

Example. An employer holds a retirement party for a long-time employee. The event includes dinner and various presentations by the employee's coworkers and company management. A formal program is printed for the event, and an employee with a visual disability requests a copy of the program in large print. The employer must provide this accommodation, absent undue hardship.

An employer will not be excused from providing an employee with a visual disability with a necessary accommodation because the employer has contracted with another entity to conduct the event.

Example. An employer offers its employees a training course on organization and time management provided by a local company with which the employer has contracted. An employee who is blind wants to take the course and asks that materials be made available in Braille. The employer claims that the company conducting the training is responsible for providing what the blind employee needs, but the company responds that the responsibility lies with their employer. Even if the company conducting the training has an obligation, under Title III of the ADA, to provide "auxiliary aids and services," which would include providing written materials in Braille, this fact does not alter the employer's obligation to provide the employee with a reasonable accommodation for the training.

CONCERNS ABOUT SAFETY

When it comes to safety concerns, an employer should be careful not to act on the basis of myths, fears, or stereotypes about vision impairments. Instead, the employer should evaluate each individual on her skills, knowledge, experience, and how the visual disability affects her.

When May an Employer Refuse to Hire, Terminate, or Temporarily Restrict the Duties of a Person Who Has or Had a Vision Impairment Because of Safety Concerns?

An employer only may exclude an individual with vision impairment from a job for safety reasons when the individual poses a direct threat. A "direct threat" is a significant risk of substantial harm to the individual or others that cannot be eliminated or reduced through reasonable accommodation. This determination must be based on objective, factual evidence, including the best recent medical evidence.

In making a direct threat assessment, the employer must evaluate the individual's present ability to safely perform the job. The employer also must consider:

- The duration of the risk
- The nature and severity of the potential harm
- The likelihood that the potential harm will occur
- The imminence of the potential harm

The harm must be serious and likely to occur, not remote or speculative. Finally, the employer must determine whether any reasonable accommodation would reduce or eliminate the risk. Here are a few examples:

- An assembly line worker has lost much of his vision, but because he has held his job for more than ten years, he can effectively perform the job's functions using a combination of his remaining limited vision and touch. The employer's normal practice is to flash an alarm light when there is an assembly line malfunction that could cause injuries to workers. Rather than discharging the employee because he no longer is able to see the flashing light and may, therefore, be in harm's way, the employer should consider installing an audio alarm to accommodate him.
- A blind sous-chef who began working as a line cook and has worked in restaurants for 15 years in positions of increasing levels of responsibility applies for a job at a newly opened restaurant. Although it initially takes him slightly more time than other workers to learn the layout of the kitchen, once he does so he is able to move about easily and safely. The combination of his experience, his use of touch to perform some tasks that other workers perform visually, and a few simple accommodations, such as Braille labels on oven controls, enables him to use all kitchen equipment and to supervise kitchen staff. The restaurant may not

refuse to hire this chef on the grounds that he cannot work safely in a busy kitchen.

- A line cook develops a severe visual disability and has difficulty adjusting to his vision loss. As a result, he has problems navigating in the kitchen and barely avoids bumping into three different coworkers, two of whom were carrying trays of food just removed from the oven and one who was carrying a pot of boiling water. He also was warned twice about placing his hands too close to open flames and fryers filled with hot oil. Reasonable accommodations have not eliminated or reduced these problems. This individual poses a direct threat to his own health and safety and to the health and safety of others, and therefore the employer may terminate his employment as a line cook.

What Should an Employer Do When Another Federal Law Prohibits It from Hiring Anyone with a Vision Impairment?

If a federal law prohibits an employer from hiring a person with a vision impairment, the employer would not be liable under the ADA. The employer should be certain, however, that compliance with the law actually is required, not voluntary. The employer also should be sure that the law does not contain any exemptions or waivers.

Example. A courier service that uses vans and small trucks weighing less than 10,000 pounds may not use the DOT standards applicable to commercial motor vehicles weighing more than 10,000 pounds to automatically exclude applicants with a monocular vision from driver jobs. The employer may exclude a particular applicant with a monocular vision only if it can demonstrate that she would pose a direct threat.

HARASSMENT

The ADA prohibits harassment, or offensive conduct, based on disability just as other federal laws prohibit harassment based on race, sex, color, national origin, religion, age, and genetic information.

Offensive conduct may include, but is not limited to, offensive jokes, slur, epithets or name-calling, physical assaults or threats, intimidation, ridicule or mockery, insults or put-downs, offensive objects or pictures, and interference with work performance. Although the law does not prohibit simple teasing, offhand comments, or isolated incidents that are not very serious, harassment is illegal when it is so frequent or severe that it creates a hostile or offensive work environment or when it results in an adverse employment decision (such as the victim being fired or demoted).

Example. A grocery store cashier with a visual disability is frequently taunted by his coworkers. They regularly ask him how many fingers they are holding up and take away his white cane and tell him to go find it. The cashier complains to his supervisor in accordance with his employer's antiharassment policy. The employer must promptly investigate and address the harassing behavior.

What Should Employers Do to Prevent and Correct Harassment?

Employers should make clear that they will not tolerate harassment based on disability or on any other basis. This can be done in a number of ways, such as through a written policy, employee handbooks, staff meetings, and periodic training. The employer should emphasize that harassment is prohibited and that employees should promptly report such conduct to a manager. Finally, the employer should immediately conduct a thorough investigation of any report of harassment and take swift and appropriate corrective action.

RETALIATION

The ADA prohibits retaliation by an employer against someone who opposes discriminatory employment practices, files a charge of employment discrimination, or testifies or participates in any way in an investigation, proceeding, or litigation related to a charge of employment discrimination. It is also unlawful for an employer to retaliate against someone for requesting a reasonable accommodation. Persons who believe that they have been retaliated against may file a charge of retaliation.

How to File a Charge of Employment Discrimination

AGAINST PRIVATE EMPLOYERS AND STATE/LOCAL GOVERNMENTS

Any person who believes that her or his employment rights have been violated on the basis of disability and wants to make a claim against an employer must file a charge of discrimination with the EEOC. A third party may also file a charge on behalf of another person who believes she or he experienced discrimination. For example, a family member, social worker, or other representatives can file a charge on behalf of someone with a vision impairment. The charge must be filed by mail or in-person with the local EEOC office within 180 days from the date of the alleged violation. The 180-day filing deadline is extended to 300 days if a state or local antidiscrimination agency has the authority to grant or seek relief as to the challenged unlawful employment practice.

The EEOC will send the parties a copy of the charge and may ask for responses and supporting information. Before the formal investigation, the EEOC may select the charge for EEOC's mediation program. Both parties have to agree to mediation, which may prevent a time-consuming investigation of the charge. Participation in mediation is free, voluntary, and confidential.

If the mediation is unsuccessful, the EEOC investigates the charge to determine if there is "reasonable cause" to believe discrimination has occurred. If reasonable cause is found, the EEOC will then try to resolve the charge with the employer. In some cases, where the charge cannot be resolved, the EEOC will file a court action. If the EEOC finds no discrimination, or if an attempt to resolve the charge fails and the EEOC decides not to file suit, it will issue a notice of a "right to sue," which gives the charging party 90 days to file a court action. A charging party can also request a notice of a "right to sue" from the EEOC 180 days after the charge was first filed with the Commission, and may then bring suit within 90 days after receiving the notice.

AGAINST THE FEDERAL GOVERNMENT

If you are a federal employee or job applicant and you believe that a federal agency has discriminated against you, you have a right to file a complaint. Each agency is required to post information about how to contact the agency's EEO Office. You can contact an EEO Counselor by calling the office responsible for the agency's EEO complaints program. Generally, you must contact the EEO Counselor within 45 days from the day the discrimination occurred. In most cases, the EEO Counselor will give you the choice of participating either in EEO counseling or in an alternative dispute resolution (ADR) program, such as a mediation program.

If you do not settle the dispute during counseling or through ADR, you can file a formal discrimination complaint against the agency with the agency's EEO Office. You must file within 15 days from the day you receive notice from your EEO Counselor about how to file.

Once you have filed a formal complaint, the agency will review the complaint and decide whether or not the case should be dismissed for a procedural reason (for example, your claim was filed too late). If the agency doesn't dismiss the complaint, it will conduct an investigation. The agency has 180 days from the day you filed your complaint to finish the investigation. When the investigation is finished, the agency will issue a notice giving you two choices: either request a hearing before an EEOC Administrative Judge or ask the agency to issue a decision as to whether the discrimination occurred.

Chapter 59 | Social Security If You Are Blind or Have Low Vision

IF YOU ARE BLIND OR HAVE LOW VISION

If you are blind, there are special rules that allow you to receive benefits when you are unable to work. There are benefits provided to people who are blind under two programs: the Social Security Disability Insurance (SSDI) program and the Supplemental Security Income (SSI) program. The medical rules used to decide whether you are blind are the same for each program. Other rules are different. The different rules for each program are explained below.

You Can Get Disability Benefits If You Are Blind

You may qualify for Social Security benefits or SSI disability payments if you are blind. A person is considered to be blind if their vision cannot be corrected to better than 20/200 in their better eye or if their visual field is 20 degrees or less in their better eye for a period that lasted or is expected to last at least 12 months.

You Can Get Disability Benefits Even If You Are Not Blind

If your vision does not meet Social Security's definition of blindness, you may still qualify for disability benefits if your vision problems alone, or combined with other health problems, prevent you from working. For Social Security disability benefits, you must also

This chapter includes text excerpted from "If You're Blind or Have Low Vision—How We Can Help," U.S. Social Security Administration (SSA), January 2020.

have worked long enough in a job where you paid Social Security taxes. For SSI payments based on disability and blindness, you need not have worked, but your income and resources must be under certain dollar limits.

How You Qualify for Social Security Disability Benefits

When you work and pay Social Security taxes, you earn credits that count toward future Social Security benefits.

If you are blind, you can earn credits anytime during your working years. Credits for your work after you become blind can be used to qualify you for benefits if you do not have enough credits at the time you become blind.

Also, if you do not have enough credits to get Social Security disability benefits based on your own earnings, you may be able to get benefits based on the earnings of one of your parents or your spouse.

Disability Freeze

There is a special rule that may help you get higher retirement or disability benefits someday. You can use this rule if you are blind but are not getting disability benefits now because you are still working. If your earnings are lower because of your blindness, those years to calculate your Social Security retirement or disability benefit in the future can be excluded. Because Social Security benefits are based on your average lifetime earnings, your benefit will be higher if those years are not counted. This rule is called a "disability freeze."

You Can Get Supplemental Security Income Disability Payments

The SSI program is a means-tested program. Your income and resources must be less than certain dollar limits. The income limits vary from one state to another. You need not have worked under Social Security to qualify for SSI. Ask your local Social Security office about the income and resource limits in your state.

YOU CAN WORK WHILE RECEIVING BENEFITS

Rules, called "work incentives" make it easier for people receiving disability benefits to work.

People getting Social Security disability benefits can continue to receive their benefits when they work as long as their earnings are not more than an amount set by law.

If you are receiving Social Security disability benefits and you are blind, you can earn as much as $2,110 a month in 2020. This is higher than the earnings limit of $1,260 a month that applies to disabled workers who are not blind. The earnings limits usually change each year.

Additionally, if you are blind and self-employed, the time you spend working in your business as others do for people who are not blind is not evaluated. This means you can be doing a lot of work for your business, but still receive disability benefits, as long as your net profit averages $2,110 or less a month in 2020.

Work Figured Differently Beginning at 55 Years of Age

If you are aged 55 or older, and blind, determination rules about work for you are used that are different from the rules used for people who are not blind. Beginning at age 55, even if your earnings exceed $2,110 a month in 2020, benefits are only suspended, not terminated, if the work you are doing requires a lower level of skill and ability than what you did before you reached 55. Disability benefits for any month your earnings fall below this limit will be paid. Different work incentives apply to people getting SSI.

SPECIAL SERVICES FOR PEOPLE WHO ARE BLIND OR HAVE LOW VISION

Some services and products are designed specifically for people who are blind or have low vision.

Social Security Notices

You can choose to receive notices in one of the following ways:

- Standard print notice by first-class mail
- Standard print notice by certified mail
- Standard print notice by first-class mail and a follow-up telephone call

- Braille notice and a standard print notice by first-class mail
- Microsoft Word file on a data compact disc (CD) and a standard print notice by first-class mail
- Audio CD and a standard print notice by first-class mail
- Large print (18-point size) notice and a standard print notice by first-class mail

You have several options for choosing how you want to receive notices from us:

- Visit the website at www.socialsecurity.gov/notices and follow the steps provided.
- Call the toll-free at 800-772-1213. If you are hard-of-hearing, you may call the TTY number at 800-325-0778.
- Write or visit your local Social Security office.

Publications Available in Alternative Formats

All publications are made available in multiple formats, including Braille, audio cassette tapes, compact discs, or enlarged print on request. Also, most of the publications are available in audio format on the website, www.socialsecurity.gov/pubs.

To request copies of these publications in alternative formats, you can:

- Visit the website, www.socialsecurity.gov/pubs/alt-pubs.html, to order online
- Call the toll-free at 800-772-1213. If you are hard-of-hearing, you may call the TTY number, 800-325-0778.
- Mail, call, or fax your request to the Braille Services Branch at the Social Security Administration:

Social Security Administration Office of Printing and Alternative Media Services

6401 Security Boulevard
Room 1305 Annex Building
Baltimore, MD 21235

Phone number: 410-965-6414
TTY number: 800-325-0778
Fax number: 410-965-6413

CONTACTING SOCIAL SECURITY

There are several ways to contact SSA, such as online, by phone, and in person. For more than 80 years, Social Security has helped secure today and tomorrow by providing benefits and financial protection for millions of people throughout their life's journey.

Visit the Website

The most convenient way to conduct Social Security business from anywhere is online at www.socialsecurity.gov. You can:

- Apply for Extra Help with Medicare prescription drug plan costs
- Apply for most types of benefits
- Find copies of the publications
- Get answers to frequently asked questions

When you create a, My Social Security account, you can do even more.

- Review your Social Security Statement
- Verify your earnings
- Print a benefit verification letter
- Change your direct deposit information
- Request a replacement Medicare card
- Get a replacement SSA-1099/1042S
- Request a replacement Social Security card, if you have no changes and your state participates.

Call U.S. Social Security Administration (SSA)

If you do not have access to the Internet, many automated services by telephone are offered, 24 hours a day, 7 days a week. Call the toll-free at 800-772-1213 or at the TTY number, 800-325-0778, if you are hard-of-hearing.

A member of the staff can answer your call from 7 a.m. to 7 p.m., Monday through Friday, if you need to speak with someone.

Schedule an Office Visit

You can find the closest office location by entering your ZIP code on the office locator webpage.

If you are taking documents for review, remember that they must be original or certified copies that are certified by the issuing agency.

Chapter 60 | **Current Vision Research**

Chapter Contents

Section 60.1 | Delayed Treatment Safe for Some People with Diabetic Eye Disease

This section includes text excerpted from "Delayed Treatment Safe for Some People with Diabetic Eye Disease," National Institutes of Health (NIH), May 7, 2019.

Almost 15 percent of people in the United States live with diabetes—a disorder in how the body uses glucose, a sugar that serves as the body's fuel. The condition can potentially damage many parts of the body, especially if left untreated.

People with diabetes may develop a problem in their eyes called "diabetic macular edema" (DME). This is a swelling or thickening of the macula, an area in the center of the retina—the part of the eye that senses light. It is caused by damage to the small blood vessels of the retina. DME is the most common cause of vision loss among people with diabetes.

If doctors detect vision loss caused by DME early, treatment can slow or stop it. But, it has not been clear if treatment should be given to people with DME who still have good vision.

To better understand the appropriate timing for treatment, a team led by Dr. Carl Baker from the Paducah Retinal Center in Kentucky enrolled about 700 people into a clinical trial. All participants had DME but still had a normal or near-normal vision. The team randomly assigned participants into three groups.

One group received injections into the eye with a drug that prevents vision loss. The second group underwent a treatment called "photocoagulation," which uses lasers to seal leaky blood vessels in the eye. The third group received no immediate treatment, but had their eyes checked at 8 and 16 weeks after study entry, and then every 16 weeks. If vision loss began to develop in participants in this group over 2 years of follow-up, they immediately began drug injections.

Due to progressive vision loss, 25 percent of people in the photocoagulation group and 34 percent of people in the observation group started drug injections. At the end of the study, rates of vision loss were about the same between the 3 groups, regardless of what treatment they started with. After 2 years, the average vision was 20/20 in all groups—the same as at the start of the study.

Increases in pressure within the eye were more common in the drug injection group than in the observation group. Other side effects did not differ between the groups.

"We now know that in patients with good vision and DME, similar to those enrolled in this trial, it is an acceptable strategy to closely monitor patients, and initiate treatment only if their vision starts to show signs of decline," Baker says.

Participants in the trial had good control of their blood sugar, which helps prevent diabetic eye disease, and came in for regular checkups. The researchers caution that delaying treatment may not be as safe for people who have trouble managing their blood sugar or coming in for regular eye exams.

Section 60.2 | **Immune System Can Slow Degenerative Eye Disease**

This section includes text excerpted from "Immune System Can Slow Degenerative Eye Disease, NIH-Led Mouse Study Shows," National Institutes of Health (NIH), June 17, 2019.

A study shows that the complement system, part of the innate immune system, plays a protective role to slow retinal degeneration in a mouse model of retinitis pigmentosa, an inherited eye disease. This surprising discovery contradicts previous studies of other eye diseases suggesting that the complement system worsens retinal degeneration. The research was performed by scientists at the National Eye Institute (NEI), part of the National Institutes of Health (NIH), and appears in the *Journal of Experimental Medicine.*

Retinitis pigmentosa is an incurable and unpreventable blinding eye disease that affects 1 in 4,000 people.

"Much research is devoted to studying therapies that attempt to alter the immune system's role in inherited diseases such as retinitis pigmentosa because such treatments would have broad applicability, regardless of a patient's causative mutation," said the study's principal investigator Wai T Wong, M.D., Ph.D., chief of the Neuron-Glia Interactions in Retinal Disease Section at NEI.

In previous studies, activation of the complement system mediates some aspects of inflammation and worsens damage in age-related macular degeneration (AMD), a leading cause of blindness in people aged 65 years and older.

"The current study involving retinitis pigmentosa underscores the notion that the complement system may, in fact, exacerbate or curb retinal degeneration depending on the context. Appreciating this complexity is important for guiding the development of therapies that target the complement immune system to treat degenerative diseases of the retina," Dr. Wong said.

Sean Silverman, Ph.D., an NEI postdoctoral researcher in Dr. Wong's lab and the lead author of the study, and colleagues monitored the genetic expression of the complement system in a transgenic mouse model of retinitis pigmentosa. They found that the upregulation of complement expression and activation coincided with the onset of photoreceptor degeneration. Furthermore, this upregulation occurs in the exact location of the degeneration.

"Having found complement at the scene of the crime, we then wanted to know whether it was helping or hurting the degenerative process," Dr. Wong said.

Using the retinitis pigmentosa mouse model, the researchers examined the role of C3 and CR3, the central component of complement and its receptor, by comparing mice with genetically ablated C3 or CR3 to mice with normal expression. They found that the absence of C3 or CR3 made degeneration worse. Rod photoreceptors, the light-sensing cells that die off first in retinitis pigmentosa, were precipitously lost along with a surge in the expression of neurotoxic inflammatory cytokines.

They pieced together that C3 gets secreted by microglia, trash-collecting cells in a healthy retina clears away dead cells by phagocytosis to keep the tissue working properly. Once secreted, C3 lands on dead photoreceptors labeling them for destruction and removal. The receptor, CR3, recognizes the C3 markers and conveys the information to microglia. "Breakdown of this C3-CR3 interaction results in a decreased ability of microglia to phagocytose dead photoreceptors, which then accumulate in the retina, stimulating greater inflammation and degeneration," Dr. Wong said. "Degeneration accelerates pretty quickly."

When placed alongside each other in a dish, microglia from C3- or CR3-ablated retinas turned out to be toxic to photoreceptors.

Taken together, the results show that in the context of retinitis pigmentosa, complement activation is actually helpful for clearing away dead cells and maintaining a state of homeostasis, a physiological balance, in the retina.

However, in the context of AMD, harmful effects observed from complement activation have spurred clinical trials testing complement inhibitors. "Our findings suggest that this approach may be appropriate for some disease scenarios, but may induce complex responses in other disease scenarios by inhibiting helpful and homeostatic functions of inflammation," Dr. Wong said.

Further research is needed to complete the picture of how, and under what circumstances, complement activation has beneficial or harmful effects on photoreceptors and disease progression.

Section 60.3 | **Patch Replaces Damaged Retinal Cells**

This section includes text excerpted from "Patch Replaces Damaged Retinal Cells," National Institutes of Health (NIH), January 29, 2019.

Macular degeneration is a leading cause of vision loss among people over 50 years of age. This disease damages an area near the center of the retina, the light-sensitive tissue in the eye. Retinal pigment epithelial (RPE) cells gradually waste away and die. These pigmented cells support and nurture light-sensing cells known as "photoreceptors," so these cells also eventually die. The disease makes the center of your vision blurry, distorted, or dark.

Researchers have tried to treat macular degeneration by replacing dying RPE cells with healthy ones derived from stem cells. But, the new cells have a hard time growing without support structures. If the cells are from another person, the patient's immune system might reject the new cells. Another potential problem is that the previous techniques used cells that were prone to having cancer-causing genomic alterations.

A team led by Dr. Kapil Bharti at the National Institutes of Health's (NIH) National Eye Institute (NEI) set out to develop a treatment for macular degeneration that used RPE cells derived from a patient's own healthy cells. They also designed a scaffold to support healthy RPE cells and promote their attachment inside the eye. The work was also funded by the NIH Common Fund.

The research team collected cells from blood that was donated by three people with macular degeneration and converted them into induced pluripotent stem cells (iPSCs). These cells can theoretically be coaxed into becoming any other cell type. Next, the team programmed the iPSCs to become RPE cells. The cells were grown in a single layer on a biodegradable polymer scaffold. The researchers designed a tool that enabled them to slip the patch between damaged retinal pigment cells and photoreceptors in the eyes of rats and pigs.

Ten weeks after the patches were inserted, imaging studies showed integration of the cells into the animal retinas. Lab tests confirmed that the transplanted cells expressed the gene for RPE65, a mark of mature RPE cells. Further tests showed that the transplanted RPE cells were helping to keep the photoreceptors healthy. In contrast, the photoreceptors died in a test of a patch without RPE cells.

Because a patient would receive RPE cells derived from their own cells, the chance that the immune system would reject them is low. In addition, the research team did not detect any known cancer-causing alterations in the iPSC-derived RPE cells.

The researchers are now planning to test the safety of this treatment in people.

Section 60.4 | **Stem-Cell Therapy for Eye Disease**

This section includes text excerpted from "NIH Discovery Brings Stem Cell Therapy for Eye Disease Closer to the Clinic," National Institutes of Health (NIH), January 2, 2018.

Scientists at the National Eye Institute (NEI), part of the National Institutes of Health (NIH), report that tiny tube-like protrusions called "primary cilia" on cells of the retinal pigment epithelium (RPE)—a layer of cells in the back of the eye—are essential for the survival of the retina's light-sensing photoreceptors. The discovery has advanced efforts to make stem cell-derived RPE for transplantation into patients with geographic atrophy, otherwise known as dry "age-related macular degeneration" (AMD), a leading cause of blindness in the United States.

"We now have a better idea about how to generate and replace RPE cells, which appear to be among the first type of cells to stop working properly in AMD," said the study's lead investigator, Kapil Bharti, Ph.D., Stadtman investigator at the NEI. Bharti is leading the development of patient stem cell-derived RPE for an AMD clinical trial launched in 2018.

In a healthy eye, RPE cells nourish and support photoreceptors, the cells that convert light into electrical signals that travel to the brain via the optic nerve. RPE cells form a layer just behind the photoreceptors. In geographic atrophy, RPE cells die, which causes photoreceptors to degenerate, leading to vision loss.

Bharti and his colleagues are hoping to halt and reverse the progression of geographic atrophy by replacing diseased RPE with lab-made RPE. The approach involves using a patient's blood cells to generate induced pluripotent stem cells (iPSCs), cells capable of becoming any type of cell in the body. iPSCs are grown in the laboratory and then coaxed into becoming RPE for surgical implantation.

Attempts to create functional RPE implants, however, have hit a recurring obstacle: iPSCs programmed to become RPE cells have a tendency to get developmentally stuck, said Bharti. "The cells frequently fail to mature into functional RPE capable of supporting photoreceptors. In cases where they do mature, however, RPE maturation coincides with the emergence of primary cilia on the iPSC-RPE cells."

The researchers tested three drugs known to modulate the growth of primary cilia on iPSC-derived RPE. As predicted, the two drugs known to enhance cilia growth significantly improved the structural and functional maturation of the iPSC-derived RPE. One important characteristic of maturity observed was that the RPE cells all oriented properly, correctly forming a single, functional monolayer. The iPSC-derived RPE cell gene expression profile also resembled that of adult RPE cells. And importantly, the cells performed a crucial function of mature RPE cells: they engulfed the tips of photoreceptor outer segments, a pruning process that keeps photoreceptors working properly.

By contrast, iPSC-derived RPE cells exposed to the third drug, an inhibitor of cilia growth, demonstrated severely disrupted structure and functionality.

As further confirmation of their observations, when the researchers genetically knocked down the expression of cilia protein IFT88, the iPSC-derived RPE showed severe maturation and functional defects, as confirmed by gene expression analysis. Tissue staining showed that knocking down IFT88 led to reduced iPSC-derived RPE cell density and functional polarity, i.e., cells within the RPE tissue pointed in the wrong direction.

Bharti and his group found similar results in iPSC-derived lung cells, another type of epithelial cell with primary cilia. When iPSC-derived lung cells were exposed to drugs that enhance cilia growth, immunostaining confirmed that the cells looked structurally mature.

The report suggests that primary cilia regulates the suppression of the canonical WNT pathway, a cell signaling pathway involved in embryonic development. Suppression of the WNT pathway during RPE development instructs the cells to stop dividing and to begin differentiating into adult RPE, according to the researchers.

The researchers also generated iPSC-derived RPE from a patient with ciliopathy, a disorder that causes severe vision loss due to photoreceptor degeneration. The patient's ciliopathy was associated with mutations of cilia gene *CEP290*. Compared to a healthy donor, iPSC-derived RPE from the ciliopathy patient had cilia that were smaller. The patient's iPSC-derived RPE also had maturation and functional defects similar to those with IFT88 knockdown.

Further studies in a mouse model of ciliopathy confirmed an important temporal relationship: Looking across several early developmental stages, the RPE defects preceded the photoreceptor degeneration, which provides additional insights into ciliopathy-induced retinal degeneration.

"The study's findings have been incorporated into the group's protocol for making clinical-grade iPSC-derived RPE. They will also inform the development of disease models for research of AMD and other degenerative retinal diseases," Bharti said.

Section 60.5 | **How Storing Corneas Affects Transplantation Success**

This section includes text excerpted from "How Storing Corneas Affects Transplantation Success," National Institutes of Health (NIH), November 21, 2017.

The cornea is the eye's clear outer covering. Certain diseases can cloud the cornea, causing reduced vision and even blindness. Replacing a cloudy cornea with a healthy cornea from a donor can restore vision. Last year, nearly 50,000 corneal transplantations were performed in the United States. The supply of donor corneas is currently sufficient for U.S. patients; however, demand is expected to increase with the aging population.

The U.S. Food and Drug Administration (FDA) has approved the use of solutions to preserve donated corneas for up to 14 days before transplantation. However, surgeons in the United States generally prefer not to use corneas stored for longer than 7 days.

To investigate how long corneas can be safely stored, a team of researchers led by Dr. Jonathan Lass of Case Western Reserve University (CWRU) School of Medicine and University Hospitals (UH) Eye Institute compared success rates of transplantation for corneas stored for 7 days or less to those stored for eight to

14 days. The study was funded by NIH's National Eye Institute (NEI). Two reports on the study's results appeared online in JAMA Ophthalmology on November 10, 2017.

The researchers evaluated three-year corneal transplantation success rates from 1,090 patients who had surgery on one or both eyes (1,330 eyes total) to restore vision loss from corneal disease. Patients were randomly assigned to receive corneas that had been either stored up to 7 days or stored between 8 and 14 days. The eye surgeries were performed by 70 surgeons across the United States.

The three-year success rates for corneas stored up to 7 days was 95 percent and for those stored between 8 and 14 days was 92 percent. However, the success rate for corneas stored between 12 and 14 days was 89 percent. The success rate for those stored between 8 and 11 days was 94 percent. Thus, most of the difference in success rates between the two main groups could be attributed to a lower success rate for corneas stored between 12 and 14 days.

In the second study report, the research team analyzed cell loss among 769 participants in the innermost layer of the cornea 3 years after transplantation. Cell loss in the innermost layer is related to the long-term failure of transplanted corneas. Three years after transplantation, corneas stored up to seven days had a 37 percent loss of cells, and those stored between 8 and 14 days had a 40 percent loss. The effect of storage time on the loss of cells at three years was comparable for corneas stored between 4 and 13 days.

Taken together, the studies support the use of corneas that have been stored up to 11 days. The results suggest that more patients would have access to vision-saving transplantations if surgeons expand the window in which donor tissues can be considered suitable.

"The current practice of surgeons to use corneas preserved for no longer than seven days is not evidence-based," Lass says, "but rather a practice based on opinion, which hopefully will change with this new evidence."

Section 60.6 | **Eye Could Provide "Window to the Brain" after Stroke**

This section includes text excerpted from "Eye Could Provide 'Window to the Brain' after Stroke," National Institutes of Health (NIH), February 7, 2018.

Research into curious bright spots in the eyes on stroke patients' brain images could onc day alter the way these individuals are assessed and treated. A team of scientists at the National Institutes of Health (NIH) found that a chemical routinely given to stroke patients undergoing brain scans can leak into their eyes, highlighting those areas and potentially providing insight into their strokes. The study was published in Neurology.

"We were kind of astounded by this—it is a very unrecognized phenomenon," said Richard Leigh, M.D., an assistant clinical investigator at the NIH's National Institute of Neurological Disorders and Stroke (NINDS) and the paper's senior author. "It raises the question of whether there is something we can observe in the eye that would help clinicians evaluate the severity of a stroke and guide us on how best to help patients."

The eyes glowed so brightly on those images due to gadolinium, a harmless, transparent chemical often given to patients during magnetic resonance imaging (MRI) scans to highlight abnormalities in the brain. In healthy individuals, gadolinium remains in the bloodstream and is filtered out by the kidneys. However, when someone has experienced damage to the blood-brain barrier, which controls whether substances in the blood can enter the brain, gadolinium leaks into the brain, creating bright spots that mark the location of brain damage.

Previous research had shown that certain eye diseases could cause a similar disruption to the blood-ocular barrier, which does for the eye what the blood-brain barrier does for the brain. Dr. Leigh's team discovered that a stroke can also compromise the blood-ocular barrier and that the gadolinium that leaked into a patient's eyes could provide information about her or his stroke.

"It looks like the stroke is influencing the eye, and so the eye is reflective of what is going on in the brain," Dr. Leigh said. "Clearly

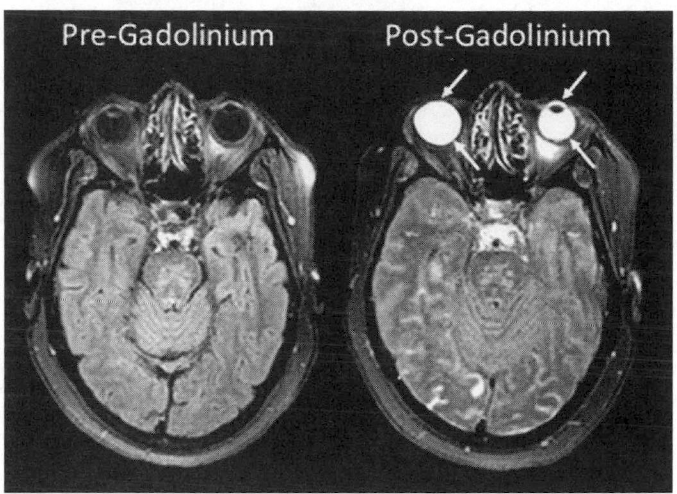

Figure 60.1. MRI Scan of a Stroke Patient

Eyes yield information about strokes: Magnetic resonance imaging (MRI) scans revealed that a chemical called "gadolinium," used to improve images, leaked into the eyes of stroke patients.

these results are preliminary, so future studies will have to be attuned to this to fully understand its impact."

The researchers performed MRI scans on 167 stroke patients upon admission to the hospital without administering gadolinium and compared them to scans taken using gadolinium 2 hours and 24 hours later. Because gadolinium is transparent, it did not affect patients' vision and could only be detected with MRI scans. Roughly three-quarters of the patients experienced gadolinium leakage into their eyes on one of the scans, with 66 percent showing it on the two-hour scan and 75 percent on the 24-hour scan. The phenomenon was present in both untreated patients and patients who received a treatment, called "tPA," to dissolve the blood clot responsible for their strokes.

Gadolinium was typically present in the front part of the eye, called the "aqueous chamber," after 2 hours, and in a region towards the back, called the "vitreous chamber," after 24 hours. Patients showing gadolinium in the vitreous chamber at the later timepoint tended to be of older age, have a history of hypertension, and have more bright spots on their brain scans, called "white matter hyperintensities," that are associated with brain aging and decreased cognitive function.

In a minority of patients, the two-hour scan showed gadolinium in both eye chambers. The strokes in those patients tended to affect a larger portion of the brain and cause even more damage to the blood-brain barrier than the strokes of patients with a slower pattern of gadolinium leakage or no leakage at all. The findings raise the possibility that, in the future, clinicians could administer a substance to patients that would collect in the eye just like gadolinium and quickly yield important information about their strokes without the need for an MRI.

"It is much easier for us to look inside somebody's eye than to look into somebody's brain," Dr. Leigh said. "So if the eye truly is a window to the brain, we can use one to learn about the other."

Despite the relationship between gadolinium leakage and stroke severity, the phenomenon was not found to be related to the level of disability the patients developed following their strokes. It also remains unclear whether gadolinium can enter the eye in healthy people.

Part 8 | **Additional Help and Information**

Chapter 61 | Glossary of Terms Related to Eyes and Eye Disorders

accommodation: The ability of the eye to increase its focusing power. As an object is viewed closer up, greater focusing power is needed to continue to see it clearly.

acuity: Clearness, or sharpness of vision.

adaptive and assistive devices: Prescription and nonprescription devices that help people with low vision enhance their remaining vision.

age-related macular degeneration: An eye disease that results in a loss of central, "straight-ahead" vision.

anterior chamber: The space in the front portion of the eye between the cornea and the iris. The space is filled with a clear fluid.

astigmatism: A distortion of the image on the retina caused by irregularities in the cornea or lens.

blood vessels: Arteries, veins, and capillaries that carry blood through the body.

cataract: A clouding of the lens. People with a cataract see through a haze.

conjunctivitis: Eye infection, pink eye, swelling and redness around your eyes.

cornea: Clear outer part of the focusing system that is located at the front of the eye.

This glossary contains terms excerpted from documents produced by several sources deemed reliable.

corneal transplant: Surgical treatment where the patient's cloudy cornea is cut away and a clear cornea, donated by someone who has died, is sewn into its place.

diabetes: A chronic disease related to high blood sugar that may lead to vision loss (diabetic retinopathy).

diabetic eye disease: A group of eye problems that people with diabetes may get. All of these eye problems can lead to vision loss or blindness.

diabetic retinopathy: Damage to the blood vessels in the retina due to diabetes.

dilate: Widening or enlargement of the pupil so that the retina is more visible

dilated eye exam: An eye examination where drops are placed in your eyes to widen, or dilate, the pupils. The eye-care professional uses a special magnifying lens to examine the retina and optic nerve for signs of damage and other eye problems.

dominant optic nerve atrophy: Hereditary damage to the optic nerve, resulting in a loss of vision.

double vision: Seeing two images of a single object instead of one.

endothelial cells: The cells that line the inner surface of the cornea in a single layer (endothelium). They are responsible for pumping fluid out of the cornea to keep it clear.

endothelium: The innermost layer of cells lining the inner surface of the cornea.

epithelium: The outermost layer of cells of the cornea and the eye's first defense against infection.

excimer laser: An ultraviolet laser used in refractive surgery to remove corneal tissue.

eyelash: The fringe of hair edging the eyelid; they close to keep particles, like dust, out of your eyes.

eyelid: The skin-covered structure that protects the front of the eye. It limits light entering the eye and spreads tears over the cornea.

fovea: The center of the macula, which gives the sharpest vision

glare: Scatter from bright light that causes discomfort and can decrease vision and the ability to perform tasks like driving.

glaucoma: A group of eye diseases in which the normal fluid pressure inside the eyes slowly rises, leading to vision loss or even blindness.

hyperopia/farsightedness: The inability to see near objects as clearly as distant objects, and the need for accommodation to see distant objects clearly.

intraocular lens: A lens that is surgically implanted inside the eye.

intraocular pressure: The pressure of fluid inside the eye.

iridotomy: Incision of the iris.

iris: The colored part of the eye; it regulates the amount of light entering the eye.

iritis: Inflammation of the front portion of the eye that can lead to scarring inside the eye and glaucoma.

keratectomy: The surgical removal of corneal tissue.

keratitis: Inflammation of the cornea.

keratoconus: A disorder characterized by an irregular corneal surface (cone-shaped) resulting in blurred and distorted images.

keratomileusis: Carving of the cornea to reshape it.

lens: The clear part of the eye behind the iris that helps to focus light on the retina. It allows the eye to focus on both far and near objects.

low vision: A visual impairment, not corrected by standard eye glasses, contact lenses, medication, or surgery, which interferes with the ability to perform everyday activities.

low vision therapist: A vision rehabilitation professional who trains people with low vision to use optical and nonoptical devices and adaptive techniques to make the most of their remaining vision.

macular: The small, sensitive area of the retina that gives central vision.

macular edema: When fluid leaks into the center of the macula, the part of the eye where sharp, straight-ahead vision occurs. The fluid makes the macula swell, blurring vision.

microkeratome: A mechanical surgical device that is affixed to the eye by use of a vacuum ring. When secured, a very sharp blade cuts a layer of the cornea at a predetermined depth.

monovision: The purposeful adjustment of one eye for near vision and the other eye for distance vision.

myopia/nearsightedness: The inability to see distant objects as clearly as near objects, because the focusing power of the eye is too strong.

occupational therapist: A rehabilitation professional who works with persons with disabilities, including low vision, to complete the everyday activities that they need for independence and quality of life.

ophthalmologist: A medical doctor who diagnoses and treats all diseases and disorders of the eye and prescribes glasses and contact lenses.

optic nerve: Bundle of more than 1 million nerve fibers that carry visual messages from the retina to the brain.

orientation and mobility specialist: A vision rehabilitation professional who trains people with low vision to move about safely in the home and travel by themselves.

posterior chamber: The space in the eye between the back of the iris and the front of the vitreous (the jelly-like substance that fills the space in the back central portion of the eyeball).

presbyopia: The inability to maintain a clear image (focus) as objects are moved closer.

pseudoexfoliation: Abnormal deposits of white, flaky material seen on the structures in the front part of the eye that may be associated with cataracts and high pressure in the eye or glaucoma.

pupil: The opening at the center of the iris. The iris adjusts the size of the pupil and controls the amount of light that can enter the eye.

refraction: A test to determine the refractive power of the eye; also, the bending of light as it passes from one medium into another.

refractive errors: Imperfections in the focusing power of the eye, for example, hyperopia, myopia, and astigmatism.

refractive surgery: General term referring to many different procedures to correct the refractive error of the eye.

retina: Light-sensitive tissue lining the back of the eyeball. It sends electrical impulses to the brain.

retinal detachment: Separation of the retina from its attachments to the back of the eyeball often resulting in loss of vision. Flashinglights, floating spots, and blank spots in vision can be symptoms of a retinal detachment.

sclera: The tough, white, outer layer (coat) of the eyeball that, along with the cornea, protects the eyeball.

Sjögren syndrome: Dry eyes and mouth.

specialist in low vision: An ophthalmologist or optometrist who specializes in the evaluation of low vision. This professional prescribes magnifying devices.

stroma: The middle, thickest layer of tissue in the cornea.

tonometry: An instrument that measures the pressure inside your eye. Numbing drops may be applied to your eye during this test.

uveitis: Inflammation of the inner eye that includes the iris, the tissue that holds the lens of the eye, and a network of blood vessels surrounding the eyeball called the choroid plexus.

visual acuity: The sharpness of vision; the measurement of the eyes ability to distinguish object details and shape.

visual acuity test: An eye chart test that measures how well you see at various distances.

vitrectomy: A surgical treatment where an ophthalmologist removes the vitreous gel and replaces it with a salt solution.

vitreous gel: Transparent, colorless mass that fills the rear two-thirds of the eyeball, between the lens and the retina.

wavefront: A measure of the total refractive errors of the eye, including nearsightedness, farsightedness, astigmatism, and other refractive errors that cannot be corrected with glasses or contacts.

Chapter 62 | **Directory of Resources Related to Eye Disorders and Vision Loss**

GOVERNMENT AGENCIES THAT PROVIDE INFORMATION ABOUT EYE CARE

Agency for Healthcare Research and Quality (AHRQ)

Office of Communications
5600 Fishers Ln.
Seventh Fl.
Rockville, MD 20847
Phone: 301-427-1104
Website: www.ahrq.gov

Americans with Disabilities Act (ADA)

Toll-Free: 800-514-0301
Toll-Free TTY: 800-514-0383
Website: www.ada.gov

Centers for Disease Control and Prevention (CDC)

1600 Clifton Rd.
Atlanta, GA 30329-4027
Toll-Free: 800-CDC-INFO (800-232-4636)
Phone: 404-639-3311
Toll-Free TTY: 888-232-6348
Website: www.cdc.gov
E-mail: cdcinfo@cdc.gov

Federal Occupational Health (FOH)

7700 Wisconsin Ave.
Ste. 600
Bethesda, MD 20814
Toll-Free: 866-4FOH-HLP (866-436-4457)
Website: foh.psc.gov

Resources in this chapter were compiled from several sources deemed reliable; all contact information was verified and updated in March 2020.

Genetic and Rare Diseases Information Center (GARD)
P.O. Box 8126
Gaithersburg, MD 20898-8126
Toll-Free: 888-205-2311
Toll-Free TTY: 888-205-3223
Fax: 301-251-4911
Website: rarediseases.info.nih.gov

MedlinePlus
U.S. National Library of Medicine (NLM)
Website: www.medlineplus.gov

National Cancer Institute (NCI)
9609 Medical Center Dr.
BG 9609, MSC 9760
Bethesda, MD 20892-9760
Toll-Free: 800-4-CANCER (800-422-6237)
Website: www.cancer.gov
E-mail: NCIinfo@nih.gov

National Center for Biotechnology Information (NCBI)
National Library of Medicine
8600 Rockville Pike
Bethesda, MD 20894
Website: www.ncbi.nlm.nih.gov
E-mail: info@ncbi.nlm.nih.gov

National Eye Institute (NEI)
Information Office
31 Center Dr.
MSC 2510
Bethesda, MD 20892-2510
Phone: 301-496-5248
Website: www.nei.nih.gov
E-mail: 2020@nei.nih.gov

National Highway Traffic Safety Administration (NHTSA)
1200 New Jersey Ave. S.E.
W. Bldg.
Washington, DC 20590
Toll-Free: 888-327-4236
Phone: 202-366-9550
Toll-Free TTY: 800-424-9153
Website: www.nhtsa.gov
E-mail: nhtsa.webmaster@dot.gov

National Human Genome Research Institute (NHGRI)
National Institutes of Health (NIH)
31 Center Dr., MSC 2152, 9000 Rockville Pike
Bldg. 31, Rm. 4B09
Bethesda, MD 20892-2152
Phone: 301-402-0911
Fax: 301-402-2218
Website: www.genome.gov

National Institute of Arthritis and Musculoskeletal and Skin Diseases (NIAMS)
Information Clearinghouse, National Institutes of Health (NIH)
One AMS Cir.
Bethesda, MD 20892-3675
Toll-Free: 877-22-NIAMS (877-226-4267)
Phone: 301-495-4484
Fax: 301-718-6366
Website: www.niams.nih.gov
E-mail: NIAMSinfo@mail.nih.gov

National Institute of Diabetes and Digestive and Kidney Diseases (NIDDK)

Health Information Center
Toll-Free: 800-860-8747
Toll-Free TTY: 866-569-1162
Website: www.niddk.nih.gov
E-mail: healthinfo@niddk.nih.gov

National Institute of Neurological Disorders and Stroke (NINDS)

NIH Neurological Institute
P.O. Box 5801
Bethesda, MD 20824
Toll-Free: 800-352-9424
Website: www.ninds.nih.gov

National Institute on Aging (NIA)

31 Center Dr., MSC 2292
Bldg. 31, Rm. 5C27
Bethesda, MD 20892
Toll-Free: 800-222-2225
Toll-Free TTY: 800-222-4225
Website: www.nia.nih.gov
E-mail: niaic@nia.nih.gov

National Institute on Deafness and Other Communication Disorders (NIDCD)

National Institutes of Health (NIH)
31 Center Dr., MSC 2320
Bethesda, MD 20892-2320
Phone: 301-827-8183
Website: www.nidcd.nih.gov
E-mail: nidcdinfo@nidcd.nih.gov

National Institutes of Health (NIH)

9000 Rockville Pike
Bethesda, MD 20892
Phone: 301-496-4000
TTY: 301-402-9612
Website: www.nih.gov

Occupational Safety and Health Administration (OSHA)

U.S. Department of Labor (DOL)
200 Constitution Ave. N.W.
Rm. N3626
Washington, DC 20210
Toll-Free: 800-321-OSHA
(800-321-6742)
Website: www.osha.gov

Office of Disease Prevention and Health Promotion (ODPHP)

Office of the Assistant Secretary for Health (OASH), Office of the Secretary
1101 Wootton Pkwy
Ste. LL100
Rockville, MD 20852
Fax: 240-453-8281
Website: health.gov
E-mail: odphpinfo@hhs.gov

U.S. Department of Education (ED)

400 Maryland Ave., S.W.
Washington, DC 20202
Toll-Free: 800-USA-LEARN
(800-872-5327)
Phone: 202-401-2000
Toll-Free TTY: 800-437-0833
Website: www.ed.gov

U.S. Department of Veterans Affairs (VA)
Toll-Free: 844-698-2311
Website: www.va.gov

U.S. Environmental Protection Agency (EPA)
1200 Pennsylvania Ave., N.W.
Washington, DC 20460
Phone: 202-564-4700
Fax: 202-501-1450
Website: www.epa.gov

U.S. Equal Employment Opportunity Commission (EEOC)
131 M St., N.E.
Fourth Fl., Ste. 4NWO2F
Washington, DC 20507-0100
Toll-Free: 800-669-4000
Phone: 202-663-4900
Toll-Free TTY: 800-669-6820
Fax: 202-419-0739
Website: www.eeoc.gov
E-mail: info@eeoc.gov

U.S. Food and Drug Administration (FDA)
10903 New Hampshire Ave.
Silver Spring, MD 20993-0002
Toll-Free: 888-INFO-FDA
(888-463-6332)
Website: www.fda.gov

U.S. Library of Congress (LOC)
101 Independence Ave., S.E.
Washington, DC 20540
Phone: 202-707-5000
Website: www.loc.gov

U.S. Social Security Administration (SSA)
Office of Earnings & International Operations (OEIO)
P.O. Box 17769
Baltimore, MD 21235-7769
Toll-Free: 800-772-1213
Toll-Free TTY: 800-325-0778
Website: www.ssa.gov

PRIVATE AGENCIES THAT PROVIDE INFORMATION ABOUT EYE CARE

All About Vision (AAV) Media, LLC.
5580 La Jolla Blvd.
Ste. 78
La Jolla, CA 92037
Phone: 858-454-2145
Website: www.allaboutvision.com

American Academy of Ophthalmology (AAO)
P.O. Box 7424
San Francisco, CA 94120-7424
Phone: 415-561-8500
Fax: 415-561-8533
Website: www.aao.org
E-mail: eyesmart@aao.org

American Diabetes Association® (ADA)
2451 Crystal Dr., Ste. 900
Arlington, VA 22202
Toll-Free: 800-DIABETES (800-342-2383)
Website: www.diabetes.org
E-mail: AskADA@diabetes.org

American Foundation for the Blind (AFB)
1401 S. Clark St., Ste. 730
Arlington, VA 22202
Phone: 212-502-7600
Website: www.afb.org
E-mail: afbinfo@afb.net

American Optometric Association (AOA)
243 N. Lindbergh Blvd.
First fl.
St. Louis, MO 63141
Toll-Free: 800-365-2219
Website: www.aoa.org

American Stroke Association
7272 Greenville Ave.
Dallas TX 75231
Toll-Free: 800-STROKES (800-787-6537)
Website: www.stroke.org
E-mail: info@stroke.org

Boston Children's Hospital
300 Longwood Ave.
Boston, MA 02115
Phone: 617-355-6000
Website: www.childrenshospital.org

Children's Glaucoma Foundation (CGF)
Two Longfellow Pl., Ste. 201
Boston, MA 02114
Phone: 617-227-3011
Website: www.childrensglaucoma.org
E-mail: info@childrensglaucomafoundation.org

The Choroideremia Research Foundation, Inc. (CRF)
23 E. Brundreth St.
Springfield, MA 01109-2110
Toll-Free: 800-210-0233
Website: www.curechm.org
E-mail: info@curechm.org

Cornea Research Foundation of America (CRFA)
9002 N. Meridian St.
Ste. 212
Indianapolis, IN 46260
Phone: 317-814-2993
Fax: 317-814-2806
Website: www.cornea.org

eMedicineHealth
c/o WebMD LLC.
1201 Peachtree St., N.E.
400 Colony Sq., Ste. 2100
Atlanta, GA 30361
Toll-Free: 866-788-3097
Website: www.emedicinehealth.com

EyeCare America®
American Academy of Ophthalmology (AAO)
P.O. Box 7424
San Francisco, CA 94120-7424
Toll-Free: 877-887-6327
Fax: 415-561-8567
Website: www.aao.org
E-mail: eyecareamerica@aao.org

Foundation Fighting Blindness
7168 Columbia Gateway Dr.
Ste. 100
Columbia, MD 21046
Toll-Free: 800-683-5555
Phone: 410-423-0600
TDD: 410-363-7139
Toll-Free TDD: 800-683-5551
Website: www.blindness.org
E-mail: info@FightBlindness.org

The Glaucoma Foundation (TGF)
80 Maiden Ln., Ste. 700
New York, NY 10038
Phone: 212-285-0080
Website: www.glaucomafoundation.org
E-mail: info@glaucomafoundation.org

Glaucoma Research Foundation (GRF)
251 Post St., Ste. 600
San Francisco, CA 94108
Toll-Free: 800-826-6693
Phone: 415-986-3162
Fax: 415-986-3763
Website: www.glaucoma.org
E-mail: grf@glaucoma.org

International Children's Anophthalmia Network (ICAN)
c/o Center for Developmental Medicine and Genetics
5501 Old York Road
Genetics, Levy 2 West Philadelphia, PA 19141
Toll-Free: 800-580-ican (800-580-4226)
Website: www.anophthalmia.org
E-mail: info@anophthalmia.org

International Foundation for Optic Nerve Disease (IFOND)
P. O. Box 777
Cornwall, NY 12518
Phone: 845-534-8606
Website: www.ifond.org
E-mail: ifond@aol.com

Lighthouse Guild
250 W. 64th St.,
New York, NY 10023
Toll-Free: 800-284-4422
Phone: 212-769-6212
Website: www.lighthouse.org

Macular Degeneration Partnership
Gavin Herbert Eye Institute (GHEI), Department of Ophthalmology
850 Health Sciences Rd.
Irvine, California 92697
Phone: 949-824-9771
Website: www.ucirvineamd.org
E-mail: tnyoung@uci.edu

National Keratoconus Foundation (NKCF)
850 Health Sciences Rd.
Irvine, CA 92697
Toll-Free: 800-521-2524
Phone: 310-623-4466
Website: www.nkcf.org

North American Neuro-Ophthalmology Society (NANOS)
5841 Cedar Lake Rd.
Ste. 204
Minneapolis, MN 55416
Phone: 952-646-2037
Fax: 952-545-6073
Website: www.nanosweb.org
E-mail: info@nanosweb.org

Ocular Immunology and Uveitis Foundation (OIUF)
Massachusetts Eye Research and Surgery Institution (MERSI)
348 Glen Rd.
P. O. Box 646
Weston, MA 02493
Phone: 781-647-1431
Website: www.uveitis.org

Prevent Blindness America
225 W. Wacker Dr.,
Ste. 400
Chicago, IL 60606
Toll-Free: 800-331-2020
Website: www.preventblindness.org
E-mail: info@preventblindness.org

Sjögren's Syndrome Foundation (SSF)
10701 Parkridge Blvd.
Ste.170
Reston, VA 20191
Toll-Free: 800-475-6473
Phone: 301-530-4420
Fax: 301-530-4415
Website: www.sjogrens.org

Stevens Johnson Syndrome Foundation
P.O. Box 350333
Westminster, CO 80035-0333
Phone: 303-635-1241
Fax: 303-648-6686
Website: www.sjsupport.org
E-mail: sjsupport@gmail.com

Wayfinder Family Services
5300 Angeles Vista Blvd.
Los Angeles, CA 90043
Toll-Free: 800-352-2290
Phone: 323-295-4555
Fax: 323-296-0424
Website: www.juniorblind.org
E-mail: info@wayfinderfamily.org

INDEX

INDEX

Page numbers followed by 'n' indicate a footnote. Page numbers in *italics* indicate a table or illustration.

A

B

C

D

E

G

H

I

J

K

L

M

N

O

P

Q

R

S

T

U

V

X

Z